NUTRITION AND MEDICAL PRACTICE

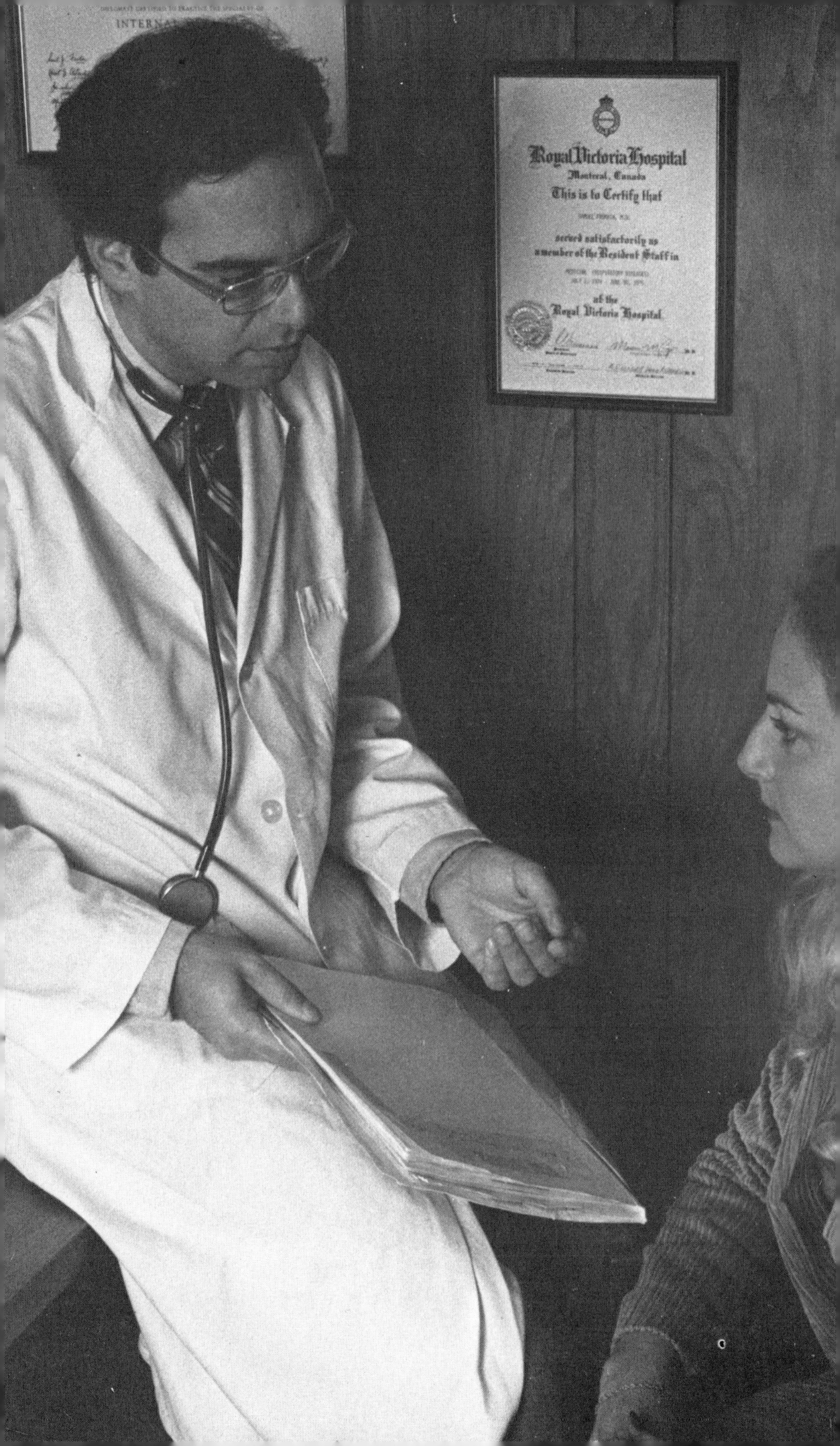
Royal Victoria Hospital
Montreal, Canada
This is to Certify that
served satisfactorily as
a member of the Resident Staff in
of the
Royal Victoria Hospital

NUTRITION AND MEDICAL PRACTICE

Editor, Lewis A. Barness, M.D.
with Yank D. Coble, Jr., M.D.
Donald I. Macdonald, M.D.
George Christakis, M.D., M.P.H.

MEMBERS OF THE FLORIDA MEDICAL ASSOCIATION

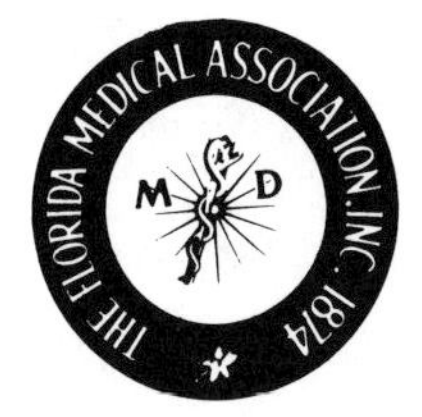

AVI PUBLISHING COMPANY, INC.
Westport, Connecticut

Cover photograph from David Attie; frontispiece courtesy of Samuel Frumkin, M.D., Internal Medicine Associates, Westport, CT. with patient.

Library of Congress Cataloging in Publication Data
Main entry under title:

Nutrition and medical practice.

Includes index.
1. Diet therapy. I. Barness, Lewis A.
[DNLM: 1. Nutrition. 2. Diet therapy. QU 145 N97094]
RM216.N83 615.8'54
ISBN 0-87055-365-8
80-25541

Printed in the United States of America by
The Saybrook Press, Inc.

Foreword

All forms of life require food materials in certain minimum amounts to insure an active life and successful reproduction. Nutrition is concerned with what these materials are, how they function, what effects they have when absent and what happens to them when ingested.

During the past two centuries such nutritional disorders as scurvy, beriberi, rickets and pellagra have been discovered, successfully treated and eradicated by physicians in developed countries. In this century, such noted researchers as Rose, Meyerhof and Krebs have contributed enormously to the field of nutrition.

Currently, research is evolving new concepts and facts so rapidly that the average practitioner can hardly keep current, even in his own field of medicine. Bona fide research by universities and governmental agencies has produced voluminous information, much of which seems contradictory and therefore tends to confuse the general public, particularly in the area of potential carcinogens.

This confusion has prompted consumer groups, politicians, and social welfarists to bring pressures and demands on medical schools and practitioners of medicine to increase their knowledge and concern in the field of nutrition.

Taking advantage of and adding to this confusion are the health food faddists and cultists, some only for monetary gain and others with a real religious zeal.

The above developments are partially responsible for the Florida Medical Association adopting Nutrition as its scientific theme for 1978–1979. Part of this theme was exhibited in a special edition of the *Journal of the Florida Medical Association, Inc.,* dedicated entirely to the subject of Nutrition. This issue of the *Journal* was so widely acclaimed across the nation that inspiration was generated to publish this in book form. The original articles published in the special issue have been updated and additional topics have been added.

This publication is thought to be extraordinary and will contribute greatly to the education of physicians, medical students and the knowledgeable public alike. It should serve as a valid reference source for many years to come.

Drs. Barness, Coble, Macdonald and Christakis have certainly selected their subject matter and contributors well and may be rightfully proud of this compendium of information.

We all wish to make a special note of thanks to Dr. J. Lee Dockery, University of Florida Medical School and Dr. Norman W. Desrosier, AVI Publishing Company, for their efforts in bringing this new book into being.

O. William Davenport, M.D.

January, 1981

Acknowledgement

The Editors gratefully acknowledge the generosity of the following who helped make this publication on Nutrition possible: Mead Johnson & Company, Evansville, Indiana; Ross Laboratories, Columbus, Ohio; University of Miami School of Medicine, Miami; University of South Florida College of Medicine, Tampa; University of Florida College of Medicine, Gainesville; Florida Pediatric Society and Florida Chapter, American Academy of Pediatrics.

Lewis A. Barness, M.D.

January, 1981

Dedication

The editors and contributors of this book wish to dedicate their efforts on its behalf to the teaching and practice of good nutrition as a fundamental of good health and a worthy endeavor in the field of medicine.

Contributors

BAKER, RUTH, R.D., M.P.H., Palm Beach County Health Department, West Palm Beach, Florida

BARNESS, LEWIS A., M.D., Professor and Chairman, Department of Pediatrics, University of South Florida College of Medicine, Tampa

BOYCE, H. WORTH JR., M.D., Director, Division of Gastroenterology, Department of Internal Medicine, University of South Florida College of Medicine, Tampa

BRAY, GEORGE A., M.D., University of California at Los Angeles School of Medicine, Harbor-UCLA Medical Center, Torrance

BRIN, MYRON, Ph.D., Department of Biochemical Nutrition, Roche Research Center, Hoffman-LaRoche Inc., Nutley, New Jersey

BRUMBACK, C.L., M.D., M.P.H., Palm Beach County Health Department, West Palm Beach, Florida

BURR, JANICE M., M.D., Co-Principal Investigator, Nutrition Division, Department of Epidemiology and Public Health, University of Miami School of Medicine, Miami, Florida

CERDA, JAMES J., M.D., Professor of Medicine and Director of the Nutrition Laboratory, University of Florida College of Medicine, Gainesville

CHRISTAKIS, GEORGE, M.D., M.P.H., Chief, Nutrition Division, Department of Epidemiology and Public Health, University of Miami School of Medicine, Miami, Florida

COBLE, YANK D. JR., M.D., Specialist in Endocrinology and Nutrition, Jacksonville, Florida

COPELAND, EDWARD M. III, M.D., Professor of Surgery, University of Texas Medical School, Houston

DARBY, WILLIAM J., M.D., Ph.D., President, The Nutrition Foundation, New York and Washington, D.C.

DAVIS, GEORGE K., Ph.D., Professor of Nutrition, I.F.A.S., University of Florida, Gainesville

DOLIN, BEN J., M.D., Private Practitioner; Associate Director of Nutritional Support Service, Methodist Hospital, Peoria, Illinois

EASTON, PENELOPE S., Ph.D., R.D., Chairman, Dietetics and Nutrition, Florida International University, Miami

GERACE, TERENCE A., Ph.D., Director of Intervention and Co-Investigator, Nutrition Division, Department of Epidemiology and Public Health, University of Miami School of Medicine, Miami, Florida

GROW, THOMAS E., Ph.D., Department of Basic Dental Sciences, University of Florida College of Dentistry, Gainesville

GUILD, RALPH T., M.D., Instructor in Gastroenterology, University of Florida College of Medicine, Gainesville

HARPER, ALFRED E., Ph.D., E.V. McCollum Professor of Nutritional Sciences, Departments of Nutritional Science and Biochemistry, University of Wisconsin, Madison

HERBERT, VICTOR, M.D., J.D., Professor and Vice Chairman of Medicine, State University of New York, Downstate Medical Center, New York

KAFATOS, ANTHONY G., M.D., M.P.H., Associate Professor, Department of Epidemiology, University of Miami School of Medicine, Miami, Florida

KAMINSKI, MITCHELL V. JR., M.D., Clinical Professor of Surgery, University of Health Sciences/Chicago Medical School, Chicago, Illinois

LEAPLEY, PATRICIA M., R.D., Diabetes Center Dietician, University of South Florida College of Medicine, Tampa

LIEBER, CHARLES S., M.D., Chief, Alcoholism Research and Treatment Center, Veterans Administration Medical Center, Bronx, New York

MacDONALD, DONALD IAN, M.D., Pediatrician, Clearwater, Florida

MAHAN, CHARLES S., M.D., Associate Professor, Department of Obstetrics and Gynecology, University of Florida College of Medicine, Gainesville

MALONE, JOHN I., M.D., Professor of Pediatrics and Co-Director of the Diabetes Center, University of South Florida College of Medicine, Tampa

MAUER, ALVIN M., M.D., Director, St. Jude's Children's Research Hospital, Memphis, Tennessee

MILLS, CHRISTOPHER B., M.D., Fellow, Metabolic Support Service, Ravenswood Hospital Medical Center, Chicago, Illinois

PONDER, DEBRA L., M.S., R.D., Doctoral Student, Department of Food and Nutrition, Florida State University, Tallahassee

RACKOW, JEANNE R., M.S., R.D., Professor of Nutrition, University of South Florida, Tampa

RIFKIN, STEPHEN I., M.D., Assistant Professor, Division of Nephrology, Department of Internal Medicine, University of South Florida College of Medicine, Tampa

ROE, DAPHNE, M.D., Division of Nutrition, Cornell University, Ithaca, New York

RUGGIERO, ROBERT P., M.D., Fellow, Metabolic Support Service, Thorek Hospital and Medical Center, Chicago

STREIFF, RICHARD R., M.D., Professor of Medicine, Veterans Administration Medical Center, Tampa, and Department of Medicine, University of Florida, Gainesville

VAN SLYKE, HEIDI, R.D., Dietitian, Victoria Hospital, Miami, Florida

WENDER, ESTHER H., M.D., Assistant Professor of Pediatrics, University of Utah College of Medicine, Salt Lake City

WILCOX, MARY ELLEN, R.D., M.Ed., Project Chief Nutritionist, Department of Epidemiology and Public Health, University of Miami School of Medicine, Miami, Florida

Contents

1

INTRODUCTION

Lewis A. Barness, M.D.

The prospect of a long, healthy and happy life is enthralling. Many feel that good nutrition is the path to this goal, and certainly the medical profession has a key role to play.

The officers of the Florida Medical Association determined that an increased focus be placed on nutritional knowledge, with particular reference to medical practice. A special issue of its Journal was to be dedicated to this subject. A group of authors was selected by the editorial board, consisting of Drs. Yank Coble, George Christakis, Donald Macdonald and myself, to address the various areas of knowledge and to point out those of which we are ignorant. Subsequently, the idea was conceived to bring together the extant material and to broaden the coverage by adding a number of new important chapters to form a textbook on the subject of nutrition and medical practice. This book is the result.

We would like to call attention to many highlights.

The chapters on nutritional evaluation and nutritional diseases should be helpful to all who are interested in preventing disease. The importance of relatively new tools for evaluation, such as skin fold thickness and immune responses, is well explained. Cancer, gastrointestinal diseases, surgical and other hospital states, as well as needs for and methods of parenteral nutrition, are excellent reading and learning articles.

One chapter included is of vital importance to all who care for the pregnant and pre-pregnant woman. Following the advice herein promises to reduce perinatal morbidity and mortality.

Fad diets, hyperactivity in relation to the diet, food additives in general, megavitamin therapy, and diet-drug interactions are still con-

Dr. Barness is Professor and Chairman of the Department of Pediatrics, University of South Florida College of Medicine, Tampa. He is a member of the FMA Ad Hoc Committee on Nutrition.

troversial, but information is given to help the reader make an informed decision.

The paper relating agriculture to medicine and nutrition can be a source of nutritional ideas. Public health problems are touched on, as are the successful WIC programs, the Multiple Risk Factor Intervention Trial, and the role of nutrition in the management of *Diabetes mellitus*.

Nutrition of children is addressed in several chapters, including that on school lunch programs. Determinants of later disease are discussed in a logical manner.

The physician who has largely an office practice will be helped, it is hoped, not only by these papers, but also by several excellent papers on the importance of dietetic support in medical practice and on how to get nutritional help at home or in the office. More intelligent use of the RDAs is made possible, and pertinent references on nutrition information are provided for the physician as well as the patient.

Special attention is given in chapters on nutritional anemias, nutrition in renal failure, and nutrition and food selection. We have also included for your ready reference an Appendix of the most recent American Dietetic Association Recommendation on Nutrition and Physical Fitness, with their permission.

No promises are made for better life, but reasons for some present diet information are offered. It may seem incongruous to write about deficiencies when the various nutritional surveys indicate that, in this country, deficiencies, except for iron, are rare or non-existent, except in association with other diseases. The next leading manifestation of malnutrition in this country is obesity, which requires not only dietary control but also increased activity.

For the areas addressed, the editors and authors trust that the information will be helpful in preventing nutritional diseases, recognizing and treating those that are present, and in preventing waste of food and money while providing bases for accepting new information as it becomes available.

2

HOW TO MAKE A NUTRITIONAL DIAGNOSIS:

A. ADULT NUTRITIONAL DIAGNOSIS

George Christakis, M.D., M.P.H.

Perhaps no other field in medicine is more annoying—and challenging—to today's practicing physician than nutrition. It is ironic that while it is public knowledge that physicians rarely receive adequate training in nutrition, patients are often walking recipes of unsavory stews of nutrition information and misinformation. While few patients would claim to be experts in the more esoteric aspects of health, the lay press, health food stores and grandma herself repeat old nutrition fables with fervor and periodically invent new ones to keep the physician off guard.

"How do I know I am in good nutritional condition?"

"I feel weak, do I need vitamins?"

"Should I take lecithin for my high cholesterol?"

"Will megavitamins help my son's depression?"

"Won't vitamin E prevent heart attacks?"

It is understandable that when barraged by such questions the physician retreats into the safer role of healer rather than educator. However, nutritional diagnoses are in fact easily missed; it is hoped that this brief outline may serve as a guide to the detection of symptoms and signs of nutritional states in adults.

Dr. Christakis is Chief, Nutrition Division, Department of Epidemiology and Public Health, University of Miami School of Medicine, Miami.

REGAINING THE LOST ART OF NUTRITIONAL DIAGNOSIS

Nutrition, in common with other aspects of clinical medicine, utilizes the history, physical examination and laboratory to provide the data on which definitive diagnosis is based. Complete nutritional assessment includes (1) dietary history which surveys dietary intakes and patterns (usually over a 24-hour period), (2) interviewing the patient for specific nutrition-related symptoms in the "Review of Systems" which has been neglected, (3) identifying the physical signs of nutritional deficiencies, and (4) utilizing the standard clinical laboratory as well as the nutrition laboratory where available.

The nutrition history has a unique advantage in being less threatening to the patient than other parts of the medical history. Patients are often anxious when they visit the office or clinic, especially for the first time. Vital questions such as "Have you coughed up blood?" "Have you noticed any blood in your stool?" or "Have you lost weight?" may put some patients on the defensive because of their ominous and threatening connotations. However, the nutrition history poses questions which relate to both the healthy as well as the sick since most of us eat at least three times daily (if not more). Asking patients, "What do you usually have for breakfast and . . . etc." helps put them at ease. They are often gratified that their doctor thinks enough about nutrition to ask them about their eating habits; it helps "break the ice" and allows the patient to approach the other parts of the medical history with greater ease, and thus perhaps greater truthfulness.

The dietary history has traditionally been an integral component of the medical history, and often documented under "Personal History" with the patient's sleep, smoking and exercise patterns. The hurried physician, however, may not secure a dietary history if he feels it may contribute little to the understanding of the patient, particularly if it does not appear to be related to the chief complaint. Unfortunately, the usefulness of the dietary history is often shrouded by somber warnings from nutritionists that most people cannot remember all they eat (probably true); that conversion from portion sizes to ounces or grams, and utilizing food composition tables to derive macro- and micronutrient composition is riddled with gross inaccuracies (which it is); and finally, that archaic nutritional chemical procedures were used in the first place to obtain nutrient data on food composition (also true).

CLINICAL SIGNIFICANCE OF DIETARY HISTORY

What then is the value of a nutrition history to the practicing physician? Several useful parameters can be targeted by even a brief, carefully structured history of eating behavior to provide the physician with clues to not only understanding his patient's nutritional patterns but revealing psychosocial dynamics related to health.

Personality Characteristics.—Use of health foods or vegetarianism may provide clues to personal philosophies and lifestyles. The obese person may hide supplies of food or candy to satisfy compulsive eating behavior; in contrast, aversion to food may be a facet of anorexia nervosa. The obese businessman may need to "throw his weight around" as a façade for personal insecurity. A mother may strictly watch her own calories and figure but surreptitiously overfeed her daughter so that she may gain weight and lose in the competition for her father's attention. Rapid weight gain in a child whose parent has died may represent a "reactive obesity," which may assist the child in negotiating this psychic trauma. Teenage obesity in a girl may be a protective barrier against social interaction with boys for which she is not psychologically prepared.

Eating Patterns.—Who cooks at home and prepares meals also provides insight into the home environment. Does sibling prepare meals because mother is alcoholic? Are tension-provoking topics discussed at mealtimes? Does husband eat out on pretext of business matters in order to escape conflicts at home? Do food allergies or preferences of other family members adversely affect the patient's diet?

The nutrition history (dietary history and review of nutritional symptoms) fulfills three clinical nutrition objectives:

1. Provides an overview of the patient's food intake and allows the physician to gauge whether there are gross macro- and micronutrient deficits or surpluses.
2. Detects nutritional symptoms associated with a primary nutrient deficiency state, or which may be secondary to another disease. The presence of these symptoms will alert the physician to the possibility of detecting signs of nutrient deficiency states when he examines the patient. Laboratory confirmation may also be required by the determination of serum levels of vitamins, trace minerals, lipids and other tests.
3. Evaluates whether the eating behavior of the patient contributes to a nutritionally determined risk factor of chronic disease. For example, obvious overeating and alcohol abuse can result in obesity and hypertriglyceridemia. Obesity is related to diabetes, osteoarthritis, cancer of the corpus uteri, and is a secondary risk factor in coronary heart disease and hypertension. Chronic high salt intake may also be a factor in hypertension. Low fiber diets appear to be epidemiologically associated with colon carcinoma; high saturated fat diets also may be related to colon and breast cancer.

A *dietary history* may be obtained, utilizing either the 24-hour dietary history or the "nutrition scan" which I use in practice. The dietary history simply documents what the patient recalls having eaten in the past 24 hours, noting whether it is representative of the patient's "usual" pattern of eating. If the patient is on a therapeutic diet, taking vitamins or "health foods" and supplements, this should be noted.

What is usually eaten for breakfast? There is the "no breakfast" breakfast characteristic of the obese who may then skip lunch (or have a light lunch), and eat continuously from 6 to 11 p.m. There is the "black coffee and cigarette" breakfast, and the 10:30 a.m. "coffee break" breakfast (i.e., donut-coffee). On weekends, the "cowboy breakfast" is often consumed, consisting of ham, eggs, and pancakes or waffles. There is also the vodka breakfast of the alcoholic "to get the day started." The presence or absence of citrus fruit or juice, a protein source (cheese, eggs or skim milk with cereal) and lipid intake (margarine, butter or cheese) can be quickly outlined. Snacks (soft drinks, pastry, etc.) should also be listed in the dietary history.

As for lunch, is it usually a sandwich or a hot meal? Is alcohol included? What is the dessert? Does he or she eat at the desk or workbench, thus reflecting the nature or extent of on-the-job stresses? Is a walk included after lunch if there is time?

Afternoon snacks should also be listed as well as number of coffee, tea or caffeinated soft drinks consumed (these may trigger cardiac arrhythmias in susceptible persons).

Are alcoholic beverages consumed while waiting for the train or bus home? What foods are eaten at supper and in what approximate portions? How much salt is added during cooking or at the table? Is TV snacking a regular pastime? Is liquor part of saying "good night?" Does the patient wake up at 2 a.m. and attack the refrigerator ("night-eating syndrome")?

The dietary history thus permits a very broad assessment of the nutritional status of the patient. For example, an elderly patient may not have consumed citrus fruits for the past four months because she has lately found them too "acid" in taste; accordingly, it would be prudent to look for perifollicular skin hemorrhages of scurvy. Again, the dietary history may record that a patient eats meat twice daily every day, loves butter and ice cream, and hates fish. The preponderance of foods high in saturated fats should pique the curiosity to order a serum cholesterol, HDL and LDL tests. If a patient eats little whole grain cereals, vegetables and legumes, drinks little water and is sedentary, the lack of dietary fiber may be a clue as to why he is chronically constipated. On the other hand, if the patient with diverticulosis is doing well on a high fiber diet, but develops occasional abdominal pain when eating vegetables or fruits that contain seeds (squash, eggplant, figs, strawberries), the dietary history will uncover this finding of possible clinical importance.

The *nutrition scan* outlines the number of meals per week that contain certain food groups and items that have particular relevance to specific nutritional diagnoses. Four questions are asked:

1. How many times a week do you have the following for breakfast in usual portions:
   a. Citrus fruit (oranges, grapefruit, whole or juice).
   b. Whole grain cereals, hot or cold.
   c. Eggs (plain, or with bacon, ham, sausages).
   d. Pancakes, waffles.
   e. Coffee, milk (whole, 2% fat or skim).
2. Of the 14 lunches and dinners you eat a week, how many are:
   a. Beef, lamb, pork or organ meats (liver, heart, kidneys).
   b. Poultry (chicken, turkey or duck).
   c. Fish, shellfish.
3. How many times a week do you eat or drink:
   a. Bread, rolls
   b. Vegetables of all types
   c. Cheese
   d. Legumes (peas, beans, chick-peas)
   e. Pasta (spaghetti, noodles)
   f. Fruit
   g. Butter
   h. Margarine
   i. Vegetable oil/salad dressings
   j. Ice cream
   k. Alcoholic beverages (beer, wine, hard liquor)
   l. Snacks (pretzels, potato chips, etc.)
   m. Cookies
   n. Nuts
   o. Raisins
   p. Soft drinks
4. How much water do you drink daily?
5. How heavily do you salt your food?

The nutrition scan is incomplete and permits only a broad view of the eating pattern of the patient. However, it takes only five minutes and can provide a rough estimate of the following:

1. Adequacy of intake of the six food groups and the major macro- and micronutrients they contain. (See Appendix B, page 386)
2. The relative proportions of saturated, monounsaturated and polyunsaturated fats in the diet.

3. Adequacy of dietary protein with regard to amount and sources from animal and/or vegetable origin.
4. Estimate of whether dietary cholesterol is excessive because of over-intake of eggs, organ meats, red meats, butter, ice cream, cheese.
5. Estimate of whether fiber is adequate through intake of whole grain cereals, vegetables and fruit.
6. Whether snacks, alcohol or salt intake are excessive.

NEED FOR INCLUSION OF NUTRITION SYMPTOMS IN "REVIEW OF SYSTEMS"

Since symptoms from primary or secondary nutritional deficiencies affect many organ systems, the physician may not include them in the Review of Systems or may list only a few under the "metabolic" category when he queries the patient. Table 2.1 provides examples of symptoms or signs of nutritional states that may be useful in practice, particularly if the physician suspects that the chief complaint may be relevant to a nutritional diagnosis.

Obviously, the symptoms and signs of nutritional deficiency overlap with many other diseases. For example, niacin deficiency and Korsakoff's syndrome in the alcoholic with thiamin deficiency mimic many organic and psychopathic disorders. Subacute combined degeneration of B_{12} deficiency and Wernicke's syndrome may mimic the onset of multiple sclerosis and other demyelinating diseases as well as the organic brain syndromes of cerebral arteriosclerosis.

PHYSICAL DIAGNOSIS OF NUTRITIONAL DISORDERS

The examination of the patient begins with inspection as he enters the office or you approach him at the hospital bed.

Do his belt marks reveal progressive weight gain? Do his clothes fit loosely and betray weight loss? Does your strict vegetarian patient have an ataxic gait of subacute combined degeneration of B_{12} deficiency (veganism)? Does the patient present with the obvious pallor of severe anemia? Does your alcoholic patient shuffle into the office because of polyneuropathy due to multiple B vitamin deficiencies? Is your postoperative patient after ten days on IV saline and glucose solutions slowly developing the moon facies of kwashiorkor (protein-calorie malnutrition)? Is his hair lusterless, "staring" or showing signs of horizontal depigmentation (flag sign)? Are the latter third of the eyebrows missing (hypothyroidism)? Does your patient show the neck, upper thorax or arm atrophy of lean muscle mass loss (protein-calorie malnu-

TABLE 2.1. EXAMPLES OF HISTORY QUESTIONS RELATED TO NUTRITIONAL DIAGNOSES

Symptom	Nutrient Deficiency or Excess to be Considered
Hair becomes thin, coarse, falls out or changes colors	Protein
Slowed speech, "thickened tongue," dysphagia	Iodine
Poor night vision, especially at twilight hours, eyes feel dry	Vitamin A
Gums bleed or skin ecchymoses occur easily	Vitamin C
Tongue sore, sensitive to hot beverages (due to filiform and/or fungiform atrophy) impaired taste, poor appetite	Nutritional anemias: iron, folic acid, riboflavin, niacin, zinc
Lips burn (due to cheilosis)	Thiamin
Fatigue, malaise, apathy, mental depression	Nutritional anemias (iron, folic acid), electrolytes (potassium and sodium), protein, hypoglycemia; multiple vitamin (especially B vitamins) and mineral deficiencies
Tingling, numbness, "burning" of hands or feet (due to polyneutritis)	Thiamin, Riboflavin
Personality changes, hyperexcitability	Niacin; electrolytes, hypoglycemia, magnesium
Headache	Hypoglycemia, hypervitaminosis A
Blurred vision (optic neuritis)	Alcohol excess, B Vitamin deficiencies
Low back pain	Folic acid, B-12 and osteoporosis related to protein, calcium and fluoride deficiencies
Exertional dyspnea, congestive heart failure, angina	Hyperlipidemias, aggravation of preexisting coronary heart disease by anemia; thiamin deficiency
Dry, scaly skin	Linoleic acid, arachidonic acid
Diarrhea	Lactose intolerance, gluten sensitivity, niacin
Stools which do not float	Fiber
Pica (compulsive eating of ice, earth, laundry starch, wall plaster)	Iron
Anorexia	Thiamine, zinc, neoplasms, especially G.I.; onset of anorexia nervosa; depression
Fatigue, malaise, lethargy, bone pain, headaches, insomnia, night sweats, loss of hair	Hypervitaminosis A
Hypercalcemia and renal damage, anorexia, nausea, weight loss, children: failure to thrive	Hypervitaminosis D
Ataxic gait	B-12, Thiamin

trition)? Do ill-fitting dentures or dental problems prevent proper chewing or limit the variety of foods habitually eaten by the patient?

The closer inspection of the patient requires skill and patience but if the more detailed and easily missed signs of nutritional deficiency diseases are carefully assessed, the more evident physical signs of other diseases are less likely to be missed.

Palpation of the hair may reveal dryness and the easy and painless pluckability of the patient with protein-calorie malnutrition. Does he have the acneiform lesions of vitamin A deficiency? As you pass your hand over the midtriceps area of the arm and "pinch" the skin to gauge the width of subcutaneous fat, can you feel the "shark-skin" (follicular hyperkeratosis) associated with vitamin A deficiency? The dry, cracked skin of the patient with niacin, linoleic acid, or protein-calorie deficiency should also be palpated. Miliary xanthomatous nodules in the simian creases of the hand are indicative of Type III hyperlipoproteinemia.

The eyelids, conjunctivae, sclera, cornea and optic nerve head may all reveal signs of malnutrition. Xanthelasma at the nasal aspect of the lids, and arcus cornealis, particularly in a young patient, may indicate severe primary Type II hyperlipoproteinemia.

Has the ocular conjunctiva lost its luster and moisture (xerosis of vitamin A deficiency)? Is a small foamy whitish lesion—Bitot's spot—present which is suggestive of vitamin A deficiency? If you're out in rural areas of developing countries and you see a person whose cornea is soft and wiggles when the eye moves, this is a medical emergency. Water soluble vitamin A will be needed immediately to prevent blindness due to corneal ulceration and possible extrusion of the lens.

Is there a fine capillary network around the cornea (riboflavin deficiency)? When you evert the lower lid to look for the pallor of iron or folic acid deficiency, can you detect small mounds of mucosal tissue or angular blepharitis also suggestive of riboflavin deficiency? Funduscopic examination may reveal the optic neuritis of thiamin deficiency.

The nose and mouth also sensitively reflect micronutrient deficiencies. Nasolabial dyssebacea and seborrhea are seen in riboflavin and pyridoxine deficiencies respectively. Inflammation of the lips (cheilosis) is a common sign of riboflavin deficiency.

The tongue, gums, and teeth also play an important role in nutritional diagnosis. Inflammation of the tongue (glossitis) with atrophy of papillae occurs in iron and/or folate deficiency; hypertrophy of papillae can be seen in riboflavin deficiency. Gums that bleed on pressure and reveal interdental hypertrophy are classical signs of scurvy.

The skeletal and neuromuscular systems also contribute to nutritional diagnosis. Osteoporosis associated with chronic protein, calcium or fluoride deficiency may be patently detectable on x-ray. The sequellae of rickets comprise the thoracic cage "rosary," bowing of the lower legs or craniotabes. Leg and thigh muscle atrophy due to thiamin or protein-calorie malnutrition is commonly seen among the elderly in long-term care institutions. Finally, thiamin, niacin, pyridoxine, protein deficiencies and nutritional anemias can also induce abnormal behavior or psychotic states.

Table 2.2 lists the physical signs of specific nutrient deficiency states according to organ systems.

TABLE 2.2. PHYSICAL SIGNS OF NUTRIENT DEFICIENCIES

Organ System	Physical Signs	Nutrient Deficiency
Hair	Becomes fine, dull, dry, brittle, stiff, straight; becomes red in Blacks, then lighter in color; may be "bleached" in Whites ("flag sign"); is easily and painlessly pluckable; outer one third of eyebrow may be sparse in hypothyroidism (cretinism, iodine deficiency or other causes)	Protein-Calorie
Nails	Ridging, brittle, easily broken, flattened, spoon shaped, thin, lusterless	Iron
Face	Brown, patchy, pigmentation of cheeks, Parotid enlargement "Moon Face"	Protein-Calorie
Eyes	Photophobia; poor twilight vision; loss of shiny, bright, moist appearance of eyes; xerosis of bulbar conjunctivae; loss of light reflex; decreased lacrimation; keratomalacia (corneal softening), corneal ulceration which may lead to extrusion of lens; Bitot's spot (frothy white or yellow spots under bulbar conjunctivae)	Vitamin A
	Palpebral conjunctivae are pale	Iron or Folate
	Circumcorneal capillary injection with penetration of corneal limbus.	Riboflavin
	Tissue at external angles of both eyes which is red and moist. Angular blepharitis (or palpebritis)	Riboflavin Pyridoxine
	Optic neuritis	B-12
Nose	Nasolabial dyssebacea (exfoliation, inflammation, excessive oil production and fissuring of sebaceous glands, which are moist and red). May be found at angles of eyes, ears or other sites	Riboflavin
	Nasolabial seborrhea	Pyridoxine
Lips	Cheilosis, inflammation of the mucus membranes of the lips and the loss of the clear differentiation between the mucocutaneous border of the lips	Riboflavin
Gums	Interdental gingival hypertrophy	Vitamin C
	Gingivitis	Vitamin A; Niacin Riboflavin
Mouth	Angular stomatitis; cheilosis; angular scars	Riboflavin
	Apthous stomatitis	Folic Acid
Tongue	Atrophic lingual papillae, sore, erythematous	Iron
	Glossitis, painful, sore	Folic Acid

Organ System	Physical Signs	Nutrient Deficiency
	Magenta in color, atrophic lingual papillae; filiform and fungiform papillae hypertrophy	Riboflavin
	Scarlet; raw; atrophic lingual papillae; fissures	Niacin
	Glossitis	Pyridoxine
Teeth	Caries	Fluoride
	Mottled enamel, fluorosis	Fluoride (excessive)
	Caries	Phosphorus
	Malposition; hypoplastic line across upper primary incisors; becomes filled with yellow-brown pigment; caries then occurs and tooth may break off	Protein-Calorie
Neck	Neck mass (goiter)	Iodine
Skin	Xerosis (dryness of skin) Follicular hyperkeratosis ("gooseflesh," "sharkskin," "sand-paper skin;" keratotic plugs arising from hypertrophied hair follicles. Acneiform lesions	Vitamin A
	Perifollicular petechiae which produce a "pink-halo" effect around coiled hair follicles. Intradermal petechiae, purpura, ecchymoses due to capillary fragility. Hemarthroses; cortical hemorrhages of bone visualizable on x-ray	Vitamin C
	Intracutaneous hemorrhages; GI hemorrhage	Vitamin K
	Pallor	Iron, folic acid
	Pallor; icterus	B-12
	Erythema early, vascularization, crusting, desquamation. Increased pigmentation (even in Blacks), thickened, inelastic, fissured, especially in skin exposed to sun; becoming scaly, dry, atrophic in intertrigenous areas, maceration and abrasion may occur. "Necklace of Casals" in neckline exposed to sun; Malar and supraorbital pigmentation	Niacin
	Edema (pitting), "Flaky paint" dermatosis, Hyperkeratosis or "Crazy pavement" dermatosis Hyperpigmentation	Protein-Calorie
	Scrotum Dermatitis, erythema, hyperpigmentation	Niacin
Vulva	Vulvovaginitis and chronic mucocutaneous candidiasis	Iron
Skeletal	Osteoporosis (in association with low protein intake and fluoride deficiency)	Calcium
	Epiphyseal enlargement, painless. Beading of ribs ("Rachitic Rosary"). Delayed fusion of fontaneles, craniotabes. Bowed legs, frontal or parietal bossing of skull. Deformities of thorax (Harrison's Sulcus, pigeon breast). Osteomalacia (adults)	Vitamin D
	Subperiosteal hematoma. Epiphyseal enlargement, painful	Vitamin C
Muscular	Hypotonia	Vitamin D
	Muscle wasting; weakness, fatigue, inactivity; loss of subcutaneous fat	Protein-Calorie
	Intramuscular hematoma	Vitamin C
	Calf muscle tenderness; weakness	Thiamin

Organ System	Physical Signs	Nutrient Deficiency
Central Nervous System	Apathy (kwashiorkor); irritability (marasmus); Psychomotor changes.	Protein
	Hyporeflexia; foot and wrist drop. Hypesthesie; parasthesia	Thiamin
	Psychotic behavior (dementia)	Niacin
	Peripheral neuropathy, symmetrical sensory and motor deficits, especially in lower extremities. Drug resistant convulsions (infants). Dementia, forgetfulness	Pyridoxine
	Areflexia. Extensor plantar responses. Loss of position and vibratory sense. Ataxia, paresthesias	B-12
	Tremor, convulsions, behavioral disturbances	Magnesium
Liver	Hepatomegaly (fatty infiltration)	Protein-Calorie
Gastro-intestinal	Anorexia, flatulence, diarrhea	B-12
	Diarrhea	Niacin, Protein-Calorie
Cardio-vascular	Tachycardia, congestive heart failure (high output type), Cardiac enlargement, electrocardiographic changes	Thiamin

ROLE OF LABORATORY IN NUTRITIONAL DIAGNOSIS

Automated laboratory determinations commonly used in community hospitals can provide clues to nutritional diagnosis. The Wintrobe indices such as the mean corpuscular volume (MCV) may be only slightly elevated yet suggest the macrocytic anemia of folic acid. The mention of a few microcytes or cells with pale centers may suggest iron deficiency. Hypersegmented neutrophils is often another sign of folic acid deficiency that may be easily missed in a perusal of laboratory data.

The serum albumin and blood urea nitrogen levels are almost routinely obtained but not always accurately interpreted. They are both key laboratory criteria of malnutrition. Serum albumin values under 3.0 gm/dl and low BUN or blood sugar values should always include protein-calorie malnutrition in their differential diagnosis.

Table 2.3 summarizes specific micronutrient or functional enzyme determinations which are valuable in nutritional diagnosis. Not all may be available in hospital or commercial laboratories.

NUTRITIONAL EVALUATION OF OBESE PATIENT

Because obesity is so common (approximately 10–15% in adolescents and 30–50% in adults) and is such an exasperating clinical problem for the patient and his physician, the following questions as part of the

TABLE 2.3. CURRENT GUIDELINES FOR CRITERIA OF NUTRITIONAL STATUS FOR LABORATORY EVALUATION

Nutrient and Units	Age of Subject (years)	Deficient	Criteria of Status Marginal	Acceptable
*Hemoglobin (gm/dl)	6–23 mos.	Up to 9.0	9.0– 9.9	10.0+
	2–5	Up to 10.0	10.0–10.9	11.0+
	6–12	Up to 10.0	10.0–11.4	11.5+
	13–16M	Up to 12.0	12.0–12.9	13.0+
	13–16F	Up to 10.0	10.0–11.4	11.5+
	16+M	Up to 12.0	12.0–13.9	14.0+
	16+F	Up to 10.0	10.0–11.9	12.0+
	Pregnant (after 6+ mos.)	Up to 9.5	9.5–10.9	11.0+
*Hematocrit (Packed cell volume in percent)	Up to 2	Up to 28	28–30	31+
	2–5	Up to 30	30–33	34+
	6–12	Up to 30	30–35	36+
	13–16M	Up to 37	37–39	40+
	13–16F	Up to 31	31–35	36+
	16+M	Up to 37	37–43	44+
	16+F	Up to 31	31–37	33+
	Pregnant	Up to 30	30–32	33+
*Serum Albumin (gm/dl)	Up to 1	—	Up to 2.5	2.5+
	1–5	—	Up to 3.0	3.0+
	6–16	—	Up to 3.5	3.5+
	16+	Up to 2.8	2.8–3.4	3.5+
	Pregnant	Up to 3.0	3.0–3.4	3.5+
*Serum Protein (gm/dl)	Up to 1	—	Up to 5.0	5.0+
	1–5	—	Up to 5.5	5.5+
	6–16	—	Up to 6.0	6.0+
	16+	Up to 6.0	6.0–6.4	6.5+
	Pregnant	Up to 5.5	5.5–5.9	6.0+
*Serum Ascorbic Acid (mg/dl)	All ages	Up to 0.1	0.1–0.19	0.2+
*Plasma vitamin A (mcg/dl)	All ages	Up to 10	10–19	20+
*Plasma Carotene (mcg/dl)	All ages	Up to 20	20–39	40+
	Pregnant	—	40–79	80+
*Serum Iron (mcg/dl)	Up to 2	Up to 30	—	30+
	2.5	Up to 40	—	40+
	6–12	Up to 50	—	50+
	12+M	Up to 60	—	60+
	12+F	Up to 40	—	40+
*Transferrin Saturation (percent)	Up to 2	Up to 15.0	—	15.0+
	2–12	Up to 20.0	—	20.0+
	12+M	Up to 20.0	—	20.0+
	12+F	Up to 15.0	—	15.0+
**Serum Folacin (ng/ml)	All ages	Up to 2.0	2.1–5.9	6.0+
**Serum vitamin B_{12} (pg/ml)	All ages	Up to 100	—	100+

TABLE 2.3. (*Continued.*)

Nutrient and Units	Age of Subject (years)	Criteria of Status: Deficient	Marginal	Acceptable
*Thiamin in Urine (mcg/g creatinine)	1–3	Up to 120	120–175	175+
	4–5	Up to 85	85–120	120+
	6–9	Up to 70	70–180	180+
	10–15	Up to 55	55–150	150+
	16+	Up to 27	27– 65	65+
	Pregnant	Up to 21	21– 49	50+
*Riboflavin in Urine (mcg/g creatinine)	1–3	Up to 150	150–499	500+
	4–5	Up to 100	100–299	300+
	6–9	Up to 85	85–269	270+
	10–16	Up to 80	70–199	200+
	16+	Up to 27	27– 79	80+
	Pregnant	Up to 30	30– 89	90+
**RBC Trans-ketolase-TPP-effect (ratio)	All ages	25+	15– 25	Up to 15
**RBC Gluta-thione Reductase-FAD-effect (ratio)	All ages	1.2+	—	Up to 1.2
**Tryptophan Load (mg Xan-thurenic acid excreted)	Adults (Dose: 100 mg/kg body weight)	25+(6 hrs.)	—	Up to 25
		75+(24 hrs.)	—	Up to 75
**Urinary Pyridoxine (mcg/g creatinine)	1–3	Up to 90	—	90+
	4–6	Up to 80	—	80+
	7–9	Up to 60	—	60+
	10–12	Up to 40	—	40+
	13–15	Up to 30	—	30+
	16+	Up to 20	—	20+
*Urinary N'methyl nicotinamide (mg/g creatinine)	All ages	Up to 0.2	0.2–5.59	0.6+
	Pregnant	Up to 0.8	0.8–2.49	2.5+
**Urinary Pantothenic Acid (mcg)	All ages	Up to 200	—	200+
**Plasma vitamin E (mg/dl)	All ages	Up to 0.2	0.2–0.6	0.6+
**Transaminase Index (ratio)				
+EGOT	Adult	2.0+	—	Up to 2.0
‡EGPT	Adult	1.25+	—	Up to 1.25

*Adapted from the Ten State Nutrition Survey
**Criteria may vary with different methodology.
+Erythrocyte Glutamic Oxalacetic Transaminase
‡ Erythrocyte Glutamic Pyruvic Transaminase

Reprinted from the American Journal of Public Health, November, 1973, Part Two, V. 63.

nutrition history may be useful in delineating pathogenic factors involved:

1. Are/were the mother and father of the patient obese?
   There is a 40% chance of obesity if one parent is obese, 80% if both.
2. Did the obesity originate in childhood; if so at what age and concurrent with what possible major life event?
   "Reactive" obesity of childhood which occurs at the time of some major event (e.g. death of a parent) may well continue through childhood.
3. Has the patient gained or lost weight in a cyclical fashion? What diets or medications have been tried?
   Crash diets, improper and unsupervised fasting and inappropriate "protein-sparing" diets require special nutritional evaluation.
4. How does the weight of the patient appear to correlate with the dietary and physical activity history?
   Onset of "middle-age" obesity usually gradual and associated with decreased activity.
5. Was the weight gain associated with marriage or pregnancy?
   In one series, 29% of women became obese at such times. Men also gain weight at the time of marriage.
6. What is the duration of the obesity?
   There may be an inverse relationship between duration and successful weight reduction.
7. Does the patient use food to negotiate psychologically stressful situations?
   Psychogenic factors are frequently related to excessive caloric intake.

The laboratory examination plays a particularly significant role in the nutritional evaluation of the obese patient. As long as the patient is obese, why not take advantage of the fact that obesity may provoke or be associated with certain metabolic abnormalities?

Laboratory or clinical determinations which may be useful include:

1. Complete blood count and serum iron to exclude polycythemia and iron deficiency.
2. One hour postprandial blood sugar level, or glucose tolerance test to rule out "chemical" diabetes.
3. Serum cholesterol, HDL and LDL cholesterol and serum triglycerides, as hypertriglyceridemia or hyperlipoproteinemias Types IIb, III, IV and V may be associated with obesity.
4. T_3-T_4 levels to exclude hypothyroidism.
5. Uric acid to exclude gout.
6. Insulin levels which may be elevated in prediabetic obese individuals.

Pulmonary function studies and resting or treadmill exercise electrocardiograms may also yield valuable clues to early respiratory or coronary dysfunction.

SUMMARY

In summary, many nutritional deficiency states are common and easily missed, particularly in their early stages. The physician has the opportunity to learn new diagnostic skills or hone those learned in the past by probing for signs and symptoms of nutritional deficiencies.

BIBLIOGRAPHY

CHRISTAKIS, G. 1973. Nutritional assessment of health programs. Am. J. Public Health *63*, Suppl. 1.

HODGES, R.E. 1980. Nutrition in Medical Practice. W.B. Saunders, Philadelphia.

McLAREN, D.S. (Editor). 1976. Nutrition in the Community. John Wiley and Sons, New York.

NATIONAL ACADEMY OF SCIENCES (NRC). 1980. Recommended Dietary Allowances, 9th Ed. Washington, D.C.

3

HOW TO MAKE A NUTRITIONAL DIAGNOSIS:

B. PEDIATRIC NUTRITIONAL DIAGNOSIS

Anthony G. Kafatos, M.D., M.P.H.

Optimal nutrition is necessary in maintaining good health which oftentimes is compromised by pediatric diseases. Optimal nutritional status can be considered more essential for the fetus, infant, child and adolescent than it is after growth has been completed. Evaluation of nutritional status at these vulnerable ages can provide valuable clinical assistance in the treatment of acute disease, assist in evaluating growth and development, and provide a possible basis for the prevention of chronic disease later in life. It is well known, for example, that various nutritional disorders act synergistically with infectious disease[1,2]. Therefore, correction of malnutrition may diminish the incidence and severity of several categories of infectious diseases. Evaluation of nutritional status will also provide very important information regarding the risk factors for chronic diseases such as coronary heart disease, hypertension, diabetes and cancer of the colon.

The process of the evaluation of nutritional status is often inadequately considered in pediatric practice despite its indisputable usefulness. It is also common in pediatric clinics or wards to find laboratory data being routinely ordered, the results of which indicate serious nutritional problems that go unrecognized or remain unresolved. These laboratory data have special significance to pediatric practice in the United States, where gross nutritional deficiencies are not common but borderline or subclinical malnutrition may be endemic in many low socioeconomic areas.

Dr. Kafatos is Associate Professor, Department of Epidemiology, University of Miami School of Medicine and Associate Director, Institute of Child Health, Athens, Greece.

On the other hand, over-nutrition and obesity are endemic in many ethnic and socioeconomic groups in the United States.

Nutritional problems likely to occur in children are dental caries; obesity; vitamin A, vitamin C, folic acid and pyridoxine deficiency; iron deficiency; hypercholesterolemia; and trace mineral deficiencies.[3,4] Severe malnutrition including protein-calorie malnutrition may also occur as a consequence of child abuse or in the failure-to-thrive infant and child.

Besides the effects of severe malnutrition on physical growth during prenatal life and early infancy, its effect on brain cell multiplication and subsequently on psychomotor development has been well established. Behavioral disorders, hyperactivity, short attention span, and other psychological and neurological problems may be related, at least in part, to the suboptimal nutritional status of the fetus and infant. Therefore, priority has to be given to utilizing all available means for early and accurate evaluation of the nutritional status of the infant and child.

In assessing the nutritional status of children, these methodologies are used: (1) dietary, (2) anthropometric measurements, (3) clinical evaluation, and (4) laboratory measurements.

DIETARY METHODOLOGY

The dietary history should be particularly useful in children who exhibit abnormal growth and development. However, even in the well-baby clinic, an evaluation of the caloric and nutrient intake will orient practicing physicians to subclinical nutritional deficiencies. For example, in a one-year-old child who consumes only evaporated or skimmed milk, it can be anticipated that iron-deficiency anemia will develop. Anemia can be detected clinically by pallor only if the hemoglobin is very low, i.e. less than 9 g/dl. It is, therefore, helpful to recognize this condition by utilizing the dietary history. Questions can be asked related to iron content of the milk. If sugar is added to milk and bottle feeding is continued after the first year, dental caries are to be expected. In cases of the failure-to-thrive syndrome, careful evaluation of caloric intake and the percentage of calories from every macronutrient may reveal dietary omissions of the mother. Determining whether the diet contains an adequate variety of foods and evaluating child-feeding practices, such as pica, assists in establishing the diagnosis.

However, the practicing physician often does not have enough time for a detailed dietary history so that he can translate food consumption information into types and amounts of nutrients with the use of food composition tables. A detailed calculation of nutrient intake is not required for every child. However, a child with retarded growth needs a careful evaluation of caloric and major nutrient intake such as protein, vitamin A and iron.

For rapid caloric and nutrient evaluation, food composition tables of the most commonly used foods are included (Appendix B.1). Qualitative information concerning adequacy of the child's diet can be obtained by asking about the frequency of intakes from all six food groups. These groups include protein-rich foods such as meat, fish, poultry; cereal grains, dairy products, vegetables, fruits and fats and oils. For routine pediatric dietary evaluation, a diet history form is available in Tables 3.1 and 3.2. The 24-hour dietary recall is the most frequently used and the most rapid method of assessing food intake. It is particularly useful for persons whose daily fluctuations of food intake is minimal, which is likely to be the case in infants. This method does not indicate trends in eating habits; however, in combination with weekly or monthly frequency of foods consumed, this can result in a realistic assessment of nutrient intake. Consecutive 24-hour dietary recalls every two weeks during clinic visits of children with inadequate growth and nutritional problems may reveal trends in their eating habits.

TABLE 3.1. DIETARY INTAKE BY FOOD GROUP/FREQUENCY OF CONSUMPTION IN A 1-WEEK PERIOD

Check the column which indicates number of times child eats foods in each group, for period of one week:

Food Group	Hardly ever or never	1	2	3	4	5	6	7	7 specify
Milk (any kind) cheese or yogurt									
Beef, pork, sausage									
Chicken									
Fish									
Eggs									
Legumes									
Fruits									
Vegetables									
Bread, crackers, rice, macaroni, spaghetti, noodles, cereals, potatoes									
Candy, soft drinks, chocolate, jam, jellies, syrup									

ANTHROPOMETRIC MEASUREMENTS

Body size, as assessed by weight and skinfold thickness, is closely related to food intake and utilization from the time of conception to the geriatric period. The rapid increase of body size of the fetus, infant, child and adolescent requires frequent and accurate evaluation. This will determine whether caloric and nutrient intake is adequate for normal growth and development. It is therefore necessary for every pediatrician

TABLE 3.2. DIET EVALUATION SCORE SHEET

Food Groups	Include 1 weekend day 1st	2nd	3rd	Average Per day	Number of servings and serving size CHILD 1–3	4–6	7–10	ADOLESCENT 11–14	15–18	Difference
Milk Group										
Milk					2/3 c	2/3 c	3/4 c	4/5 c	4/5 c	
Ice Cream										
Cheese					6 oz	8 oz	8 oz	8 oz	8 oz	
Meat Group					2 serv	2 serv	2 serv	2 serv	2+ serv	
Meat, poultry/fish					2/3 oz	3/4 oz	4/5 oz	5/6 oz	5/6 oz	
Eggs					1	1	2	2	2	
Dried beans, peas					1/2 c	3/4 c	1 c	1 c	1 c	
Bread/Cereal Group					4 sm ser	4 serv	4/5 serv	5/6 serv	6/8 serv	
(whole grain or enriched)										
Bread					1/2 sl	1 sl	1 sl	1 sl	1 sl	
Cereal					1/3 c	1/2 c	3/4 c	1 c	1 c	
Fruit & Vegetables					4 sm serv	4/5 serv	5/6 serv	6+ serv	6+ serv	
Vitamin C-good source					1/4 c	1 c	1 c	1 c	1 c	
Vitamin A-good source					2 T	2/3 wk	2/3 wk	2/3 wk	2/3 wk	
Others					4 T					
Miscellaneous										
Sweets/desserts/snack foods/chips/soft drinks										
Butter/margarine					0	2/3 T	2/3 T	4+ T	4+ T	
Recommended Allowances										
Calories					1300	1800	2400	Girls: 2400 Boys: 2800	Girls: 2100 Boys: 3000	
Protein					23 gm	30 gm	36 gm	Girls: 44 gms Boys: 44 gms	Girls: 48 gms Boys: 54 gms	

to undertake pediatric anthropometric measurements and subsequently to compare them with standards derived from the same population.[6]

The most practicable and easily obtainable anthropometric measurements are the weight, length or height, head circumference, arm circumference, midarm and subscapular skinfold thickness.[5,7] (Appendices B.2 and B.3). Measurements obtained are plotted on growth charts. To use the chart, one plots points that represent the child's age on the horizontal axis and the weight or length on the vertical axis (Appendix B.2). If individual measurements taken at one point in time are plotted in a group of children, a pattern of growth achievement for the group can be determined. Plots of measurements of children having low birth weight may be misleading if plotted against the reference growth chart, particularly during the first year of life because commonly used growth charts are based on full-term infants. If, for example, 45% of the children in a group fall below the 25th percentile of the reference chart for body length instead of the expected 25%, nutritional problems are likely to exist. Important determinants of anthropometric measurements are sex, birth weight and socioeconomic status of the families.

The interpretation of anthropometric findings in an infant or child should be based on serial observations rather than single measurements at one point in time. Two measurements over a defined period of time permit calculation of growth. Although it is recognized that weight and height of the normal infant and child do not necessarily progress in a uniform fashion along well-defined channels, the extent to which serially-made measurements may differ independently and simultaneously from such channels has never been determined. There are marked differences in rates of growth at various ages. Therefore, susceptibility of a child to nutritional deprivation will vary at different ages but is always greater during periods of more rapid growth.

Weight should be measured to the nearest 10 g for infants or 100 g for children. The scale should be calibrated every few months using reference weights. The measurements of length require great care in order to assess the linear growth of the child.

Length or height correlates better with socioeconomic status than does weight. It is not usually affected by short-term nutritional deficits and is, therefore, valuable in indicating long-standing nutritional deficiencies. Length is usually taken for children up to 36 months of age and height thereafter.

Head circumference is a good index of brain growth. It is usually taken from infants and children as a screening test for microcephaly and macrocephaly.[7]

Skinfold thickness indicates the caloric reserve of the individual. Decreased skinfold thickness (less than 5 mm) suggests protein-calorie malnutrition, and excessive thickness indicates obesity (Table 3.3). The measurement of skinfold thickness utilizing calipers correlates well with ultrasonic and electrical conductivity measurement of adipose tissue as well as with total body fat. This measure is superior to weight-for-age and weight-for-height in assessing obesity.[8,9]

The left mid-arm circumference is another convenient method to quantitate muscle development and fatness. Muscle circumference is calculated by subtracting skinfold measurements from arm circumference which indicates muscle size. Protein-calorie malnutrition and negative nitrogen balance induce muscle wasting and decreased muscle circumference.

TABLE 3.3. APPROXIMATE LIMITS FOR MID-UPPER ARM CIRCUMFERENCE AND TRICEPS FATFOLD[1]

Age	Mid-Upper Arm Circumference 3rd to 5th Percentile* Cm	Boys	Triceps Fatfold 90th to 97th Percentile**	Girls
0 mos.	9		10	
3 mos.	10		11	
6 mos.	11½		12	
9 mos.	12		13	
12 mos.	13		14	
2 yrs.	13		13	
3 yrs.	13		13	
4 yrs.	13½		13	
5 yrs.	13½		13	
6 yrs.	14	12		15
7 yrs.	14	13		16
8 yrs.	14½	14		17
9 yrs.	15	14		18
10 yrs.	16	16		20
11 yrs.	16½	17		21
12–16 yrs.	17–20	18–20		22–25

*Under this value suggests undernutrition
**Over this value suggests obesity (values in mm)

[1] Zerfas and Neumann, Pediatric Clinics of North America, 24:253, 1977.

CLINICAL EVALUATION

Clinical nutritional evaluation should be an integral part of the physical examination. It is not time consuming because general problems such as apathy, irritability, pallor, edema, obesity or emaciation are easy to detect. Specific clinical signs of primary hypovitaminoses or trace mineral deficiencies are not commonly seen in the United States but are frequently found in children of developing nations. Every practicing physician should be familiar, however, with clinical signs of malnutrition because secondary malnutrition from malignancies, gastrointestinal diseases, kidney, liver, central nervous system diseases and others are commonly seen in hospitalized children.

The effects of intrauterine malnutrition are more difficult to recognize. Low birthweight babies were considered to be premature. Objective means are available today for the accurate estimation of gestational age based on clinical criteria and not on the last menstruation.[10] The estimated gestational age and birthweight will define the percentile in which the newborn's weight is located (Appendix B.4).

Newborns subjected to intrauterine malnutrition are substantially below the 10th percentile on the growth chart. They have paper-thin skinfolds and are irritable from hypoglycemia and/or pyridoxine deficiency; convulsions may therefore occur. Small-for-gestational age babies may be due to endogenous (placental abnormalities) or exogenous (maternal malnutrition) factors. They also exhibit increased risk of perinatal asphyxia, polycythemia, hypothermia, congenital malformations, chronic intrauterine infections and massive pulmonary hemorrhage. In a similar way, preterm infants are predisposed to a large number of special risks including hyaline membrane disease, recurrent apnea, infection, hypoglycemia, hypothermia, hyperbilirubinemia, necrotizing enterocolitis, and intraventricular hemorrhage.

Post-term babies are also at special risk for perinatal asphyxia, meconium aspiration and pneumothorax. They are characteristically thin with very little subcutaneous fat; the skin is wrinkled and paper-like. Babies born to diabetic mothers are often large for gestational age and at high risk for hyaline membrane disease, hypocalcemia and hyperbilirubinemia. Early diagnosis and aggressive nutritional therapy of these high-risk newborns serve to decrease their perinatal morbidity and mortality.

The diagnosis of infants and children with growth failure should include medical history, physical examination, laboratory tests and roentgenograms to exclude infections or inflammatory diseases of kidneys, central nervous system, cardiovascular and gastrointestinal systems, etc. Attempts should be made to arrive at a definite diagnosis. On the other hand, signs of nutritional disorders in children having surgery-related or other major illnesses should be promptly recognized and corrected. Hospital malnutrition in children is often iatrogenic and may be associated with serious complications and prolong hospitalization. The prevalence of this problem, unlike that of adult hospital malnutrition, is not currently known.

Protein-calorie malnutrition due to inadequate food intake is not unusual in immigrants arriving from the Caribbean Islands and from South America. It is essential for every physician to know how to detect a child with protein-calorie malnutrition. The child with kwashiorkor is apathetic and disinterested but if disturbed during the examination may become miserable and irritable. Edema is always present in kwashiorkor because of lack of protein in the diet and very low serum albumin. The hair changes in texture and color and is easily pluckable. There is depigmentation of the skin with extensive dermatosis in areas of friction. Diarrhea, parasites, anemia and signs of vitamin and mineral deficiencies may also be present. Growth failure is common in both kwashiorkor and marasmus.

Marasmus, in contrast to kwashiorkor, is due to combined severe deficiency of both protein and calories. In the United States, marasmus can be seen in neglected children. They have severe muscle wasting and very little subcutaneous fat. In contrast to kwashiorkor, marasmic children have good appetites; they are wide-eyed and alert in appearance. Anemia, diarrhea and parasites may also be present.

SPECIFIC NUTRIENT DEFICIENCIES

Vitamin A deficiency is among the most prevalent nutritional deficiencies in developing countries of the world. In the United States, subclinical vitamin A deficiency may be detected by biochemical means.[4] Vitamin A deficiency involves nearly all organs. Prolonged deficiency causes growth failure; impaired dark adaptation and hyperkeratosis of the skin are among the first clinical signs of deficiency. Dark adaptation is difficult to measure in infants and young children. Other symptoms of vitamin A deficiency include mental retardation, dry and scaly skin, Bitot's spot on the sclera of the eye, and corneal changes that may proceed to ulceration and blindness. Cartilage and bones are often involved in addition to other epithelial and connective tissue; bone formation ceases and bone shape is abnormal.[11]

Excessive doses of vitamin A, i.e., 20,000 I.U. or more daily for more than one month, are likely to be toxic. Symptoms of vitamin A toxicity include anorexia, irritability, increased intracranial pressure, desquamation of the skin, and bone changes.[11]

The child with rickets (vitamin D deficiency) appears to be plump and well fed. He or she tends to be irritable and flabby because of decreased muscle tone. The child is late in reaching developmental milestones such as sitting, standing or walking. There is delay in teeth eruption; swelling of the epiphysis of the bones also occurs which may first be seen at the wrist. A bead-like appearance at the costochondral margin is called "rachitic rosary." Deformities of the chest include Harrison's sulcus and pigeon chest. In infants, craniotabes is often the first sign of rickets. This consists of areas of softening of the skull which usually affect the occipital and parietal bones. There is also delayed closure of the anterior fontanel. In advanced rickets, there may be bossing of the skull and bowed leg deformities. Kyphosis is a very serious deformity of the spine, and changes in the pelvic bones may result in difficulties in childbirth in women who had rickets during childhood. Tetany may occur as a result of reduced levels of serum calcium.[12]

Excessive intake of vitamin D causes infantile "idiopathic" hypercalcemia. Vitamin D toxicity follows ingestion of 3000 to 4000 I.U. of vitamin D daily. Symptoms include failure-to-thrive, vomiting, mental retardation, bony changes, elevated concentration of serum calcium, renal failure and hypertension.[12]

Vitamin E deficiency has been found in premature infants and results in increased hemolysis of erythrocytes, which can be reversed by administration of alphatocopherol.[13]

Petechial hemorrhages are the earliest clinical signs of vitamin C deficiency. Other symptoms are fatigue, irritability, tenderness of the lower extremities and swelling of joints and gums. Growth retardation and iron deficiency anemia are also common in vitamin C-deficient children. Vitamin C deficiency in premature infants causes transient tyrosinemia which, if untreated, may be related to low I.Q. status later in life. Full-blown clinical manifestations of vitamin C deficiency (scurvy) do not usually occur in infants less than three months of age.

Vitamin B_1 or thiamin deficiency is not usually found in American infants and children. Soy-based formulas, not supplemented with thiamin and which serve as the major source of calories for a long period of time, may cause thiamin deficiency. In children in developing countries having inadequate milk intake, thiamin deficiency is common. Severe vitamin B_1 deficiency causes beriberi. Infantile beriberi is characterized by dyspnea, cyanosis, cardiac failure and rapid death. In chronic forms, the infant is thin and wasted, diarrhea and vomiting may develop, and the appearance is marasmic. Edema, aphonia and convulsions may occur in the terminal stages.

Vitamin B_2 (riboflavin) deficiency of the diet causes hyporiboflavinosis. Symptoms include angular stomatitis, cheilosis, glossitis, papillary atrophy, vascularization of the cornea, photophobia and lacrimation.

Niacin deficiency (pellagra) is most likely to occur in children with cirrhosis of the liver, chronic diarrhea diseases, diabetes mellitus, neoplasia, prolonged febrile illness and after total parenteral nutrition without niacin supplements. The symptoms of niacin deficiency include abdominal pain, diarrhea, angular stomatitis, cheilosis, irritability and skin lesions (erythema, scaly, cracked skin progressing to desquamation).

Vitamin B_6 deficiency (pyridoxine) results in convulsive seizures in infants, hyperirritability and anemia.

Folic acid deficiency is responsible for megaloblastic anemia in children and infants on a solely milk diet because milk is deficient in folate.

The major minerals, sodium, chlorine, potassium, calcium, phosphorus, magnesium, sulfur and iron, will not be discussed. Most of the trace minerals, however, such as chromium, manganese, cobalt, copper, zinc, molybdenum, iodine, and selenium, are under current investigation. The only manifestation of chromium deficiency thus far documented in human subjects is impaired glucose tolerance.[14] There is no evidence of manganese deficiency in human subjects. Cobalt is an essential nutrient because it is part of vitamin B_{12}. Copper is necessary for the structure and function of various enzymes. Copper deficiency coexists with severe malnutrition associated with bone changes and growth retardation. Copper deficiency causes anemia and has also been described in premature infants.

Dietary deficiency of zinc in infants and children is associated with anorexia, retarded growth, delayed sexual maturation, lymphopenia, and abnormalities in keratinization.[15] Acrodermatitis enteropathica is due to severe zinc deficiency as a result of a genetic disorder in zinc metabolism. It is characterized by severe growth retardation and diarrhea, which does not respond to any other therapeutic measure. A characteristic exanthem is almost always present in acrodermatitis enteropathica. All symptoms disappear quickly following the administration of zinc 10–20 times above the recommended daily dietary allowances.

LABORATORY STUDIES

A number of hematological and biochemical measurements are useful in determining nutritional status of infants and children including albumin, hemoglobin, red blood cell indices, serum transferrin saturation, serum proteins, serum vitamins and minerals. Homeostatic mechanisms control levels of certain components independently of short-term dietary influences. Such components include hemoglobin, protein, cholesterol, and vitamin A. In contrast, blood levels of water-soluble vitamins, such as ascorbic acid, may fluctuate with dietary intake. These relationships should be taken into account in selecting biochemical determinations to be carried out and in evaluating the results in relation to dietary intake.

Criteria used to establish that a population of children is normal involve the development of standards for that population. Children having values two standard deviations below the mean of the population are considered abnormal. Existing standards of selected measurements are presented in Chapter 2.

Certain biochemical tests such as white blood cell pyruvate kinase and adenylate kinase may predict fetal malnutrition before the 32nd week of pregnancy. Cord blood total cholesterol and low density lipoprotein cholesterol give an accurate diagnosis of the genetic hypercholesterolemias. As in the adult, skin testing (Candida, PPD) for immune response and decreased lymphocyte count may indicate underlying malnutrition.

CONCLUSION

Nutritional adequacy is a basis for the function and growth of every cell in the human body. Over-consumption or under-consumption of nutrients, defects in absorption, excretion or metabolism, may lead to nutritional disorders. Dietary and laboratory methodologies assist in the diagnosis of these nutritional disorders in the preclinical stage for early correction. Advanced nutritional disorders are characterized by specific clinical signs. The use of anthropometry will greatly assist the pediatric nutritional diagnosis in cases of primary or secondary malnutrition.

Finally, a dietary history assessment in every pediatric clinic visit will reveal feeding and eating practices of the child which serve as a nutrition education tool for optimal growth and maintenance of good health.

REFERENCES

1. SCRIMSHAW, N.S.; TAYLOR, C.E., and GORDON, J.E.: Interactions of Nutrition and Infection, WHO Monograph, Geneva 1968.
2. HUGHES, W.T.; PRICE, R.A.; SISKO, F.; HORVAN, S.; KAFATOS, A.G.; SCHONLAND, M., and SMYTHE, P.M.: Protein-Calorie Malnutrition. A Host Determinant for Pneumocystis Carinii Infection, Am. J. Dis. Child 128:44, 1974.
3. TEN-STATE NUTRITION SURVEY, 1968–1970. Health Services and Mental Health Administration, Center for Disease Control, Atlanta, Georgia. U.S. Govt. Printing Office, 1973.
4. KAFATOS, A.G., and ZEE, P.: Nutritional Benefits From Federal Food Assistance. A Survey of Pre-School Black Children From Low-Income Families in Memphis, Am. J. Dis. Child. 131:265, 1977.
5. ZERFAS, A.J., and NEUMANN, C.G.: Office Assessment of Nutritional Status, Pediatric Clin. N. Amer. 24:253, 1977.
6. CHRISTAKIS, G. (ed.): Nutritional Assessment in Health Programs, J. Am. Public Health (suppl.) 63, Part 2, November, 1973.
7. NELLHAUS, G.: Head Circumference From Birth to 18 Years, Pediatrics 41:106, 1968.
8. BOOTH, R.A. *et al.*: Measurement of Fat Thickness in Man: A Comparison of Ultrasound, Harpenden Calipers and Electrical Conductivity, J. Nutr. 20:719, 1966.
9. PARVIZKOVA, J.: Total Body Fat, Skinfold Thickness in Children, Metabolism 10:794, 1961.

10. DUBOWITZ, L., and DUBOWITZ, V., and GOLDBERG, C.: Clinical Assessment of Gestational Age in the Newborn Infant, J. Pediat. 77:1, 1970.
11. OOMEN, H.A.P.C.: Vitamin A Deficiency, Xerophthalmia and Blindness, In Nutrition Reviews, Present Knowledge in Nutrition. The Nutrition Foundation, Inc. New York/Washington, 1976.
12. OMDAHL, J.L., and DELUCA, H.F.: Vitamin D- in Modern Nutrition, in Health and Disease. Ed. by R. S. Goodhart and M.E. Shils. Lea & Febiger, Philadelphia, 1973.
13. OSKI, F.A., and BARNESS, L.A.: Vitamin E Deficiency: A Previously Unrecognized Cause of Hemolytic Anemia in Premature Infants, J. Pediat. 70:211, 1967.
14. GURSON, C.T., and SANER, G.: Effects of Chromium on Glucose Utilization in Marasmic Protein-Calorie Malnutrition, Am. J. Clin. Nutr. 24:1313, 1971.
15. HAMBRIDGE, K.M.: The Role of Zinc and Other Trace Metals in Pediatric Nutrition and Health, Ped. Clin. North America, 24:95, 1977.

4

REVOLUTION IN OBSTETRICS: PREGNANCY NUTRITION

Charles S. Mahan, M.D.

Doctors, nurses, and the people they help take care of have all seemed to develop their own particular, and at times unusual, views of how and what and how much pregnant women should eat. Over the past four decades, theories on feeding pregnant women have jumped from pushing red meat, to no meat, to starvation, and currently to a total reversal of the latter. In the past five years there has been a strong interest developing in all aspects of nutrition by the public and professionals alike. In many areas of medicine, this interest has raised more questions than there are answers available. In this short treatise, an attempt will be made to contrast the older ideas of the past decade, about some of the more common prenatal nutrition problems, to ideas that have sprung up recently. For more detailed information on these and some of the less common nutrition problems in pregnancy, references 1–4 are good general works to consult.

PRECONCEPTION NUTRITION

In the past, often the first opportunity the physician had to give nutrition counseling was at the first prenatal visit or perhaps at the time of confirmation of pregnancy when a pregnancy test was done. Today we are encouraging women to make preconception visits to their physicians so that all possible health problems that might influence the pregnancy

Dr. Mahan is Associate Professor, Department of Obstetrics and Gynecology, University of Florida College of Medicine, Gainesville, and also Director of the Division of Ambulatory Services for Women. He serves as Director of the North Central Florida Maternal and Infant Care Project.

can be reviewed. This serves as a time not only to screen for any possible genetic problems that the prospective family may have but also to review many facets of the person's nutritional status. This would include smoking and alcohol intake, both of which should be stopped before pregnancy begins. Contraceptive techniques that would affect nutrition include the intrauterine device, which usually causes increased blood loss during periods and may therefore cause an increased iron loss. Oral contraceptives may decrease the amount of folic acid available in the mother early in pregnancy if they were taken close to the time of conception with no replacement of folic acid by supplements. It is now thought that oral contraceptives should be stopped at least three months before conception, not only for nutritional reasons but for teratogenic reasons. Other general aspects of diet and nutrition need to be reviewed at this time including a look at the patient's weight. Women who are overweight may be successful in reducing before pregnancy is attempted, but if this is done they should be back on a regular diet the month before they attempt to conceive. Patients who are underweight have the more serious problem as far as a prognosis for pregnancy outcome and should be strongly encouraged to supplement their diet to try to gain enough weight to be within normal range for their height at the time pregnancy begins.

MATERNAL WEIGHT GAIN

In the past pregnant women were instructed, sometimes in an overbearing fashion, to limit their weight to a total gain of 15–18 lb during their whole pregnancy. Usually no adjustments were made for the prepregnancy weight and often the obese woman was told to use pregnancy as an opportune time to lose weight. In the past the standard urinalysis done at the time of each prenatal visit included sugar and albumin testing but not testing for ketones.

Now, studies have shown that in general "bigger babies are better babies." Most nutrition experts in the United States have now recommended that the normal weight gain for pregnancy for women of normal height should range between 20–30 lb. The average weight gain in Scandinavian countries, which have better perinatal outcomes than the United States, is between 30–35 lb, so we still may be shooting rather low in our country. If people have low prepregnancy weights for their heights they are encouraged to gain much more than the average woman in pregnancy.

The ideal weight gain curve in pregnancy is shown in Figure 4.1. As can be seen from that figure, most of the extra calories that need to be taken in and, hopefully, most of the weight gain, will occur in the last two trimesters of pregnancy. This is especially important in the last trimester

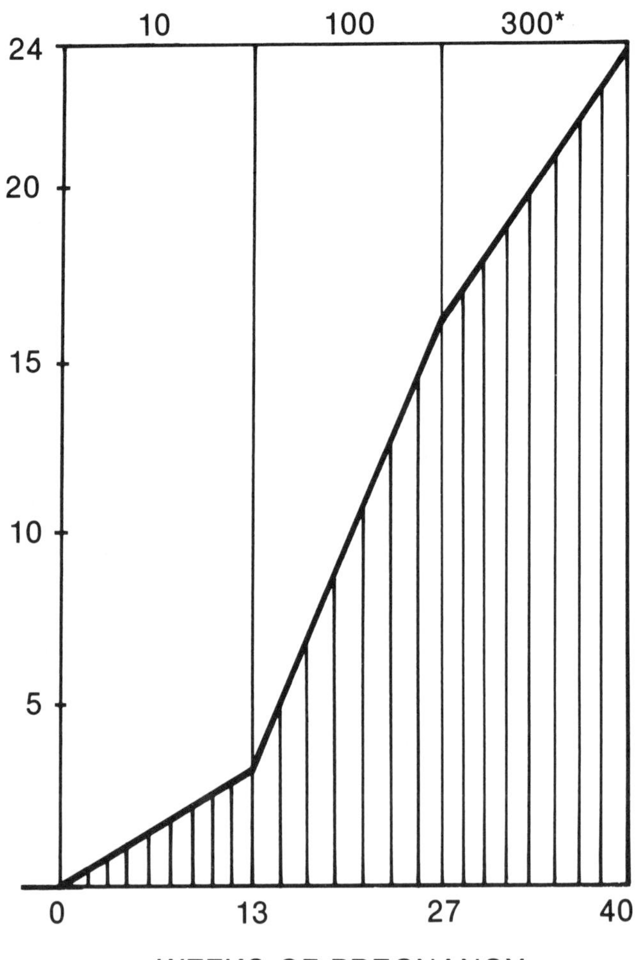

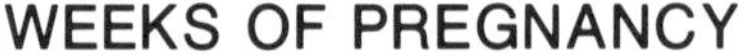

FIG. 4.1. THE IDEAL WEIGHT GAIN CURVE FOR PREGNANCY IN A WOMAN OF NORMAL HEIGHT. THE STAR IS BESIDE THE NUMBERS OF EXTRA CALORIES NEEDED PER DAY IN EACH TRIMESTER OF PREGNANCY.

since much of the brain growth of the new individual will occur in the last three months of intrauterine life and the first three months in the outside world. This makes the brain very vulnerable to malnutrition during this six month period of time.

Ketone testing is usually available on the same dip sticks that are used to test urines at each prenatal visit for sugar and protein. Testing for ketones is important since ketonuria, especially in the third trimester of pregnancy when the brain is most actively growing, is usually a sign of starvation ketosis which may cause direct brain damage.[5]

The finding of ketone bodies in the urine should be taken seriously and the mother's diet should be reviewed to be sure that she is not missing meals and is taking in adequate amounts of calories. Occasionally hospitalization is mandatory to correct the ketosis through intravenous feedings and to help the mother with her diet under closer observation. The ketone bodies that appear in the urine during the first trimester as a result of nausea and vomiting in pregnancy have not been found to be as important in affecting pregnancy outcome as those later in gestation when brain growth is occurring.

One of the most important topics to be covered at the first prenatal visit with the physician is the expected ideal weight gain during the pregnancy for that particular patient. Using her prepregnancy weight, she should be given a definite range to shoot for, as far as expected weight at the end of the pregnancy. If the patient has any high-risk nutritional problems uncovered at the first prenatal visit or if any develop during the pregnancy, it may be important to refer the patient to a registered nutritionist if the physician does not have time to take a 24-hour recall diet history and do in-depth diet counseling.

THE TEEN-AGE MOTHER

In the past, due to her late entrance into the prenatal system, and possibly because of the physicians' fears of the possible development of toxemia, teenagers either have had no nutritional advice or were advised on low salt, low calorie diets.

Recent studies done at the University of Florida College of Medicine have confirmed that most of the pregnancy problems encountered by the young pregnant teenagers (those under 16) are either directly or indirectly related to their nutritional status. These teenagers have a much higher incidence of toxemia of pregnancy, premature labor and delivery, and postpartum infections than more mature mothers.[6]

Teenagers bring many problems unique to their age group into a pregnancy. Some of the problems include the fact that many teenage girls are on self-imposed weight loss diets even if their weights are normal for their heights; teenage girls typically eat very little red meat; teenage girls typically eat plenty of junk food. In addition to the tremendous caloric requirements of pregnancy, teenagers also bring into pregnancy the added caloric requirements of their rapid growth at this particular age, so good dietary management is essential to a good outcome for both mother and baby.

Teenagers who are pregnant need special dietary management, preferably by a registered nutritionist, but the doctor and nurse are important in emphasizing the importance of proper diet to the teenager since their words often carry more weight to the teenager than the nutritionist's. The nutritionist will often do a diet history by a 24-hour recall of food intake and then outline a nutritious diet for the teenager that takes into account the needs for the particular trimester of pregnancy she is in plus her growth needs. The nutritionist then usually tells the teenager that if she will follow the diet carefully she can eat any junk food she wants on top of the diet. This added touch of liberalism at the end is often what it takes to convince a recalcitrant teenager to take the outlined nutrition program seriously. Because of their rapid growth, teenagers often need foods that are high in vitamins and iron and foods that will supply extra calcium.

Teenagers typically may be deficient in vitamins A, B, C, D and perhaps folic acid. In addition to dietary supplements, it may be important to place teenagers on standard oral preparations of prenatal vitamins with folic acid and oral iron supplementation so they are getting at least 60 mg of elemental iron per day.

THE OBESE MOTHER

In the past many obese women were counseled that pregnancy was a good time to lose weight, and some doctors even provided amphetamines to these women to help this weight loss.

On the basis of recent nutritional research, proper management of the obese pregnant woman now includes impressing her with the fact that she should gain at least 25–30 lb for the pregnancy so that she will keep a good caloric balance and not start breaking down her fats due to starvation with subsequent ketosis. It is stressed to her that her obesity does make her high-risk for other problems during pregnancy such as dystocia, malpresentation, hemorrhage, etc., but that it is important to have an excellent nutritional intake for the best fetal outcome and that we will try to help her lose weight when pregnancy and/or lactation is done with. We do encourage these women to breast feed since that has been shown to help women lose weight faster in the postpartum period and we stress to the women that obesity is a form of malnutrition.

UNUSUAL DIETS

Vegans (vegetarians) and their fetuses can get through pregnancy in good health but it may take more effort and more thorough counseling than many doctors are able to give. In these situations it is important for the vegan to get counseling from a registered nutritionist.

If the mother is a strict vegan and takes in no animal-derived foods, she can suffer deficiencies of certain nutrients such as iron, zinc, chromium and vitamin B_{12} (which is not present in plants) which may lead to health problems in herself and her baby.[8] Vitamin and iron supplements may be very important for vegan mothers.

Pica is the regular and excessive ingestion of foods and substances that have no nutritional value. The practices of nibbling on refrigerator freezer ice, red clay, laundry starch, etc., are seen more commonly in poor rural women of the south. Currently, most nutritionists think that pica is a result of iron deficiency (and of course can make it even worse) and is mainly a problem because the abnormal substance ingested ruins the appetite for nutritious foods. Pica is treated by intensive, convincing dietary counseling, stressing outcomes for mother and baby and attempting to change eating habits. Iron and vitamin supplements are usually important in these cases.

ALCOHOL AND OTHER VICES

In the recent past we have told women to stop smoking completely in pregnancy and to cut down on their alcohol intake to less than three ounces of whiskey a day with no particular limits on the amount of wine and beer except to avoid becoming drunk.

Recently the medical literature has been flooded with reports outlining the various and sundry horrors of the fetal alcohol syndrome. The problems being discovered in the babies range from severe anomalies to intrauterine growth retardation. The severity of the effects on the baby seems to be related to the amount of alcohol ingested but at the present time there is some concern that any amount of alcohol can cause potential damage at any time in pregnancy. Current advice then is to cut out alcohol intake completely during pregnancy.

Both alcoholics and smokers may, in addition to the direct toxic effects of the substances they are taking in, have a related decrease in appetite and therefore fail to eat. Also, these habits may cause them to spend scarce dollars on cigarettes and whiskey instead of purchasing nutritious foods. Heavy smoking and drinking may also cause problems with the absorption or metabolism of certain important nutrients.

There is some evidence that heavy caffeine intake (over eight cups of coffee per day) can lead to poor pregnancy outcomes.[7]

ANEMIAS, IRON AND VITAMINS

One area in which very little has changed over the past ten or 15 years is the area of iron and vitamin supplementation to the pregnant woman. This has become a routine in prenatal care in most parts of the country even though there is still great argument as to whether such supplements are needed for the majority of women.

Most upper middle class women with good incomes and excellent diets who enter pregnancy with no nutritional risk problems and have a normal weight gain throughout pregnancy do not need prenatal vitamins with folic acid supplementation. However, teenagers of all social classes, indigent women and women with nutritional high-risk problems as outlined in this paper should have supplementation with a standard prenatal vitamin preparation with at least 300–500 micrograms of folic acid in it.

Ninety-five percent of all anemias seen in pregnancy are primarily due to iron deficiency. Most anemias are seen in populations of low-income women, and since most of these women are being supplemented with prenatal vitamins with folic acid, it is a rare event to diagnose a folic acid deficiency anemia in the present day. Iron deficiency in pregnant women can usually be diagnosed, not with expensive laboratory tests, but with a therapeutic trial of oral iron. If oral treatment (which is just as effective as parenteral iron treatment) slows down or stops a falling hematocrit within 3–4 weeks after beginning administration is considered diagnostic of an iron deficiency anemia and no further workup is needed. Because many women have a chronic iron deficit due to reproductive events, menstrual loss, etc., we think it is important for them to stay on low dose iron supplementation for 3–4 months after each pregnancy to build up their reserves. Again, this is probably not necessary in people with an entirely normal nutritional history and excellent nutrition intake.

It must continually be stressed to the patient that iron and vitamin supplements, while they may be helpful, are certainly no substitute for a good balanced intake of food.

SALT INTAKE, DIURETICS AND TOXEMIA

In the past we often gave pregnant women one gram sodium diets at the first sign of any ankle edema in the late second trimester. We also commonly gave diuretics to primagravidas to "prevent" preeclampsia. If high blood pressure developed, in spite of our diuretic therapy, we often increased the dosage of diuretics, put the patient on a one-gram sodium diet and were careful to give her no salt in her intravenous fluids when she was hospitalized. As a result we saw many mothers and babies suffering from hyponatremia; the preeclampsia usually stayed the same or got worse; the diuretics occasionally caused platelet problems with subsequent bleeding in the babies and occasionally hemorrhagic pancreatitis in the mother.

Modern obstetric research has still not found the cause of toxemia but it has shown that salt has little or no relationship to the development of preeclampsia. Pregnant women need at least a two-gram sodium intake each day to maintain normal growth for themselves and their babies. We know that ankle and leg edema is a normal physiologic change in pregnancy and this is now treated, if it is bothersome to the mother, with support stockings or bed rest but not with salt restriction or diuretics. Mothers are now advised to salt their food to their taste during pregnancy.

There is some evidence to show that the incidence of toxemia is decreased with better protein and calorie nutrition and that women with good nutrition and adequate weight gain have few cases of toxemia unless chronic hypertension or renal disease preexisted.

Diuretics are presently indicated in pregnancy only for congestive heart failure and other rare problems.

MOTHER WITH DIABETES

In the past, insulin-dependent diabetic mothers were given 1800 calorie ADA diets, and it was thought to be safer to manage their insulin so that their blood sugars remained on the high side to avoid insulin reactions. The majority of them were given low salt diets and diuretics to prevent toxemia which was more common in diabetic pregnancies, and usually delivery was planned strictly at 37 weeks of gestation.

Currently it is thought that pregnant diabetic women should have at least 2000 to 2200 calories per day in their diets (Table 4.1). This complicated diet problem should be handled by a registered nutritionist with strong support by the physician and nurse.

Modern management of diabetes in pregnancy includes "tight" control of food intake and insulin administration so that the woman's blood sugars are kept in the normal range at all times. This avoids two problems that are dangerous to the baby—ketosis and high blood sugar levels. Ketosis as reflected by acetonuria, whether due to fasting and subsequent starvation or to poor control of diabetes, can be damaging to the fetus as mentioned previously. On the other hand, very high levels of glucose in the mother pass freely to the baby across the placenta and cause overgrowth (macrosomia) which can lead to dystocia and/or possible deterioration of fetal status.

TABLE 4.1. DIET FOR THE PREGNANT DIABETIC

2000–2200 calories per day or 35 calories per kg of ideal body weight

	Percent of total calories
Carbohydrates	45–55
Fats	25–30
Protein	20–25
	Percent of total calories
Breakfast	25
Lunch	30
Dinner	30
Bedtime snack	15

Most perinatal centers now deliver diabetic mothers when fetal maturity tests show that the baby can survive outside the uterus. These are balanced against the results of modern methods of monitoring the in-utero well-being of the fetus (nonstress tests, stress tests, HPL, estriol) which may show early fetal deterioration. None of the above technology is as important to successful outcome of the diabetic pregnancy as careful nutritional and insulin management. Properly managed, the babies of diabetic mothers should have the same perinatal mortality rate as babies of mothers without diabetes.

INTRAUTERINE GROWTH RETARDATION

In the past, when mothers produced babies that weighed less than 2500 grams at term, people remarked how tough these little wrinkled babies were and how well they survived compared to babies born prematurely at similar weights.

In the past few decades we have learned, to our dismay, that these small, "tough" babies often remain stunted in growth and never catch up. Worse than that, they have a much higher chance than the average size baby of developing mental retardation and severe learning disabilities as they grow older. Intrauterine retardation (IUGR) is much more commonly found in impoverished mothers or women with chronic hypertension. It is important that women in these categories plus women with a past history of IUGR get very early prenatal care which includes help with good diet management. The uterus should be watched and measured carefully for normal growth, and if it deviates from the normal growth pattern serial sonograms should be obtained. In addition to eating a regular diet for pregnancy, these women, especially if they were underweight for their height prenatally, may benefit from eating canned protein-calorie supplements such as are currently given to patients with advanced malignancies, although no good studies have been done to prove that this is helpful. Bed rest, intrauterine monitoring, and possible early delivery when the fetal lungs are mature are also steps in the modern management of IUGR.

Malnutrition is an important element in intrauterine growth retardation but very often other factors are also involved and must be carefully considered.

THE MOTHER IN POVERTY

In the past women in poverty often got little or no prenatal care, often had no source of adequate nutrition, and had no access to government programs which would help supplement their diets.

Now, programs for indigent persons such as the North Central Florida Maternal and Infant Care and Adolescent Pregnancy Team Projects have been able to provide resources for prenatal care for indigent women in some parts of the United States. Until 1975 the North Central Florida program still had no way of increasing the nutritional status of those women who needed it (but couldn't afford it) other than by helping them spend what food dollars they had more wisely through nutritional counseling. In mid-1975 our Projects began participating in the U.S. Department of Agriculture's WIC Program (Special Supplemental Food Program for Women, Infants and Children) and in one year we noted an increase in the baby weights of mothers in the participating counties in the program compared to the weights of babies of mothers in counties not participating. Two years after the WIC program started, the perinatal mortality rate of the North Central Florida Projects fell to a new low of eight deaths per 1,000 live births. More detailed studies are underway to try to confirm this relationship, but this is typical of findings with WIC programs in other parts of the United States, and of reports on food supplement programs in Canada.

Mothers in poverty are at a much higher risk for most of the nutrition problems mentioned in this article than are upper middle class mothers. Many experts think that elimination of poverty problems would wipe out 80–90% of all high-risk pregnancies. However, since poverty will likely be with us for some time, American obstetrics is starting to reorder its priorities and place more emphasis on this high risk group. The WIC program seems an important step and deserves the support of the health care professional.

Certainly, people working with low income populations need to be acutely aware of the many subtle and varied health problems that malnutrition may cause in these people. Since many of them are cared for by the public health sector, public health nutritionists are currently in great demand and can be a vital force in correction of many of these problems.

DIAGNOSIS OF NUTRITIONAL PROBLEMS IN PREGNANCY

History

1. Short pregnancy interval—less than two years between conception of this pregnancy and last delivery or cessation of breast-feeding.
2. Poor obstetrical history—premature or growth retarded infants, excess pregnancy wastage, etc.
3. Recent use of oral contraceptives, IUD or induced abortion.

4. Present pregnancy: any of problems outlined in above pages plus unwanted pregnancy (may be tipoff to poor motivation) plus any woman planning to breast feed.

Physical Examination

1. Weight—under or over normal range of weight for height. Any deviations during pregnancy from set standards of weight.
2. Skin-fold thickness done with calipers. This can be a useful tool for differentiating caloric vs fluid weight.
3. Height of uterine fundus in centimeters with tape or calipers.
4. Skin turgor and color.

Laboratory

1. Routine hematocrit—every other visit.
2. Blood work to diagnose anemia (Table 4.2).
3. Urine for sugar and ketones—each visit.
4. Fasting and one hour post-glucose load (50 g) blood glucose as screen for diabetes.

TABLE 4.2. MOST VALID TESTS FOR DIAGNOSIS OF PREGNANCY ANEMIAS.

Serum iron less than 40mcg%
Total iron binding capacity (TIBC) more than 350 mcg%
Saturation less than 15%
Serum folate less than 3 nanograms/ml.

CONCLUSION

As can be learned from the previous discussion, prenatal nutrition is important to the quality of pregnancy outcome. Medical, dental and nursing schools and schools of public health are attempting to upgrade their nutrition teaching so that an updated, comprehensive overview of the subject can be presented to the students in an interesting and exciting way so that they in turn can present it to their patients in an interesting and convincing fashion.

If all of this comes about, we can presume that future visits of a woman to her prenatal care-giver will be highlighted by uplifting discussions of the positive aspects of nutrition and its relationship to quality outcome of her pregnancy and not to the old saw: "Oh dear, you've gained over a pound in the last two months, Ms. Svelte! You must stop eating so much!"

REFERENCES

1. NATIONAL ACADEMY OF SCIENCES, COMMITTEE ON MATERNAL NUTRITION, MATERNAL NUTRITION AND THE COURSE OF PREGNANCY. Washington, D.C., 1970.
2. MOGHISSI, K.S., and EVANS, T.N.: Nutritional Impacts on Women, Harper and Row, Hagerstown, MD., 1977.
3. WORTHINGTON, B.; VERMEERSCH, J., and WILLIAMS, S.: Nutrition in Pregnancy and Lactation, C.V. Mosby Co., St. Louis, 1977.
4. PITKIN, R.M.: Nutritional Support in Obstetrics and Gynecology, Clin. Ob & Gyn, 19:489, 1976.
5. CHURCHILL, J. A., and BERENDES, H.W.: Intelligence of Children Whose Mothers had Acetonuria During Pregnancy. Perinatal Factors Affecting Human Development, Washington, D.C., 185:30, 1969.
6. SPELLACY, W.N.; MAHAN, C.S., and CRUZ, A.C.: The Adolescents' First Pregnancy.
7. WEATHERSBEE, P.S.; OLSEN, L.K., and LODGE, C.P. JR.: Caffeine and Pregnancy, Postgrad. Med., 62:64, Sept. 1977.
8. HIGGINBOTTOM, M.S.; SWEETMAN, L., and NYHAN, W.C.: B-12 Deficiency Syndrome in a Breast-Fed Infant of a Vegan, New England J. Med., 299:317, 1978.
9. NUTRITION SURVEILLANCE. DHEW. Center for Disease Control, Page 9, June 1976. (Issued June 1977).

5

NUTRITIONAL CONCEPTS IN THE TREATMENT OF CANCER

Edward M. Copeland III, M.D.

Surgery, radiation therapy and chemotherapy predictably increase nutrient requirements and at the same time interfere with the patient's ability to eat. Surveys of protein-calorie malnutrition in major metropolitan hospitals have indicated that 40% of the malnourished patients have cancer.[1] Because of this high incidence, the practicing oncologist must not only recognize the malnourished patient who presents for oncologic therapy and be able to initiate measures to replenish the patient before proceeding with therapy but must also attempt to prevent further nutritional depletion during treatment.

Weight loss in the untreated cancer patient usually can be correlated with a decrease in food intake or a decrease in assimilation of ingested foods. These decreases can be secondary to gastrointestinal tract obstruction, malabsorption or pain, each a result of the anatomical location of the cancer. When cancer is initially diagnosed, patients rarely have lost more than 5% of their body weight since a palpable mass, gastrointestinal symptoms or pain usually stimulate the patient to seek early medical assistance. Consequently, complications of inanition are not often significant problems for patients undergoing initial treatment for cancer. Malnutrition usually results from the intensive effort to eradicate the tumor either by surgery, radiation therapy or chemotherapy. Each of these therapeutic steps is predicated upon recovery from the preceding step and unless adequate nutrient intake in ensured,

Dr. Copeland is Professor of Surgery at the University of Texas Medical School at Houston, and the University of Texas System Cancer Center, M.D. Anderson Hospital and Tumor Institute, Houston.

the patient is at risk for protein-calorie malnutrition. The potential benefits of antineoplastic therapy can be lost because of induced malnutrition.

No doubt, the malignant process does alter host metabolic demands. The theory that malnutrition in the cancer patient results from competition for nutrients between the host and cancer has been supported by clinical observations and experimental results. Patients with oat-cell carcinoma of the lung lose weight rapidly and out of proportion to the volume of malignant tissue. Cancer cells are thought to incorporate and concentrate amino acids and glucose better than normal cells. Once amino acids are within the cancer cell, they apparently are not available for participation in the turnover of the host's amino acid pool (the cancer acts as a "nitrogen trap"[2]). Protein-calorie malnutrition has occurred in tumor-bearing rats even though the animals remained in positive nitrogen balance.[3] The theoretical explanation of this observation was that energy for tumor metabolism was derived from host protein stores through gluconeogenesis, resulting in protein-calorie depletion, and the nitrogen liberated from gluconeogenesis was utilized by the tumor for protein synthesis and thus not available for use by the host's body. Anaerobic glycolysis is thought to predominate in cancer cells because of their enzymatic makeup and limited oxygen supply. The end product of anaerobic glycolysis is lactic acid, and the production of this compound results in lowering of the pH within the tumor environment. The cancer cells have a limited capacity for metabolism of lactic acid, and lactic acid generated from anaerobic glucose metabolism by tumor cells must enter the bloodstream and be resynthesized into glucose by the liver. This recycling process has the potential to produce an energy drain upon the host. Two moles of adenosine triphosphate are liberated by the anaerobic metabolism of glucose by the tumor, but six moles of adenosine triphosphate are required by the host to regenerate glucose from lactic acid.

The concepts of recycling lactate by the host and of trapping nitrogen by the tumor have been used by some investigators to explain the syndrome of cancer cachexia. Although these mechanisms may account for some of the weight loss encountered in cancer patients, the majority of weight loss can be accounted for by a decrease in nutrient intake. The basal metabolic rates for cancer patients do not appear to be elevated; however, the voluntary intake of nutriments does seem to progressively fail to meet nutritional demands as tumor bulk increases.[4] Nevertheless, so long as the cancer patient can ingest adequate nutriments to meet the metabolic demands of both himself and the tumor, host nutritional status will remain relatively normal.

The gastrointestinal tract is the ideal conduit for digesting and assimilating nutrients, but the cancer patient subjected to a wide variety of therapies is often unable to take food by mouth. Appetite is poor, absorption is inadequate and pain, nausea and diarrhea make eating a normal diet almost impossible. Nasogastric tube feedings may be successful in some cases, and feeding by gastrostomy tube or jejunostomy tube can restore nutritional status in patients with obstructive lesions of the esophagus, stomach or pancreas. Unfortunately, nutritional supplementation via the gastrointestinal tract can be time-consuming, and the operative insertion of feeding tubes can impose on the patient an acute surgical stress that further delays nutritional restoration. Delivery of adequate nutriments to the gut does not always result in rapid nutritional restoration of the starving patient because malnutrition may have resulted in malabsorption.[5] In the severely malnourished patient, the columnar gastrointestinal mucosal cells become cuboidal, and the brush border is reduced in height. Gastrointestinal motility diminishes and overgrowth of facultative and anaerobic bacteria occurs. Absorption of glucose, protein and fat may be greatly impaired. These morphologic, absorptive and environmental abnormalities are reversible after protein-calorie replenishment, but the process is slow because the enteral nutriments are partially malabsorbed initially. The oncologist needs to replenish the cancer patient as quickly as possible so that oncologic therapy can either be begun or resumed in an attempt to cure the patient or to achieve major palliation.

When the gastrointestinal tract is unavailable for use, a logical alternative is intravenous hyperalimentation (IVH), an established technique of parenteral nutritional support. Vitamins, minerals, amino acids and glucose are provided in amounts necessary to maintain anabolism and reverse negative nitrogen balance. Since 1971, our group has advocated the use of intravenous hyperalimentation for malnourished patients who have malignant lesions potentially responsive to oncologic treatment and who cannot be fed enterally. Cancer patients have been safely and effectively treated with IVH for prolonged periods of time, tumor growth has not been stimulated, the risk of catheter-related sepsis has been negligible when aseptic catheter care techniques were followed carefully, nutritional replenishment has occurred often within 10 to 20 days of initiating IVH and immunocompetence has been restored. Patients can be maintained on IVH during antineoplastic therapy. Morbidity may be reduced, the chance for a favorable response to oncologic therapy is increased, and there is a much greater likelihood that the well-nourished patient will advance to the next stage of oncologic treatment.

PRACTICAL CLUES TO DIAGNOSIS AND MANAGEMENT OF MALNUTRITION

A set of complex tests are not always necessary for the diagnosis of malnutrition. Nutritional depletion is defined by our team as a recent, unintentional loss of 10 percent or more of body weight, a serum albumin concentration of less than 3.4 g%, and/or a negative reaction to a battery of recall skin test antigens. Patients who satisfy two of these three criteria and who have a reasonable chance of responding to appropriate oncologic therapy are candidates for IVH. Similarly, patients who are incapable of adequate enteral nutrition because of the malnutrition imposed by previous oncologic therapy are candidates for nutritional rehabilitation with IVH, and nutritionally healthy patients whose treatment plan necessitates multiple courses of chemotherapy, possibly combined with radiation therapy or surgery, are IVH candidates if maintenance of a state of optimum nutrition during therapy, is necessary to maximize their chance for response to treatment, and to improve their quality of life.

Although weight loss is a good indicator of nutritional status, it can be deceiving. Consider a female patient with gastric carcinoma who weighs 146 pounds on admission to the hospital but weighed 186 pounds three months ago. She has lost more than 10% of her usual body weight during the time interval because pain after eating, nausea and hematemesis have resulted in a reduced food intake, but her weight is still greater than her ideal weight. On evaluation, her serum albumin level is 3.4 g%. She is a candidate for operation, but should she receive preoperative nutritional repletion with intravenous hyperalimentation? In this clinical situation, the third criterion, reactivity to a battery of skin test antigens, becomes important in detecting nutritional status. Malnutrition has been shown to depress cell-mediated immunity.[6] A positive response to skin tests indicates that this patient has an intact cell-mediated immune response; consequently, nutritional status would be considered adequate, preoperative intravenous hyperalimentation would not be utilized and surgery could be safely undertaken. If skin test responses had been negative, nutritional replenishment preoperatively for at least 7–10 days would be indicated, hopefully until skin test reactivity became positive. Hyperalimentation would then be continued postoperatively until the patient was able to eat normally.

Another example to consider is a woman 5′4″ tall and weighing 130 pounds, somewhat over ideal weight, who also has a partially obstructing carcinoma of the gastric antrum and has lost 35 pounds in the last four months. Her serum albumin is 3.1 g% on initial evaluation and her skin test reactions are all negative. This patient, while of normal weight for her height, is semistarved and at risk for postoperative complications, particularly pneumonia, poor wound healing and wound infection. Surgery should be postponed until the patient can be nutritionally replenished with intravenous hyperalimentation. Because of the magnitude of weight loss and the low serum albumin concentration, IVH would still be initiated even if skin test reactions had been positive.

There are many tests for evaluating nutritional status, and most tests for nutritional assessment can be correlated with somatic compartments. For example, the fat compartment can be evaluated by measuring the triceps skin fold thickness, the visceral protein compartment by measuring serum albumin concentration and also by skin testing for delayed hypersensitivity, and the skeletal muscle compartment by measuring upper arm circumference and creatinine-height index. All of these tests are important, but the practicing physician without the aid of an organized nutritional support service cannot always perform all available tests. From the standpoint of practicality, currently we rely on percent weight loss, serum albumin concentration and reactivity to skin test antigens.

Depending upon the patient's initial nutritional status and the magnitude of planned therapy, either maintenance or anabolic levels of calories and protein will be required. A simple way to calculate calorie and protein needs is to supply calories at 35 kcal/kg/day if maintenance levels are necessary or 45 kcal/kg/day if anabolism needs to be promoted. Nitrogen (protein in grams ÷ 6.25) should be given in a ratio of about 1 gram per 150 nonprotein calories.

Nitrogen balance studies determine the need for additional protein and calorie intake to offset body protein losses and to meet energy demands. Since amino acids are distinguished from other nutrients by the presence of nitrogen, nitrogen balance is commonly used as a nutritional index. When cumulative nitrogen output exceeds nitrogen input for several days, the patient may become protein-calorie malnourished, but as a single test nitrogen balance cannot assess the nutritional status of the patient.

INTRAVENOUS HYPERALIMENTATION

At many institutions, intravenous hyperalimentation is the responsibility of a team of people including a physician team leader, registered nurses, pharmacists, dietitians and rehabilitation therapists. Solutions for intravenous hyperalimentation generally contain 3.5 to 5% amino acids and 20 to 30% dextrose. The osmolarity of this solution is between 1800–2400 mOsm necessitating infusion via a large bore, central vein rather than a peripheral vein. Most often the subclavian vein is catheterized percutaneously via the infraclavicular approach so that the tip of the feeding catheter can be placed in the middle of the superior vena cava. Nutrients delivered through this catheter are diluted rapidly in the vena cava, resulting in less risk of inducing thrombophlebitis than if the infusion was into a smaller vessel such as the internal jugular vein. Accurate positioning of the catheter tip within the middle of the superior vena cava is verified by obtaining a chest roentgenogram prior to beginning the hypertonic IVH solutions. A constant rate of infusion is necessary to promote proper utilization of the administered glucose, amino acids, minerals and vitamins. Initially, 1000 ml is delivered in 24 hours to confirm the patient's ability to effectively metabolize the infused glucose. In the absence of hyperglycemia and glycosuria, the flow rate may be increased to 1000 ml every 12 hours. Pancreatic islet cells will again need the opportunity to adapt with an increased insulin output in response to the increased glucose infusion, but within the first 3–5 days the average adult usually will tolerate a daily ration of 3000 ml of IVH solution. Extremely wasted patients, however, may tolerate only 2000 ml per day until partial nutritional rehabilitation has been attained. The abrupt cessation of IVH may lead to insulin shock or reactive hypoglycemia. For this reason, IVH should be tapered off during the 24–48 hour period prior to completely discontinuing it. Generally the patient can be expected to gain 5–10 pounds during a three week interval of IVH. The initial 3–4 pound weight gain will be rehydration, but then the patient should gain lean body mass at a rate of about one-half pound per day. Body weight gain greater than one pound per day should be considered fluid retention, and the IVH delivery rate should be slowed or a diuretic administered.

During IVH the patient's metabolic status should be constantly reviewed in order to detect any need to alter the flow rate or composition of the nutrient solution. Important factors to examine on a regular basis are daily weights, fractional urine sugar concentration every six hours, daily intake and output, serum electrolytes, blood urea nitrogen and blood sugar levels three times a week, serum levels of albumin, magnesium, phosphorus, calcium and creatinine once a week, liver function tests, coagulation parameters and complete blood count once a week, and patient reevaluation for any temperature elevation. The nurse assigned to the hyperalimentation team changes the patient's catheter dressing and IVH delivery tubing three times a week, each time repreparing the skin with ether or acetone and an antiseptic solution. An antimicrobial ointment and a sterile dressing are reapplied to cover the catheter-skin entrance site. Proper technique must be utilized always and, doing so, a single feeding catheter can remain in place for prolonged periods of time without complications.

The patient who develops a fever during IVH is presumed to have catheter-related sepsis unless another primary focus of infection is apparent. Diagnosis of catheter-related sepsis is confirmed by a blood culture and a catheter culture positive for the same organism. The catheter should be removed immediately and the temperature usually returns to normal within 24–48 hours after catheter removal if the catheter was the source of the infection. If a primary focus of infection other than the catheter is identified and blood cultures are negative, the primary focus should be treated appropriately and the catheter left in place. Any positive blood culture, however, is an unequivocal indication for catheter removal. Twenty-four to forty-eight hours after temperature has returned to normal and blood cultures have become negative, the feeding catheter can be reinserted into the superior vena cava usually through the opposite subclavian vein.

The IVH delivery system should not be used indiscriminately. Blood, blood products and medications should be infused via an alternate vein whenever possible. A simultaneous peripheral intravenous infusion is often necessary to administer antibiotics, supplemental fluids, or chemotherapeutic agents. The incidence of catheter-related sepsis in our series of patients has ranged from 1 to 6%, with the highest rate of sepsis occurring in patients with cancer of the head and neck because they generally have open wounds or tracheostomy and pharyngostomy stomas nearby that may constantly contaminate the catheter dressings.[7]

CLINICAL MATERIAL

In the past seven years, more than 1000 patients have received IVH as adjunctive nutritional therapy at the M.D. Anderson Hospital and Tumor Institute. From the Anderson series, 406 consecutive cancer patients have been reviewed.[8] Treatment categories were chemotherapy—43%; general surgery—24%; head and neck surgery—10%; radiotherapy—10%; fistulas—6%; and supportive care—7%. Hyperalimentation was infused for an average of 23.9 days; the average weight gained by these patients during IVH was 5 pounds; and 488 subclavian vein feeding catheters were utilized. Pathogenic organisms were grown from 4.4% of the catheters; however, simultaneous positive blood and catheter cultures were obtained in only 2.3% of the patients.

Intravenous hyperalimentation was used as an adjunct to chemotherapy in 175 patients, the average period of IVH infusion was 22.8 days and the average weight gain was 5.6 pounds. Whether mucositis and the symptoms of nausea and general malàise were induced during IVH administration depended upon the chemotherapeutic regimens employed. Gastrointestinal symptoms secondary to 5-fluorouracil administration were reduced, whereas vinblastine and bleomycin continued to cause severe stomatitis. Leucocyte depression below 2500 cells/mm^3 occurred in 51.5% of patients for an average duration of 7.7 days. Neither the nadir nor duration of leucocyte depression appeared to be affected by IVH, and catheter-related sepsis occurred in only 1.4% of patients. A 50% or greater reduction in measurable tumor mass was obtained in 27.8% of patients, and responding patients survived an average period of 8.2 months compared to a survival time of 1.9 months for nonresponding patients. In a group of patients with non-oat cell carcinoma of the lung, there appeared to be a positive correlation between good nutritional status and potential for response to chemotherapy. Nutritionally healthy patients or malnourished patients who were nutritionally replenished with IVH prior to and during chemotherapy were noted to have significantly better chemotherapy response rates than were malnourished patients who were not nutritionally replenished.[9]

Some degree of radiation enteritis or stomatitis often must be accepted for an adequate tumor dose of radiation therapy to be delivered to a malignancy that lies within or near the alimentary tract. Thirty-nine patients required treatment with IVH to complete a planned course of radiotherapy.[10] IVH was utilized for an average period of 30.7 days, average weight gain was 7.8 pounds, 95% of the patients completed their planned radiation therapy course, and 54% of the patients responded with a greater than 50% reduction in measurable tumor volume. As with the chemotherapy patients, those patients who responded to radiation therapy were able to maintain the weight gained during IVH after it was discontinued, but nonresponding patients promptly lost weight.

Of 100 patients who received IVH as nutritional support for a general or thoracic surgical procedure, 52 underwent curative resections, including total gastrectomies, esophagectomies, and abdominal perineal resections, and 34 patients underwent diagnostic or palliative procedures involving major surgical intervention. Overall, IVH was infused for an average period of 24.2 days, the average weight gain during IVH was 4.2 pounds, and the mortality rate was only 4%. IVH was used for an average period of 12.3 days preoperatively and 13.9 days postoperatively. In those patients who received IVH both pre- and postoperatively, weight gain and a rise in serum albumin concentration were attained almost exclusively during the preoperative period. Because there were so few surgical complications in this group, we recommend that nutritional rehabilitative measures be instituted before operation instead of waiting until a catastrophic postoperative complication has occurred. Three patients had pharyngeal incompetence after a major head and neck surgical procedure. Pharyngeal incompetence was thought to be secondary to muscle weakness and reversible muscle injury. Nutrition was maintained with IVH and deglutitory muscular rehabilitation was begun. Weight gain of as much as 26 pounds was achieved, and with concomitant return of general body muscle strength and tone, swallowing function returned after 18 to 48 days of IVH.

The experience with management of fistulas in cancer patients was rewarding. These fistulas presented several unique problems. Cancer was either discovered in the fistulous tract, the fistula involved an area of irradiated bowel or abdominal wall, or the patient's life expectancy was so short that the physician thought that the time needed to heal the fistula was not justified. Twenty-three patients were in these categories. Spontaneous closure of the gastrointestinal fistula occurred in 44% of the patients. After closure each patient was eventually discharged from the hospital and was able to lead a productive life for at least a short period of time. In two patients, spontaneous closure occurred even though gastrointestinal cancer was present in biopsies from the fistulous tract. Results of spontaneous closures of enterocutaneous fistulas arising from irradiated bowel were not good. Although spontaneous closure was achieved in several patients, each fistula eventually reopened and the patient either died or required a surgical remedy. The current recommendation for malnourished patients who have radiation-related fistulas of the gastrointestinal tract is to prepare them for the surgical procedure by utilizing IVH preoperatively for 14 to 21 days to stimulate weight gain and induce anabolism.

Malnutrition leads to immunosuppression as does chemotherapy, surgery and radiation therapy. In an attempt to define what part malnutrition plays in immune suppression associated with cancer therapy, 65 patients who were candidates for IVH were chosen for study.[11] These patients were tested with a battery of recall skin test antigens prior to and during nutritional replenishment with IVH. On initial evaluation, 46 patients had negative reactions to skin tests, and 29 (63%) converted skin tests to positive during an average period of 13.6 days of IVH. In the chemotherapy group, 16 of 21 negative reactors converted skin tests to positive in an average of 11.6 days. A significant reduction in tumor volume in response to chemotherapy occurred only in patients with positive skin test reactions. Death occurred only in patients with negative skin test reactions and was usually secondary to fungal sepsis. Those surgery patients who maintained positive skin test reactivity or converted skin tests to positive preoperatively had an uncomplicated postoperative recovery period. Surgery patients whose skin tests remained negative throughout IVH or converted to negative during IVH either expired postoperatively or had a prolonged postoperative course with multiple complications. In the radiotherapy patients, conversion of skin test reactions to positive during IVH was more difficult to achieve than in either the surgery or chemotherapy patient groups. Radiotherapy usually was being delivered to the thymus or large segments of bone marrow or blood (mediastinum, heart or pelvis) and radiotherapy to these areas probably reduced the number or efficacy of circulating T-lymphocytes responsible for delayed cutaneous hypersensitivity. Although skin test reactivity did not convert to positive in the radiotherapy group, there were few complications and nutritional rehabilitation with

IVH was considered adequate. In these 65 patients, IVH was responsible for nutritional repletion and probably was responsible for the return of positive skin test reactivity in the majority of negative reactors. Certain chemotherapeutic drugs, radiation therapy, and the physiologic events associated with operative trauma may be innately immunosuppressive; nevertheless, this study indicated that much of the immune depression identified was secondary to malnutrition coincident with and often caused by the various therapeutic modalities. Restoring immune competence by nutritional repletion was desirable in these cancer patients since positive reactors had a better tumor response to chemotherapy and better tolerated oncologic treatment.[12]

CONCLUSION

The malnourished cancer patient can be safely and effectively replenished with intravenous hyperalimentation for prolonged periods of time. Its use has allowed specific antineoplastic therapy to be administered to malnourished patients who otherwise might not have been acceptable candidates for intensive oncologic therapy. The risk of sepsis is negligible when aseptic catheter care techniques are carefully followed. Catheter-related sepsis in our hands has been about 2.3% and somewhat higher in patients with head and neck malignancies. Nutritional replenishment is rapid, often achieved within 10 to 20 days. If proper muscle rehabilitation is undertaken, the patient gains lean body mass during the infusion of amino acids, glucose, electrolytes, minerals and vitamins. Nutritional repletion often results in the return of immunocompetence and is associated with a reduction in sepsis, proper wound healing and an apparent increase in tumor response to chemotherapy. Tumor growth has not been stimulated by nutritional repletion. Experiments done in our laboratories to evaluate tumor growth, body weight and immunocompetence in rodents receiving either a normal diet or intravenous hyperalimentation revealed that IVH did not support tumor growth any better than did a normal diet, and for both diets, maintenance of body weight and immunocompetence were similar. Physicians can practice good nutritional management in any hospital by exercising clinical judgment and using a few simple indices of nutritional status. An extensive nutritional battery is not needed in every case. Knowing the patient's disease, the treatment the patient has already received and the treatment the patient is going to get will determine the future risk of malnutrition. Couple this information with the patient's current weight, his change from usual body weight, his serum albumin concentration, and the reactivity to a battery of recall skin test antigens, and a reliable method for determining nutritional therapy is obtained. Cancer cachexia should no longer be a contraindication to adequate oncologic therapy.

REFERENCES

1. BISTRIAN, B.R.; BLACKBURN, G.L.; HALLOWELL, E., and HEDDLE, R.: Protein Status of General Surgical Patients, J. Am. Med. 230:858, 1974.
2. MIDER, E.B.; TESLUK, H., and MORTON, J.J.: Effect of Walker Carcinoma 256 on Food Intake, Body Weight and Nitrogen Metabolism of Growing Rats, Acta Union Int. Cancer 6:409, 1948.
3. SHERMAN, C.D.; MORTON, J.J., and MIDER, G.B.: Potential Sources of Tumor Nitrogen, Cancer Res. 10:374, 1950.
4. MORRISON, S.D.: Control of Food Intake During Growth of a Walker 256 Carcinosarcoma, Cancer Res. 33:526, 1973.
5. VITERI, F.E. and SCHNEIDER, R.E.: Gastrointestinal Alterations in Protein-Calorie Malnutrition, Med. Clin. N. America 58:1487, 1974.
6. CHANDRA, R.K.: Rosette-forming T. Lymphocytes and Cell-Mediate Immunity in Malnutrition, British M. J. 3:608, 1974.
7. COPELAND, E.M.; MACFADYEN, B.V., JR.; MCGOWN, C., and DUDRICK, S.J.: The Use of Hyperalimentation in Patients With Potential Sepsis, Surg. Gynec. Obst. 138:377, 1974.
8. COPELAND, E.M. and DUDRICK, S.J.: Nutritional Aspects of Cancer. Hickey, R.C. (ed.), In: *Current Problems in Cancer*, Year Book Medical Publishers, Inc., Chicago, Illinois, Vol. 1, No. 3, September, 1976.
9. COPELAND, E.M.; MACFADYEN, B.V., JR.; LANZOTTI, V., and DUDRICK, S.J.: Intravenous Hyperalimentation as an Adjunct to Cancer Chemotherapy, Am. J. Surg. 129:167, 1975.
10. COPELAND, E.M.; SOUCHON, E.A.; MACFADYEN, B.V., JR., RAPP, M.A., and DUDRICK, S.J.: Intravenous Hyperalimentation as an Adjunct to Radiation Therapy, Cancer 39:609, 1977.
11. COPELAND, E.M.; DALY, J.M.; OTA, D.M., and DUDRICK, S.J.: Nutrition, Cancer and Intravenous Hyperalimentation, Cancer 43:2108–2116, 1979.
12. COPELAND, E.M.; MACFADYEN, B.V., JR., and DUDRICK, S.J.: Effect of Intravenous Hyperalimentation on Established Delayed Hypersensitivity in the Cancer Patient, Ann. Surg. 184:60, 1976.

6

HOME MANAGEMENT OF NUTRITION FOR PATIENTS RECEIVING CANCER THERAPY

Debra L. Ponder, M.S., R.D. and Heidi Van Slyke, R.D.

In the past few years, the nutritional aspects of cancer therapy and metabolism have become major areas of interest and research. Much of the existing information deals in theory and not practice. The purpose of this paper is to present guidelines from which the practitioner can assess the nutritional status and nutrient requirements of a patient being treated for a malignancy on an outpatient basis. This review also describes factors which influence the nutritional status of the cancer patient and outlines methods of management.

Nutritional support measures should be implemented and continued on an outpatient basis to prevent the nutritional deterioration which often accompanies malignancy and its treatment.[1] The patient and family should be informed early that nutrition is an important and integral component of the management of the disease which will require his/her active participation.

Overweight or obese patients may be pleased with the new body image resulting from their initial weight loss. Convincing these patients of the importance of increased energy intake to prevent excessive weight loss can be difficult. The goal of any nutritional support measures is weight stabilization or a weight gain of 1 to 2 lb per week (if necessary).

Ms. Ponder is a Doctoral Student in the Department of Food and Nutrition, Florida State University, Tallahassee.
Ms. Van Slyke is a dietitian at Victoria Hospital, Miami, Fla.

Indications that nutritional rehabilitation or support improve the results of cancer therapy are present in current literature.[1-4] Some of these advantages which have been suggested are as follows: (1) better tolerance to chemotherapy with fewer toxic side effects, increased positive response rates with decreased intervals between dosages; (2) increased immunocompetence; (3) improved quality of life and sense of well being, and (4) a possible positive tumor response where the patient otherwise may not have responded due to malnutrition.[3] The increased tumor cell mitosis produced by adequate nutrition may maximize the efficacy of chemotherapeutic programs.[1]

NUTRITIONAL ASSESSMENT

A brief, yet informative, nutritional assessment may be completed by the physician in less than ten minutes. This involves determining (1) the percentage of weight loss over a specific time period and (2) the presence of a decreased food intake due to hypogeusia, anorexia, or alimentary tract difficulties (Table 6.1). The percentage weight loss is significant in overweight as well as underweight patients. A patient exhibiting significant weight loss and decreased food intake should be assessed further to determine the degree to which the patient is nutritionally depleted.

The baseline food intake may be difficult to assess for the office physician who is without the services of a registered dietitian. Ideally, a 24 hour recall would be obtained and analyzed to determine calorie and protein intake. The recall would also be scanned for any gross nutrient deficiencies.

An alternative method available for evaluating the adequacy of the 24 hour recall is the Food Selection Check List (Table 6.2). This can be completed by the patient while waiting to see the physician. This list is based on the basic four food groups with the addition of fat sources.

The food selection checklist is based on a point system. For example, the suggested requirements for the milk and milk products group are three servings per day. For each serving chosen, five points are obtained. The total number of points is 100 when three selections are made from the milk and milk products, five fruits and vegetables, six breads and cereals, three meats or protein sources, and three fats and oils. A miscellaneous group is included (sugars, desserts, alcoholic beverages). No points are given for these substances since they provide energy-rich foodstuffs with low nutrient densities. Their use is recommended only after the requirements for the preceding food groups have been met.

The Nutritional Care Flow Sheet (Table 6.1) reflects the nutritional assessment process. The three basic categories of depletion are (I) mild or greater than 75% of normal, (II) moderate or 60% to 75% of normal, and (III) severe or less than 60% of normal. These categories provide a broad range from which the nutritional support therapy should be designed. The percentage of normal is derived from averaging (1) the percentage of usual weight, (2) the percentage of ideal body weight, and (3) the percentage of the recommended amounts of calories and protein consumed based on recommended levels.* For example, a patient with (1) a present weight less than 60% of his ideal and usual weight, (2) a serum albumin† less than 2.8 g per 100 ml; (3) a calorie and protein intake less than 60% of the estimated requirements, is considered severely depleted. Nonvolitional nutritional support measures such as intravenous hyperalimentation (IVH), enteral tube feedings, and defined formula diets (DFD) should be considered. It is postulated that severely undernourished patients exhibiting a severe degree of depletion may not be capable of the normal digestive and absorptive functions of the gastrointestinal tract. For this reason defined formula diets may be required. Few patients receive IVH or enteral nutrition by a tube on an outpatient basis. However, these alternatives must be considered when a patient is severely depleted or the situation is extended where the diet is inadequate and further plans for treatment are considered.

On the other hand, a patient with a present weight, serum albumin concentration, and calorie/protein intake greater than 75% of normal should be supplemented with a nutritional formula to compensate for any calorie deficit present. Most patients being treated on an outpatient basis can be maintained through volitional measures—energy rich foodstuffs, commercially prepared nutritional supplements, and/or defined formula diets.

FACTORS WHICH INFLUENCE FOOD INTAKE

Chemotherapy

The primary nutritional problem in cancer is the decline of food intake. Anticancer therapies frequently interfere with food intake in addition to disease-induced anorexia. Anticancer therapies may also cause epithelial denudation of the absorptive gut, autonomic disturbances producing

*Others use a different classification for mild (90%) to moderate (60–90%) depletion. The standards on which the nutritional assessment parameters are based were derived from normal healthy subjects. Thus, a broader classification is necessary for oncology patients since there are no specific standards for this group.

†Albumin synthesis in the patient with a malignancy appears to be lower than normal with an increased turnover rate. Some part may be due to the poor nutrition of the host versus the malignant process itself.[5] For this reason, 3.5 g per 100 ml is not used in the nutritional assessment process.

TABLE 6.1. NUTRITIONAL CARE FLOW SHEET

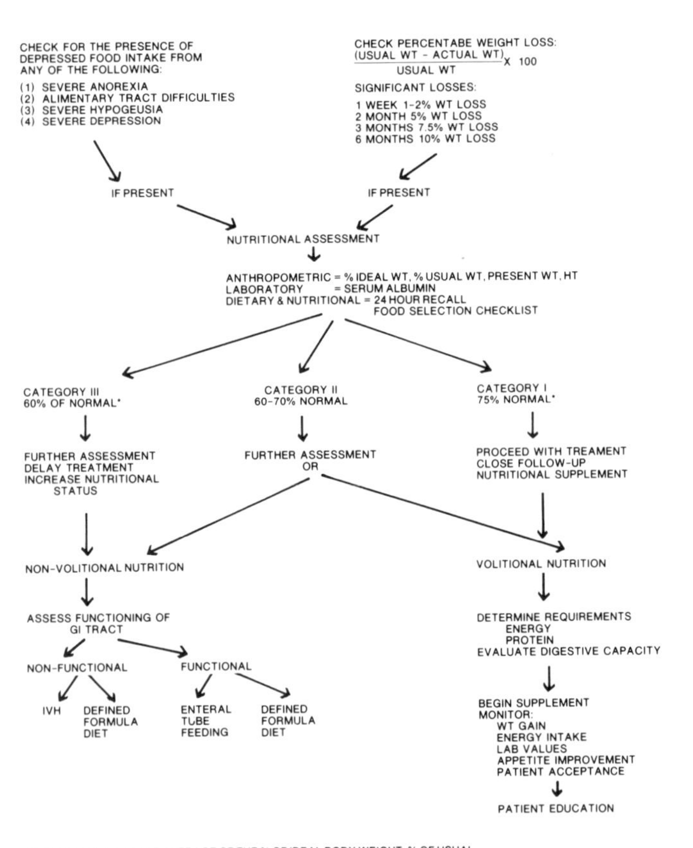

nausea and vomiting, distortion of taste perception from the anticholinergic (dry mouth) action of some chemotherapeutic agents and from vitamin deficiencies resulting from antivitamin actions of some chemotherapeutic agents.[8] Psychological distress can also contribute to a transient anorexia in the cancer patient.[9]

Stomatitis and absorptive changes in the gut mucosa should be recognized as potential side effects of most chemotherapeutic agents. Dose-limiting oral mucosal toxicities occur after actinomycin D, methotrexate, and methylglyoxal bisguanylhydrazone.[10] Oral mucosal toxicity has also been observed after azaserine, daunorubicin, adriamycin, and 5-fluorouracil.[10]

There are few dietary measures which compensate for the alimentary tract changes previously mentioned. Popsicles, ice chips, or slushes made

TABLE 6.2. FOOD SELECTION CHECKLIST

REQUIREMENTS	FOOD GROUP	CREDIT POINTS	#/DAY	SCORE (PERCENTAGES)
3	Milk & Milk Products	Total 15		
	Milk (1 cup)	5		
	Skim Milk (2 cups)	5		
	Hard Cheese (1½ oz)	5		
	Cottage Cheese (¾ cup)	5		
	Yogurt (1 cup)	5		
	Ice Cream/Pudding (½ cup)	5		
5	Fruits & Vegetables	Total 25		
	Whole Fruit (1)	5		
	Juice (½ cup)	5		
	Berries (½ cup)	5		
	Vegetable (½ cup)	5		
6	Breads & Cereals	Total 30		
	Dry Cereal (¾ cup)	5		
	Cooked Cereal (½ cup)	5		
	Breads (1 slice, 1 roll)	5		
	Pasta (½ cup)	5		
	Potatoes (1 medium)	5		
	Peas, Beans, Corn (½ cup)	5		
3	Meats	Total 15		
	Meats, Fish, Poultry (3 oz)	5		
	Eggs (2)	5		
	Hard Cheese (2 oz)	5		
3	Fats & Oils	Total 15		
	Butter, Margarine, oil (1 tsp)	5		
	Mayonnaise (1 tsp)	5		
	Salad Dressings	5		
TOTAL		100		100%

MISCELLANEOUS*

Cakes	Hard Candy	Honey/Sugar
Cookies	Alcoholic Beverages	
Jello	Pies	

*These are Energy-rich foodstuffs with low nutrient densities. Their use is recommended only after the preceding groups have been considered.

from frozen juices provide a source of carbohydrate calories and are soothing to the ulcerated mucosa. The best accepted supplements for use in frozen or clear liquids include glucose polymers (Polycose, Controlyte). Fruit-flavored and albumin-based supplements (Precision LR, Citrotein) are also well accepted when mixed in gelatin, sodas, or juices.

The effect of providing intact nutrient sources in patients with abnormal absorptive/digestive capacities due to toxicity from chemotherapeutic agents is questionable. Defined-formula diets are available which contain purified amino acids or hydrolyzed protein with amino acid supplements as their protein source, glucose oligosaccharides as the carbohydrate source, and small amounts of polyunsaturated long-chain fats or medium-chain triglycerides as the fat sources. These require minimal digestive/absorptive capacity and are generally well tolerated for short periods of time. These are best accepted when served as ices, in mixture gelatin, or mixed with juices, water, or soda. These formulas are low residue; thus fecal volume is markedly reduced. Preparations with purified amino acids tend to produce a bitter taste response and may not be well accepted. Defined formula diets frequently have osmolalities of 450 or more, thus requiring slow ingestion. (See Table 6.3).

Nausea and vomiting which accompany chemotherapy are treated primarily through the use of antiemetic drugs 30 minutes preceding a meal. The phenothiazine antiemetics have been significantly effective.[10] Few dietary manipulations have proven effective in decreasing nausea and vomiting. However, serving cold foods in place of hot foods (the aroma of hot foods may stimulate nausea), small frequent meals, serving no liquids 30 minutes pre- or postprandial, and serving lemons or dill pickles to patients without stomatitis may help reduce nausea.

Taste Acuity

Taste alterations are frequently demonstrated in cancer patients. Clinical evidence from studies conducted by DeWyss[11] showed that dys-

TABLE 6.3. PATIENT EDUCATION MATERIALS

1) "Nutrition for Patients Receiving Chemotherapy and Radiation Treatment". Available through local American Cancer Society Chapters (free).

2) "A Guide to Good Nutrition During and After Chemotherapy and Radiation". Sandra Aker, R.D., Gail Tilmont, and Vangee Harrison: Medical Oncology Unit: Dietary Department. Fred Hutchinson Cancer Research Center, 1124 Columbia Street, Seattle, Washington 98104 ($2.00 per copy).

3) "Food for Those Who Hesitate — Tips That They Might Tolerate". Jane E. Helsen, R.D., Cancer Information Center, Duke University Comprehensive Cancer Center, 200 Atlas Street, Durham, North Carolina 27705 (free).

4) "Nutritional Guide for Patients Receiving Upper and Lower Abdominal Radiation Therapy". C. Persighel, R.N., Mountain States Tumor Institute, Department of Patient and Family Support, 151 E. Bannoch, Boise, Idaho 83702 ($1.00 per copy).

5) "Home Care Guide for Patients with Head and Neck Disease". University of Wisconsin Clinical Cancer Center, Public Affairs Office, 1900 University Avenue, Madison, Wisconsin 53705 (free).

6) "Health Through Nutrition: A Comprehensive Guide for Cancer Patients". E.H. Rosenbaum, M.D., C. Stitt, R.D., H. Drasin, M.D., I.R. Rosenbaum. Life, Mind, and Body (Alchemy Books), 1515 Scott Street, San Francisco, California 94115.

geusia can be demonstrated in cachectic cancer patients characterized by a reduced threshold to bitter tastes (characterized by amino groups) and an increased threshold to sweets. Patients who reject meat (beef, pork) because of changes in taste sensation may be able to tolerate milk, cheese, eggs, fish, and poultry as suitable protein sources. For patients to detect a "sweet" taste increased concentration of sugar in foodstuffs may be necessary. The preference for sucrose appears to decrease in the later stages of the disease process.

An association between zinc and gustatory function has been suggested for some time. Henkin reported that some disorders of taste can be corrected with the administration of oral zinc sulfate; however, a clinical trial of this material in the anorectic patient has not been conducted.[2,12] More recent studies have indicated the following: (1) Zinc depletion in humans with decreased intestinal absorption seems to be definitely related to hypogeusia and (2) not all cases of hypogeusia are related to zinc deficiency.[13]

Decreased salivation or a "dry mouth" may indicate the need for texture modifications to include foods of a liquid consistency (soups, puddings, gelatins, cottage cheese). Fresh lemon juice or lemonade may help stimulate salivation. Sour balls also help relieve the "dry mouth" and contribute carbohydrate calories.

Radiotherapy may result in serious nutritional consequences. Patients receiving radiotherapy to the head and neck region frequently exhibit the following symptoms: sore throat, pain on swallowing, dry mouth, lack of appetite, and altered taste.[14] In the presence of ulcerated gastrointestinal mucosa tart or acid foods such as citrus juices frequently cause a burning sensation. Consistency modifications may be necessary. Chemical irritants (pepper, caffeine, chili powder, alcohol) are frequently eliminated as well as thermal irritants (extremes in temperature).[15]

The irradiation of the salivary glands and resultant changes in the quantity and quality of saliva are factors in the origin of dental caries in these patients. The sucrose content of the diet may need to be reduced while the high-protein, high calorie content of the diet is maintained. Solid sweets (candy), retentive sweets (cakes and jellies), and sugar in solutions (soft drinks, presweetened beverages) are avoided. Artificial sweeteners are often used in place of sugar.[15]

FORMULATING THE DIET PRESCRIPTION

The first step in formulating the diet prescription involves calculating the calorie and protein requirements. The adult requires 30–35 calories per kilogram of ideal body weight to meet calorie requirements.[1,6] Some patients may require up to 45 calories per kilogram of ideal weight.[1]

Protein requirements range from 1.2 to 1.5 grams per kilogram of ideal body weight.[1,6] The patients should be informed that adequate calorie and protein intakes are the priorities of their diet.

Vitamin and mineral supplementation are suggested in the patient who is unable to consume adequate amounts of the basic four food groups. A multiple vitamin with mineral preparation, when taken in the recommended dosage, is advisable in any patient with transient episodes of inadequate oral intake. Cancer patients frequently demonstrate deficiencies of folic acid, ascorbic acid and pyridoxine.[7]

The patient must be included in the diet prescription process. The means by which the additional (calories/protein) nutrients are provided should be decided by the patient. Some patients prefer nutritionally complete supplemental formulas; other patients may prefer energy-rich foodstuffs* such as double-strength milk, cream based soups, ice cream sodas, etc.

The volume of commercially prepared nutritional formulas required to meet the estimated energy requirements is easier to determine than the specific types and amounts of energy-rich foodstuffs which would supply the additional calories. However, energy-rich foodstuffs are preferred by many patients.

Effective Means of Nutritional Support

Due to the effects of the cancer treatment and the disease process itself, determining an acceptable means of maintaining adequate nutritional status may present a challenge to the patient as well as to the physician. The alternatives for nutritional support measures are volitional feedings (liquid formulas, high calorie foodstuffs) and nonvolitional feedings (enteral tube feedings, intravenous hyperalimentation). The quantity of regular foodstuffs needed to achieve the estimated calorie requirements may be intimidating to the anorexic patient. For this reason, energy and nutrient dense formulas are chosen as a means for providing additional calories and protein.

The nutritional supplement chosen should provide the percentage of calories remaining from the Food Selection Check List. For example, completion of the Food Selection Check List reveals a 75% intake of estimated food requirements. Thus, a 25% calorie deficit is established. The patient's ideal weight for height† is 70 kilograms or 154 pounds. The estimated calorie requirements = 2450

$$35 \text{ Kcal} \times 70 \text{ Kg} = 2450 \text{ calories}$$

*Recipes for energy-rich foodstuffs may be obtained from the patient education materials included in Table 3.
† Derived from Metropolitan Life Insurance Tables.

Twenty five percent of the estimated calorie requirements (2450) equals 600 calories; thus, 600 calories of a nutritional supplement should be provided daily in addition to the amounts ingested as listed on the Food Selection Check List.

The calories per ml of supplement are listed on the Nutritional Formula Composition Chart (Table 6.4).

The patient whose assessment parameters fall in category II should be assessed further (details on more quantitative measures of nutritional assessment can be found in reference 6). If further assessment is not possible, more aggressive means of nutritional support (IVH, enteral tube feedings, DFD) may be considered. In either case, nutritional rehabilitation is a priority. The patient requires close follow-up to determine the efficacy of the nutritional support measures selected. Biweekly office visits should include weight determination and a detailed food record with the quantity of supplemental formula ingested. A multivitamin/mineral preparation is suggested. Any alterations in digestive/absorptive capacity should be considered with the appropriate selection of nutrient sources.

Patients should receive nutritional supplements separate from their normal meals. Patients presenting with progressive anorexia may ingest more calories via the supplemental formula alone. Amounts ranging from 100 to 200 ml per hour during waking hours (9 a.m.–8 p.m.) can provide 1800 to 3600 calories respectively.*

Patients whose nutritional assessment places them in category III should probably be admitted to an acute care hospital where IVH or enteral tube feedings can be instituted. (For further information see references 16, 17). Patients who are in the terminal stages of their disease may require supportive care only.

Behavioral techniques used in adults with cancer seem to have little effect on their food intake. Attention should be given to the creation of a pleasant atmosphere around meals. The family should encourage the patient to eat and show concern with his/her food preferences. The value of social interaction with a family member or friend during meal times is sometimes immeasurable.[9]

CONCLUSION

Nutritional support in the cancer patient is an important adjunct to therapy. All patients deserve the improved sense of well-being which frequently accompanies nutritional support.

---

*Calculations were based on a calorically dense formula providing 1.5 Calories per cc.

TABLE 6.4. COMMERCIALLY PREPARED NUTRITIONAL PRODUCTS PER 1000 KILOCALORIES

1. Intact Protein (Meat and/or Milk Base)[T]

Product	Complete-B	Formula 2	Magnacal B[+]	Low-Pro[+] Carnacal	Carnation Instant Breakfast[ø]
Manufacturer	Doyle	Cutter Labs	Hospital Diet. Products	Hospital Diet. Products	Carnation
Packaging	400 ml cans 250 ml bottles	200 ml jars	360ml bottles	360ml bottles	6 envelopes/box
Caloric Density (cal/ml)	1.00	1.00	1.50	1.02	1.08
Osmolality mOs m/liter	490	435–510	725	575	**
Volume to Meet 100% RDA's in ml's	1600	2000	1000	1000	1373
% Calories derived from protein	16.0	15.0	13.3	8.4	20.5
% Calories derived from Carbohydrate	48.0	38.3	43.2	53.5	54.8
% Calories derived from Fat	36.0	46.7	43.5	38.1	24.7
Lactose, g	24.4	37.5	**	**	84.0
Calories/Nitrogen, g	131.25	142.16	390.49	270.93	88.06
Protein, g Protein source	40.0 Nonfat dry milk; Beef	37.5 Nonfat dry milk, beef, wheat, and egg yolk	33.0 Puree beef, Soy Protein	21.5 Nonfat dry milk Puree Beef	58.0 Whole milk; nonfat dry milk; soy Prot. Na caseinate

* Changes in product composition occur periodically. Contact the manufacturer or sales representative for current product information.
[T] All formulas are low lactose, low residue unless otherwise specified
+ Some of a variety of formulas offered by Hospital Diet Products Corporation
ø Vanilla flavor used; whole milk added
øø Vanilla flavor used
++ Chocolate flavor used
*** Calculations based on 1 - 5 oz serving

TABLE 6.4. *(Continued)*

1. Intact Protein (Meat and/or Milk Base)[T]					
Carbohydrate, g Carbohydrate source	120.0 Maltodestrin; vegs, frts; Lactose; sucrose	122.5 Lactose; Sucrose Vegs. Or. Jce.	407.0 Corn syrup solids, Fruits, Vegs.	134.0 Corn syrup solids; frts. veg.	135.0 Sucrose; Corn Syrup Solids; Lactose
Fat, g Fat source	40.0 Corn oil; Beef fat	40.0 Beef Fat Corn oil; Egg yolks	48.2 Soy oil, mono & di-glycerides	44.0 Soy oil, mono & di-glycerides	31.0 Whole milk; Fat
mEq Na/l	67.82	22.96	31.5	18.6	**
mEq K/l	33.33	37.95	27.0	26.6	**
Function	Unflavored; ready to use meat base blenderized tube feeding formula for patients requiring total nutritional support. Moderate residue.	Orange flavored ready to use meat base blenderized oral and tube feeding for pts. requiring total nutritional support. Moderate residue.	Ready to use meat & milk base blenderized formula for pts. requiring total or supplemental nutritional support. Moderate residue.	Low-protein content of high biological value; cholesterol. Ready to use supplemental or complete nutritional support formula	Various flavors mixed with whole milk for oral supplementation
Flavors	Unflavored	Orange	Vanilla	Vanilla	Chocolate; Eggnog; Chocolate Malt; Vanilla; Strawberry
Availability	Hospital Pharmacy Drug Stores	Hospital Pharmacy Drug Stores	Special order- HDP Corporation (Toll-Free) 800-854-0128	Special order- HDP Corporation (Toll-Free) 800-854-0128	Grocery Stores

* Changes in product composition occur periodically. Contact the manufacturer or sales representative for current product information.
T All formulas are low lactose, low residue unless otherwise specified
+ Some of a variety of formulas offered by Hospital Diet Products Corporation
* Vanilla flavor used; whole milk added
** Vanilla flavor used
++ Chocolate flavor used
*** Calculations based on 1 - 5 oz serving

TABLE 6.4. *(Continued)*

1. Intact Protein (Meat and/or Milk Base)[T]

Product	Nutrament[φφ]	Meritene Liquid[φφ]	Meritene + Milk[φ]	Nutri-1000	Sustacal Liquid
Manufacturer	Drackett Products	Doyle	Doyle	Cutter Labs	Mead-Johnson
Packaging	360 ml cans	240 ml & 300 ml cans	1, 4½, 25 lb cans 100 lb. cartons	300 ml & 960 ml cans	240 ml; 360 ml & 960 ml cans
Caloric Density (cal/ml)	1.00	1.00	1.10	1.06	1.06
Osmolality mOs m/liter	**	560 Vanilla; 610 Chocolate; 617 Eggnog	690	503	625
Volume to Meet 100% RDA's in ml's	1080	1200	1095	1920	1080
% Calories derived from protein	19.2	24.7	25.9	15.1	24.1
% Calories derived from Carbohydrate	53.8	47.5	44.6	38.2	55.4
% Calories derived from Fat	27.0	27.0	29.5	46.7	20.5
Lactose, g	**	56.7	97.5	50.1	0
Calories/Nitrogen, g	116.41	76.04	71.65	140.47	78.59

* Changes in product composition occur periodically. Contact the manufacturer or sales representative for current product information.
T All formulas are low lactose, low residue unless otherwise specified
\+ Some of a variety of formulas offered by Hospital Diet Products Corporation
φ Vanilla flavor used; whole milk added
φφ Vanilla flavor used
++ Chocolate flavor used
*** Calculations based on 1 - 5 oz serving

TABLE 6.4. *(Continued)*

1. Intact Protein (Meat and/or Milk Base)[T]					
Protein, g Protein source	48.0 Ca & Na caseinate; Skim milk; Soy Pro. Isolate	60.0 Na caseinate; Conc. Skim milk	69.0 Whole milk; nonfat dry milk	40.0 Na caseinate Skim milk	61.0 Na & Ca Caseinates; Soy Protein Isolate
Carbohydrate, g Carbohydrate source	156.0 Sucrose Corn Syrup Solids	115.0 Lactose; Corn Syrup Solids Sucrose	119.0 Lactose; Corn Syrup Solids	101.0 Corn syrup Solids; Sucrose; Lactose	140.0 Sucrose; Corn Syrup Solids
Fat, g Fat source	30.0 Partially Hydrogenated Soybean Oil	30.0 Vegetable Oil; Monodi-glycerides	35.0 Whole Milk	55.0 Corn Oil	23.0 Partially Hydrogenated Soy Oil
mEq Na/l	**	39.13	40.26	22.96	40.78
mEq K/l	**	51.28	75.92	37.95	53.46
Function	Various Flavors for oral supplemental or total nutritional support	↑Pro., ↑Cal for oral supplementation or full liquid diets	↑Pro., ↑Cal oral supplementation or complete liquid diet	Nutritionally complete for oral supplementation or tube feeding	↑ Protein nutritionally complete for oral supplementation or total nutritional support
Flavors	Vanilla; Chocolate Dutch Chocolate Strawberry; Chocolate Marshmallow	Vanilla, Chocolate; Eggnog	Plain; Chocolate; Eggnog	Vanilla; Chocolate	Vanilla; Chocolate; Eggnog
Availability	Grocery Stores	Hospital Pharmacy Drug Stores	Hospital Pharmacy Drug Stores	Hospital Pharmacy Drug Stores	Hospital Pharmacy Drug Stores

* Changes in product composition occur periodically. Contact the manufacturer or sales representative for current product information.
T All formulas are low lactose, low residue unless otherwise specified
\+ Some of a variety of formulas offered by Hospital Diet Products Corporation
ø Vanilla flavor used; whole milk added
øø Vanilla flavor used
++ Chocolate flavor used
*** Calculations based on 1 - 5 oz serving

TABLE 6.4. *(Continued)*

1. Intact Protein (Meat and/or Milk Base)[T]

Product	Sustacal + Milk[+]	Sustacal Pudding[++]	Sustagen + Water[øø]
Manufacturer	Mead-Johnson	Mead-Johnson	Mead-Johnson
Packaging	1.9 oz packets; 3.8 lb cans	5 oz tins***	1 lb & 5 lb cans
Caloric Density (cal/ml)	1.50	1.80	1.00
Osmolality mOs m/liter	760	N.A.	721
Volume to Meet 100% RDA's in ml's	1080	N.A.	1050
% Calories derived from protein	24.1	11.0	23.9
% Calories derived from Carbohydrate	55.4	53.0	68.4
% Calories derived from Fat	20.5	36.0	7.7
Lactose, g	90.0	9.0	57.3

* Changes in product composition occur periodically. Contact the manufacturer or sales representative for current product information.
[T] All formulas are low lactose, low residue unless otherwise specified
\+ Some of a variety of formulas offered by Hospital Diet Products Corporation
ø Vanilla flavor used; whole milk added
øø Vanilla flavor used
++ Chocolate flavor used
*** Calculations based on 1 - 5 oz serving

TABLE 6.4. *(Continued)*

1. Intact Protein (Meat and/or Milk Base)[T]			
Calories/Nitrogen, g	78.87	195.87	79.46
Protein, g Protein source	61.0 Whole Milk; Nonfat Dry Milk	6.8 Nonfat Milk	105.0 Nonfat Milk; Ca Caseinate; powdered Whole Milk
Carbohydrate, g Carbohydrate source	140.0 Sucrose; Lactose; Corn Syrup Solids	32.0 Sucrose; Lactose; Modified Food Starch	300.0 Corn syrup Solids Dextrose (Choc. flavor-Sucrose)
Fat, g Fat source	23.0 Cow's Milk	9.5 Partially Hydrogenated Soy oil	15.0 Powdered Whole Milk Fat (Choc. Flavor-cocoa)
mEq Na/l	40.78	5.22	52.17
mEq K/l	67.1	7.44	82.05
Function	Nutritionally Complete for oral supplementation.	As a nutritional supplement. Provides an alternate to liquids	Total nourishment for tube or oral feedings
Flavors	Vanilla; Chocolate	Vanilla; Chocolate, Butter-scotch	Vanilla; Chocolate
Availability	Hospital Pharmacy Drug Stores	Hospital Pharmacy Drug Stores	Hospital Pharmacy Drug Stores

* Changes in product composition occur periodically. Contact the manufacturer or sales representative for current product information.
[T] All formulas are low lactose, low residue unless otherwise specified
+ Some of a variety of formulas offered by Hospital Diet Products Corporation
ø Vanilla flavor used; whole milk added
øø Vanilla flavor used
++ Chocolate flavor used
*** Calculations based on 1 - 5 oz serving

TABLE 6.4. *(Continued)*

2. Intact Protein Isolates[T]

Product	Ensure	Ensure Plus	Ensure Osmolite	Isocal	Lolactene
Manufacturer	Ross	Ross	Ross	Mead-Johnson	Doyle
Packaging	240 ml bottles & cans 960 ml cans (powder)	240 ml cans 240 ml bottles	240 ml bottles & cans 960 ml cans	240 ml bottles & cans 960 ml cans	
Caloric Density (cal/ml)	1.06	1.50	1.06	1.06	0.8 (std. dilution)
Osmolality mOs m/liter	450	600	300	300	670
Volume to meet 100% RDA's in ml's	1920	1920	2000	1920	1150
% Calories derived from Protein	14.0	14.7	14.0	12.9	26.0
% Calories derived from Carbohydrate	54.5	53.3	54.6	50.2	53.0
% Calories derived from Fat	31.5	32.0	31.4	36.9	21.0
Lactose, g	0	0	0	0	4.0
Calories/Nitrogen g	154.22	145.11	154.39	169.85	69.98

* Changes in product composition occur periodically. Contact the manufacturer or sales representative for current product information.
[T] All formulas are low lactose, low residue unless otherwise specified
\+ Some of a variety of formulas offered by Hospital Diet Products Corporation
ø Vanilla flavor used; whole milk added
øø Vanilla flavor used
\++ Chocolate flavor used
*** Calculations based on 1 - 5 oz serving

TABLE 6.4. *(Continued)*

2. Intact Protein Isolates[T]					
Protein, g Protein source	37.0 Na & Ca caseinates; Soy Protein Isolate	55.0 Na & Ca caseinates; Soy Protein Isolate	37.0 Na & Ca caseinates; Soy Protein Isolate	34.0 Na & Ca caseinate; Soy Protein Isolate	66.2 Na caseinate; Nonfat Dry Milk
Carbohydrate, g Carboydrate source	145.0 Corn Syrup Solids; Sucrose	200.0 Corn Syrup Solids; Sucrose	143.0 Hydrolyzed Corn Syrup	132.0 Corn Syrup	132.4 Corn Syrup Solids
Fat, g Fat source	37.0 Corn Oil	53.0 Corn Oil	38.0 Coconut Oil (MCT) Corn Oil, Soy Oil	44.0 Soy Oil; MCT Oil	23.5 Vegetable Oil; Mono-diglycerides
mEq Na/l	32.17	46.09	23.43	22.96	47.90
mEq K/l	32.56	48.72	26.90	33.82	79.00
Function	Complete Balanced nutrition for oral supplementation or tube feeding	↑ cal ↑ pro balanced liquid nutrition for oral supplementation or tube feeding	Isotonic nutritionally complete residue food for supplemental or total feeding, oral or tube	Complete Isotonic balanced tube feeding formula lactose free	Nutritionally complete lactose residue for supplemental or total feeding, oral or tube
Flavors	Vanilla; Black walnut, Flavoring Packets: Orange, Pecan, Cherry, Strawberry, Lemon, Chocolate	Vanilla, Flavoring Packets: Orange, Cherry, Pecan, Strawberry, Lemon, Chocolate	Unflavored; flavoring Packets: Orange, Pecan, Lemon, Strawberry	Unflavored	Vanilla
Availability	Hospital Pharmacy Drug Store	Hospital Pharmacy Drug Store	Hospital Pharmacy Drug Store	Hospital Pharmacy Drug Store	Hospital Pharmacy Drug Store

* Changes in product composition occur periodically. Contact the manufacturer or sales representative for current product information.
[T] All formulas are low lactose, low residue unless otherwise specified
\+ Some of a variety of formulas offered by Hospital Diet Products Corporation
ø Vanilla flavor used; whole milk added
øø Vanilla flavor used
++ Chocolate flavor used
*** Calculations based on 1 - 5 oz serving

TABLE 6.4. ***(Continued)***

2. Intact Protein Isolates[T]

Product	Nutri-1000 LF	Precision HN	Precision-Isotonic	Precision LR
Manufacturer	Cutter Labs	Doyle	Doyle	Doyle
Packaging	300 ml & 960 ml cans	2.93-oz Packets	2.06-oz Packets	3-oz Packets
Caloric Density (cal/ml)	1.06	1.05 (std. dilution)	1.0 (std. dilution)	1.11 (std. dilution)
Osmolality mOs m/liter	304	560	300	520-orange flavor
Volume to Meet 100% RDA's in ml's	1920	3000	1500	1900
% Calories derived from Protein	15.1	16.7	12.0	9.5
% Calories derived from Carbohydrate	38.2	82.9	59.9	89.9
% Calories derived from Fat	46.7	0.4	28.1	0.6
Lactose, g	0	0	0	0

* Changes in product composition occur periodically. Contact the manufacturer or sales representative for current product information.
[T] All formulas are low lactose, low residue unless otherwise specified
+ Some of a variety of formulas offered by Hospital Diet Products Corporation
ᵠ Vanilla flavor used; whole milk added
ᵠᵠ Vanilla flavor used
++ Chocolate flavor used
*** Calculations based on 1 - 5 oz serving

TABLE 6.4. *(Continued)*

2. Intact Protein Isolates[T]				
Calories/Nitrogen, g	140.47	188.90	182.33	241.15
Protein, g Protein source	40.0 Na & Ca caseinates; Soy Protein Isolate	44.0 Egg albumin	29.0 Egg albumin	26.0 Egg albumin
Carbohydrate, g Carbohydrate source	101.0 Corn Syrup Solids; Sucrose	218.0 Maltodextrin; Sucrose	144.0 Glucose; oligosaccharides; Sucrose	249.0 Maltodextrin; Sucrose
Fat, g Fat source	55.0 Corn & soybean oil (partially saturated)	0.5 Soy oil	30.0 Vegetable oil	0.8 Soy oil
mEq Na/l	31.26	43.48	34.78	30.43
mEq K/l	37.95	23.08	24.62	22.31
Function	Nutritionally complete for oral supplementation or tube feeding. Lactose free food.	Nutritionally complete ↑nitrogen ↓residue food for oral or tube feeding	Nutritionally balanced isotonic formula for oral or tube feeding	Nutritionally complete ↓residue food for oral or tube feeding
Flavors	Vanilla; Chocolate	Citrus Fruit	Vanilla	Cherry, Lemon, Lime, Orange
Availability	Hospital Pharmacy Drug Store	Hospital Pharmacy Drug Store	Hospital Pharmacy Drug Store	Hospital Pharmacy Drug Store

* Changes in product composition occur periodically. Contact the manufacturer or sales representative for current product information.
[T] All formulas are low lactose, low residue unless otherwise specified
+ Some of a variety of formulas offered by Hospital Diet Products Corporation
° Vanilla flavor used; whole milk added
°° Vanilla flavor used
++ Chocolate flavor used
*** Calculations based on 1 - 5 oz serving

TABLE 6.4. *(Continued)*

3. Protein Hydrolysates or Crystalline Amino Acids[T]

Product	Flexical	Vipep	Vital	Vivonex	Vivonex HN
Manufacturer	Mead-Johnson	Cutter Labs	Ross	Eaton	Eaton
Packaging	2-oz tin; 1 lb cans	80 g packets	2.75-oz packet	80 g packets	80 g packets
Caloric Density (cal/ml)	1.00 (std. dilution)	1.00 (std. dilution)	1.00 (std. dilution)	1.00 (std. dilution)	1.00 (std. dilution)
Osmolality mOs m/liter	550	520	450	550-Unflavored 580–610-Flavored	810-Unflavored 850–910-Flavored
Volume to Meet 100% RDA's in ml's	2000	2000	1500	1800	3000
% Calories derived from Protein	9.0	10.0	16.7	8.2	18.26
% Calories derived from Carbohydrate	61.0	68.0	74.0	90.5	80.96
% Calories derived from Fat	30.0	22.0	9.3	1.3	0.78
Lactose, g	0	0	0.5	0	0
Calories/Nitrogen, g	254.44	231.75	120.54	277.83	126.34
Protein, g Protein source	22.5 Hydrolyzed casein, pure crystalline amino acids	25.0 hydrolyzed fish proteins, essential amino acids	42.0 soy, meat, whey hydrolysates, Free amino acids	21.0 Pure crystalline amino acids	42.0 Pure crystalline amino acids

* Changes in product composition occur periodically. Contact the manufacturer or sales representative for current product information.
[T] All formulas are low lactose, low residue unless otherwise specified
\+ Some of a variety of formulas offered by Hospital Diet Products Corporation
\# Vanilla flavor used; whole milk added
\## Vanilla flavor used
\++ Chocolate flavor used
*** Calculations based on 1 - 5 oz serving

TABLE 6.4. *(Continued)*

3. Protein Hydrolysates or Crystalline Amino Acids[T]					
Carbohydrate, g Carbohydrate source	152.5 Corn Syrup Solids; Tapioca starch	175.5 Corn Syrup Solids; sucrose; K gluconate; corn starch Tapioca flour	185.0 Maltodextrin, oligo & Polysaccharides	230.0 Glucose, oligosaccharides	210.0 Glucose, oligosaccharides
Fat, g Fat source	34.0 Soy oil, MCT oil	25.0 MCT oil, Corn oil	10.0 Sunflower oil	1.5 Safflower oil	1.0 Safflower oil
mEq Na/l	15.2	32.6	16.7	37.4	33.5
mEq K/l	32.0	21.8	29.9	30.0	18.0
Function	↓ residue, chemically defined diet for pts. with minimum digestive activity & levels of fecal residue. Nutritionally complete for oral (poor acceptance) or tube feeding	short chain peptide formula ↓residue chemically defined diet for pts. with minimum digestive activity & levels of fecal residue. Nutritionally complete for oral (very good acceptance) or tube feeding	↓ residue, hydrolyzed protein diet for pts. with minimum digestive activity & levels of fecal residue. Nutritionally complete for oral (excellent acceptance) or tube feeding	low residue. Chemically defined diet for pts. with minimum activity & levels of fecal residue. Nutritionally complete for oral (very poor acceptance) or tube feeding	low residue ↑ nitrogen diet for pts. with minimum digestive activity & levels of fecal residue. Nutritionally complete for oral (very poor acceptance) or tube feeding
Flavors	Unflavored	Custard, orange & strawberry	Banana, Flavor packets: lemon, cherry, orange, strawberry, pecan	Orange-Pineapple, strawberry, grape, lemon-lime, vanilla	Orange-Pineapple strawberry, grape, lemon-lime, vanilla
Availability	Hospital Pharmacy Drug Store	Hospital Pharmacy Drug Store	Hospital Pharmacy Drug Store	Hospital Pharmacy Drug Store	Hospital Pharmacy Drug Store

* Changes in product composition occur periodically. Contact the manufacturer or sales representative for current product information.
[T] All formulas are low lactose, low residue unless otherwise specified
\+ Some of a variety of formulas offered by Hospital Diet Products Corporation
ø Vanilla flavor used; whole milk added
øø Vanilla flavor used
++ Chocolate flavor used
*** Calculations based on 1 - 5 oz serving

TABLE 6.4. *(Continued)*

4. Feeding Modules—Supplementary Feeding— Value Per Unit Serving*								
Product	Amin-Aid	Cal-Power	Casec	Citrotein	Controlyte	dp High p.e.r. Pro.	Gatorade	Gevral
Manufacturer	McGraw	General Mills	Mead-Johnson	Doyle	Doyle	General Mills	Stokley	Lederle
Protein, g	6.6 g	0	4.0	7.67	0.04	5	0	15.6
Carbohydrate, g	118 g	34.2	0	23.3	72.0	0.5	11.0	7.05
Fat, g	22 g	0	0	0.33	24.0	0.2	0	0.52
Sodium, mEq	<2.0	0.6	0.10	5.65	0.65	0.52	5.56	0.43
Potassium, mEq	<2.0	**	N.A.	3.33	0.10	0.23	0.62	0.26
Amount per Unit Serving	1 packet with 250 ml $H_2O \rightarrow$ 340 ml	60 ml-(2 oz) 136.8 kcal	1 or more packed Tb (4.7 g)	1–1.18 oz packet with 6 oz H_2O, 127 kcal	100 g mixed with 120 ml H_2O 504.15 kcal	1 Tb (6 g) 24 kcal.	8-fl. oz (240 ml), 44 kcal.	⅓ cup (26 g) 95.6 kcal
Usage	↑ cal essential amino acid supplement for renal failure therapy	Conc. source of CHO	Protein supplement low in Na	Protein & Cal. vitamin & mineral supplement	conc. source of prot. low electrolyte source	Protein & low electrolyte source	calorie & electrolyte source	↑ protein, vitamin & mineral supplement. Good oral acceptance
Product	Hy-Cal	Lipomul-Oral	Lonalac	Lytren	MCT Oil	Microlipid	Polycose Liquid	Polycose Powder
Manufacturer	Beecham Massengill	Upjohn	Mead-Johnson	Mead-Johnson	Mead-Johnson	Hosp. Diet Products	Ross	Ross
Protein, g	0	0	9.5	0	0	0	0	0
Carbohydrate, g	72.0	0	28.9	63.25	0	0	62.4	7.52
Fat, g	0	20.0	0.4	0	8.3	15.0	0	0
Sodium, mEq	0.71	**	1.1	25.0	N.A.	N.A.	3.25	0.38

TABLE 6.4. *(Continued)*

4. Feeding Modules—Supplementary Feeding— Value Per Unit Serving*								
Potassium, mEq	0.02	**	7.6	20.75	N.A.	N.A.	0.07	0.01
Amount per Unit Serving	4 oz bottle 288 kcal.	2 Tb (30 ml) 180 kcal	8 oz (240 ml) 158 kcal (4 Tbs.)	4 oz (120 ml)	1 Tb (115 kcal)	1 fl oz 135 kcal.	4 fl oz bottles 250 kcal.	1 Tb (8 g) 32 kcal.
Usage	↑CHO source of kcal, ↓protein ↓electrolyte	Conc. fat source (Corn Oil)	Protein Supplement for low Na diets	Electrolyte supplement	fat source for malab-sorption of long chain triglycerides	Concentrat-ed fat source	concentrat-ed CHO source, ↓protein, added to beverages	↑CHO source of kcal. ↓pro-tein added to foods or beverages
Product	Sumacal							
Manufacturer	Hosp. Diet Products							
Protein, g	0							
Carbohydrate, g	15–21							
Fat, g	0							
Sodium, mEq	0.33							
Potassium, mEq	0.03							
Amount per Unit Serving	1 fl. oz 60–83 kcal depending on flavor							
Usage	CHO source of calories							

*Feeding modules serve as building blocks which can be structured or arranged according to the patient's need. Modular supplements provide carbohydrate, protein, fat, vitamins, minerals, and electrolytes as separate components. Product information changes periodically. For current information contact the manufacturer.
**Information not available.

Effective means of nutritional support should begin with the initial diagnosis of the disease and can be obtained on an outpatient basis through the use of (1) nutritional supplements, (2) close follow-up with positive reinforcement, (3) informative patient education materials and (4) volitional and nonvolitional feeding techniques. Preceding the formulation of the diet prescription, the degree of depletion (mild, moderate, severe) should be determined. Any dietary alterations should take into consideration the patient's individual tolerances and preferences.

REFERENCES

1. BLACKBURN, N.L. *et al.*: Nitrogen, Electrolytes and Minerals in Cancer, Cancer Research 37:2348–2353, 1977.
2. SCHEIN, P.S.; MACDONALD, J.S.; WATERS, C., and HAIDAIC, D.: Nutritional Complication of Cancer and its treatment, Seminars in Oncology 2, No. 4:337–347, 1975.
3. COPELAND, E.M., *et al.*: Intravenous Hyperalimentation as an Adjunct to Cancer Chemotherapy, Am. J. Surg. 129:167–173, 1975.
4. DUDRICK, S.J.: Informal Discussion: Summary of Nutritional Management, Cancer Research 37:2462–2468, 1977.
5. MUNRO, H.N.: Tumor-Host Competition for Nutrients in Cancer Patient, J. Am. Diet. Asso. 71:380–384, 1977.
6. BLACKBURN, A.L., *et al.*: Nutritional and Metabolic Assessment of the Hospitalized Patient, J. Parent. Enteral Nutri. 1, No. 1:11–22, 1977.
7. BERTINO, J.R.: Nutrients, Vitamins, and Minerals as Therapy, Nutrition Today 13:28, 1978.
8. MORRISON, S.D.: Origins of Anorexia in Neoplastic Disease, Am. J. Clin, Nutr. 31:1104–1107, 1978.
9. HOLLAND, J.C. *et al.*: Psychological Aspects of Anorexia in Cancer Patients, Cancer Research 37:2425–2428, 1977.
10. OHNUMA, T. and HOLLAND, J.C. JR.: Nutritional Consequence of Cancer Chemotherapy and Immunotherapy, Cancer Research 37:2395–2430, 1977.
11. DEWYSS, W.D.: Abnormalities of Taste as a Remote Effect of a Neoplasm, Ann. N.Y. Acad. Sci. 230:427, 1974.
12. HENKIN, R.I.; SCHECHTER, P.J.; FRIEDEWALD, W.I.; DEMETS, D.L., and RAFF, M.: A Double Blind Study of the Effects of Zinc Sulfate on Taste and Smell Dysfunction, Am. J. Med. Sci. 272:285, 1976.
13. CATALANOTTO, F.A.: The Trace Metal Zinc and Taste, Am. J. Clin. Nutr. 31:1098–1103, 1978.
14. DONALDSON, S.: Nutritional Consequences of Radiotherapy, Cancer Research 37:2395–2406, 1977.
15. HEGEDUS, S. and PELHAM, M.: Dietetics in a Cancer Hospital, J. Am. Diet. Asso. 67, No. 3:235–239, 1975.
16. FISCHER, J., ed. Total Parenteral Nutrition, Boston: Little, Brown, and Company, 1976.
17. SHILS, M.: Enteral Nutrition by Tube, Cancer Research 37:2432–2439, 1977.

7

NUTRITIONAL ASSESSMENT

A GUIDE TO DIAGNOSIS AND TREATMENT OF THE HYPERMETABOLIC PATIENT

Mitchell V. Kaminski Jr., M.D., Robert P. Ruggiero, M.D., and Christopher B. Mills, M.D.

Recognition of protein-calorie malnutrition may be obvious in the patient who evidences a 30% weight loss due to an obstructing esophageal carcinoma or the patient with multiple fistulae and intra-abdominal abscess after major colonic surgery. The established benefit of metabolic support of such patients has been well documented.[1,2] However, the early recognition of malnutrition and identification of the patient population at risk of progressing into a nutritional bankruptcy is a new challenge to the surgeon involved in day to day patient care.

The hypermetabolic state is a normal endogenous response of the individual to various forms of stress (surgery, trauma, infection, multiple organ failure). The degree of hypermetabolism is dependent upon the extent and severity of injury with the spectrum encompassing routine elective surgery (hernia, cholecystectomy) with no change in metabolic rate to the patient with a massive burn when metabolic rate may double (Fig. 7.1). The metabolic rate will also be influenced by other factors, including fever, pain, and anxiety. The physiologic metabolic response to

---

Dr. Kaminski is Clinical Professor of Surgery, University of Health Sciences/Chicago Medical School, and Director, Midwest Nutrition, Education and Research Foundation, Chicago.

Dr. Ruggiero is a Fellow, Metabolic Support Service, Thorek Hospital and Medical Center, Chicago.

Dr. Mills is a Fellow, Metabolic Support Service, Ravenswood Hospital Medical Center, Chicago.

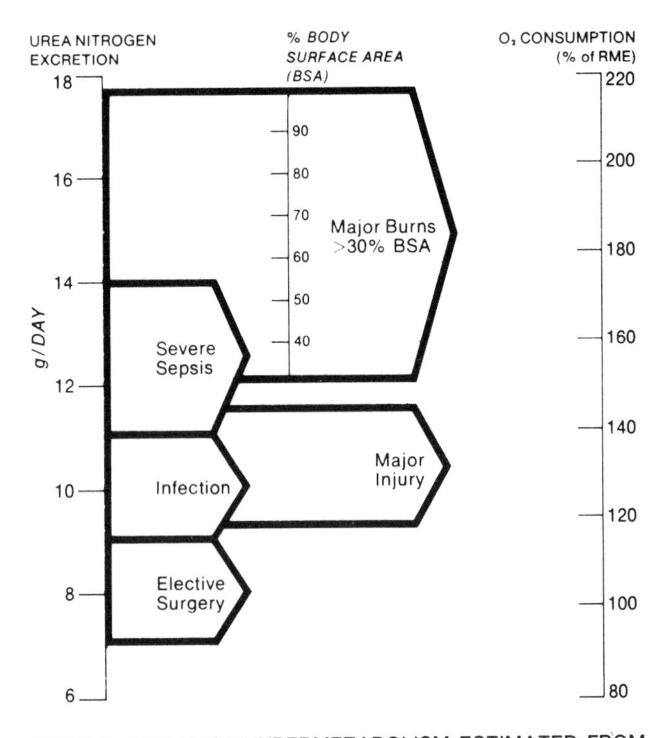

FIG. 7.1. RATES OF HYPERMETABOLISM ESTIMATED FROM URINARY UREA NITROGEN EXCRETION. (DUKE, J., ET AL., SURGERY 68:168–174, JULY 1970. RUTTEN, P., ET AL., J. SURG. RES. 18:477–483, MAY 1975.)

stress is beneficial and can be life-saving ("flight, fight, fright") when considered in short time spans. When the process becomes prolonged, the induced catabolic state becomes an impediment to normal healing and immune competence. The physiologic catabolic response to severe stress will be discussed as well as the present means of recognizing and dealing with these patients at an early state of malnutrition before they progress into a nutritionally induced "poor surgical risk" category.

METABOLIC RESPONSE TO STRESS

Stress, in the form of trauma, shock, major surgery and pain, causes multiple interrelated changes in the individual. The stressful stimuli pass via afferent fibers to the hypothalamus, resulting in increased autonomic sympathetic activity.[3] This stimulates pancreatic cells, elevating serum glucagon and suppressing serum insulin.[4] There is also adrenal medullary stimulation with resultant epinephrine release. Elaboration of growth hormone is noted as well as ACTH which will result in increased cortisol levels[5] (Fig. 7.2). The physiologic milieu of these anti-insulin hormones results in proteolysis, gluconeogenesis, lipolysis, ketogenesis and glycogenolysis. This is an immediate response necessary to meet sudden increases in substrate and energy requirements.

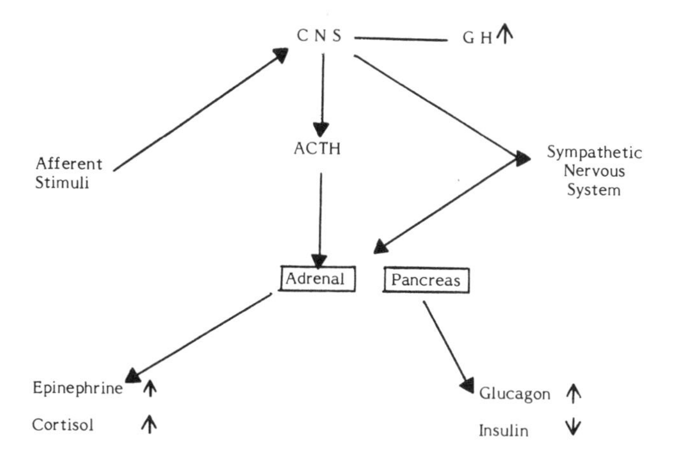

Kaminski et al.

FIG. 7.2. NEUROENDOCRINE MEDIATORS OF THE STRESS RESPONSE

The effects of glucagon and the catechols are mediated through the adenylcyclase receptor producing instantaneous changes in metabolism (Fig. 7.3). Cortisol and growth hormone exert their effect by directly stimulating intracellular protein synthesis of cyclic AMP dependent enzymes.[6] Thus, their effects upon metabolism are not instantaneous but become maximal within several days.

This catabolic or mobilizing response mediated by prostration and anti-insulin hormones results in *somatic* proteolysis with release of amino acids which sustain new *visceral* protein synthesis and provide carbohydrate intermediates and glucose precursors. Glycogen and fat are mobilized for energy substrate purposes with fatty acids providing two carbon fragments for tissue energy requirements.

In terms of effect at the adenylcyclase receptor, insulin is superior to the anti-insulin hormones. Thus, the establishment of a hormonal milieu of elevated insulin levels may be of benefit in counteracting the catabolic stress response. Insulin reverses many of the changes ascribed to the anti-insulin hormones, i.e. amino acid influx into muscle will exceed efflux, protein synthesis is increased, glycolysis is stimulated and glyco-

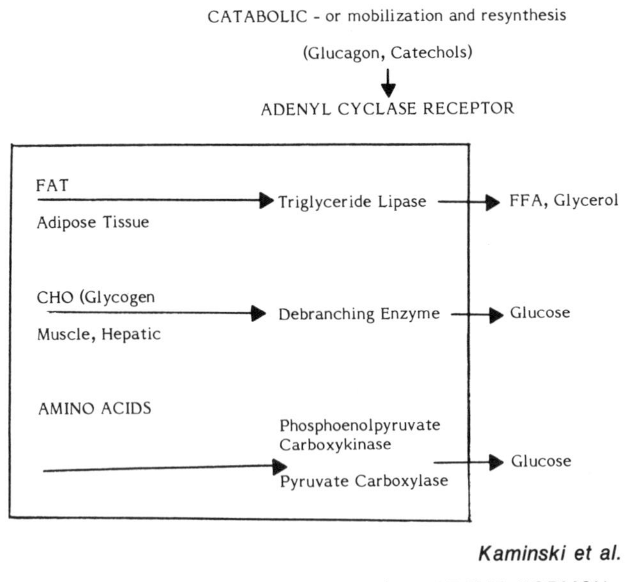

Kaminski et al.

FIG. 7.3. SUBSTRATE AVAILABILITY (CATABOLIC HORMONAL MILIEU)

gen repletion occurs (Fig. 7.4). Free fatty acid and triglyceride uptake will be enhanced with resultant increased fat synthesis.[7] These effects of insulin are also enhanced by the anabolic effects of growth hormone upon protein, if sufficient calories are provided.

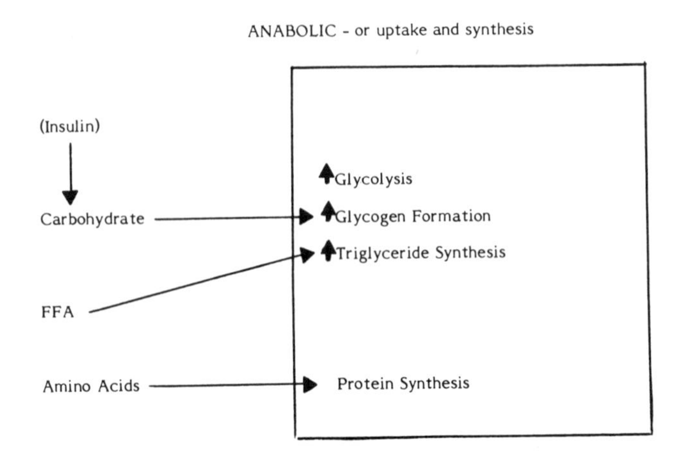

Kaminski et al.

FIG. 7.4. ANABOLIC EFFECTS OF INSULIN

NUTRITIONAL ASSESSMENT

The recognition of the patient with protein-calorie malnutrition is based on objective measurements. This same assessment profile is then used to follow and document repair of the patient's nutritional status throughout therapy. Unfortunately, all too frequently the malnutrition documented is an iatrogenic state secondary to prolonged intravenous feeding of hypocaloric glucose solutions. The major objective is to recognize protein-calorie malnutrition at an early stage and to provide the stressed individual with sufficient protein and energy substrates to assure optimal response to therapy, support recovery, and decrease morbidity and mortality.

The patient's protein status, not his fat or glycogen stores, directly affects his ability to respond to stress; therefore, nutritional assessment focuses on the protein compartments, both somatic (muscle) and visceral (all other proteins).[8] Several indices are measured for each compartment (Fig. 7.5).

SOMATIC PROTEIN COMPARTMENT

1. Body Weight—This should be recorded on the basis of actual weight and not the patient's assumed weight. Measured against ideal height/weight tables (Table 7.1), the percent ideal weight may be calculated.
   This, and the percent change in weight are extremely important. Patients with an unintentional 15% to 20% loss of body weight prior to elective surgery should undergo some form of metabolic support before proceeding with surgery. Preoperative weight loss of greater than 20% has been associated with a mortality of 33% in patients undergoing gastric surgery for peptic ulcer disease.[9]
2. Muscle Mass and Fat Stores—Specific estimates of the somatic muscle compartment are made from the creatinine height index and anthropometric measurements of the upper arm.
   A. Triceps Skinfold (TSF)—This is a measure of fat stores (nonprotein caloric reserves) determined with calipers by pulling the skin away from the triceps muscle.
   B. Arm Muscle Circumference (AMC)—This is an estimation of muscle mass which is calculated from mid-arm circumference (MAC) using the formula [(MAC) — (0.314 × TSF) = AMC]. The result is then compared to standards (Table 7.2).
   C. Creatinine/Height Index (CHI)—This is a sensitive measurement of the somatic compartment based on the constant efflux of creatinine from all active muscle.[10] When compared to ideal height tables (Table 7.1), a percent deficit is calculated.

ANERGIC METABOLIC PROFILE

PATIENT ROOM

DATE

	Parameters	Value	DEFICIT Severe	Mod	Mild	Adequate
	SOMATIC PROTEINS					
MARASMUS	WEIGHT/HEIGHT					
	TRICEPS SKINFOLD mm					
	ARM MUSCLE CIRCUMFERENCE cm					
	CREATININE/HEIGHT INDEX					
KWASHIORKOR	VISCERAL PROTEINS					
	ALBUMIN					
	TRANSFERRIN					
	TOTAL LYMPHOCYTE COUNT					
	CELL MEDIATED IMMUNITY					

NITROGEN IN gm/day ____
NITROGEN OUT gm/day − ____
NITROGEN BALANCE gm/day ☐

NUTRITIONAL STATUS	DEGREE
☐ ADEQUATE	☐ NONE
☐ MARASMUS	☐ MILD
☐ KWASHIORKOR	☐ MODERATE
☐ MARASMUS–KWASHIORKOR MIX	☐ SEVERE

Standards	Severe	Moderate	Mild
SOMATIC PROTEINS –% DEFICIT	> 30%	>15-30%	> 5-15%
ALBUMIN (gm%)	< 2.5	<3.0-2.5	< 3.5-3.0
TRANSFERRIN (mg%)	< 160	<180-160	< 200-180
LYMPHOCYTE COUNT	< 900	<1500-900	< 1800-1500
CELL MEDIATED IMMUNITY – mm	< 5 - 0	<10-5	< 15-10

FIG. 7.5 THE ANERGIC METABOLIC PROFILE (AMP)

VISCERAL PROTEIN COMPARTMENT

1. Serum Albumin and Transferrin—Deficits in these two serum proteins reflect an impairment in hepatic synthesis due to limited substrate supply, as in malnutrition or the postoperative state.

   As with the somatic proteins, a 5% to 15% deficit is consided mild, a 15% to 30% deficit moderate, and a deficit over 30% severe (Table 7.3).

TABLE 7.1. IDEAL WEIGHT AND CREATININE/HEIGHT INDICES

Height ft	Height in.	cm	Medium Frame Ideal Weight lb	Medium Frame Ideal Weight kg	Total MG Creatinine 24 hr	MG Creatinine/CM Body Ht/24 Hr
4′	10″	147.3	101.5	46.1	830	5.63
4′	11″	149.9	104	47.3	851	5.68
5′	0″	152.4	107	48.6	875	5.74
5′	1″	154.9	110	50	900	5.81
5′	2″	157.5	113	51.4	925	5.87
5′	3″	160	116	52.7	949	5.93
5′	4″	162.6	119.5	54.3	977	6.01
5′	5″	165.1	123	55.9	1006	6.09
5′	6″	167.6	127.5	58	1044	6.23
5′	7″	170.2	131.5	59.8	1076	6.32
5′	8″	172.7	135.5	61.6	1109	6.42
5′	9″	175.3	139.5	63.4	1141	6.51
5′	10″	177.8	143.5	65.2	1174	6.60
5′	11″	180.3	147.5	67	1206	6.69
6′	0″	182.9	151.5	68.9	1240	6.78

WOMEN

Height ft	Height in.	cm	Medium Frame Ideal Weight lb	Medium Frame Ideal Weight kg	Total MG Creatinine	MG Creatinine/CM Body Ht/24 Hr
5′	2″	157.5	124	56	1288	8.17
5′	3″	160	127	57.6	1325	8.28
5′	4″	162.6	130	59.1	1359	8.36
5′	5″	165.1	133	60.3	1386	8.40
5′	6″	167.6	137	63	1426	8.51
5′	7″	170.2	141	63.8	1467	8.62
5′	8″	172.7	145	65.8	1513	8.76
5′	9″	175.3	149	67.6	1555	8.86
5′	10″	177.8	153	69.4	1596	8.98
5′	11″	180.3	158	71.4	1642	9.11
6′	0″	182.9	162	73.5	1691	9.24
6′	1″	185.4	167	75.6	1739	9.38
6′	2″	188	171	77.6	1785	9.49
6′	3″	190.5	176	79.6	1831	9.61
6′	4″	193	181	82.2	1891	9.80

MEN

TABLE 7.2. ANTHROPOMETRIC STANDARDS

	Triceps Skinfold (mm)	Arm Muscle Circumference (cm)
Male	12.5	25.3
Female	16.5	23.2

Percent deficit in anthropometric measurements =

$$100 - \frac{\text{actual value}}{\text{standard value}}$$

2. Immune Competence—
   A. Total Lymphocyte Count = $\text{Total WBC} \times \frac{\%\ \text{lymphocytes}}{100}$
   B. Cell Mediated Immunity—The patient's T-lymphocyte function is assessed weekly by measurement of the area of induration resulting from intradermal injection of mumps, *candida*, PPD and SK/SD. Immune competence is characterized by a reaction of 10 mm induration to one or more antigens.

Once the nutritional assessment is performed and the need for metabolic support is determined, these same criteria are followed to assess the patient's response and document the efficacy of the nutritional therapy. Weekly nitrogen balance studies should be performed, which involves a 12 or 24 hour urine specimen with a determination of urinary urea nitrogen:

$$\text{NITROGEN BALANCE} = (\text{nitrogen in}) - (\text{nitrogen out})$$

$$= \frac{\text{Protein intake g/24 hours}}{6.25} - (\text{UUN} + 3)$$

UUN = g urinary urea nitrogen/24 hours
3 = consideration for other nonurea nitrogen loss

The hypermetabolic patient with no deficit to repair would be managed with the goal of a nitrogen balance of −1 to +1. In attempting deficit repair, a nitrogen balance of +4 to +6 is the goal of therapy. If balance studies are in a range of less than −2, the planned therapy must be reevaluated and appropriate changes made.

The basic challenge for the surgeon is to recognize those patients who present for elective surgery with a nutritional deficit. The nutritional assessment can be utilized for this purpose. If moderate to severe deficits are noted preoperatively, then nutritional repletion, enteral or parenteral, should be instituted prior to surgical intervention. The malnourished, anergic patient should be aggressively hyperalimented prior to elective therapy to attempt restoration of immune competence and initiate repair of noted deficits. If no preoperative nutritional deficit is determined, then postoperative nutritional assessment must be considered if the postoperative course is prolonged in any way. The patient who is unable to resume full oral intake by five to seven days postoperatively would certainly be a candidate for repeat nutritional assessment and support.

Beyond this point of five to seven days, the hypermetabolic, catabolic response in conjunction with starvation (inadequate protein-calorie in-

TABLE 7.3. SEVERITY OF VISCERAL PROTEIN DEFICITS

	Severe	Moderate	Mild
Serum albumin (g%)	< 2.5	< 3.0 – 2.5	< 3.5 – 3.0
Transferrin (mg%)	160	< 180 – 160	< 200 – 180
Total lymphocyte count	900	< 1500 – 900	< 1800 – 1500
Cell-mediated immunity	5mm	< 10 – 5mm	15 – 10

take) leads to a progressive deterioration of protein reserves with impairment of wound healing and immunologic response. Inadequate protein-calorie intake may also be complicated by factors such as fever and infection which increase metabolic demands above those necessary for normal recovery. One should refrain from the natural tendency to delay "one more day" in these patients because this only increases the patient's nutritional deficit.

The use of small feeding tube jejunostomies, as advocated by Page *et al.*,[11] is one method of nutritional support which should strongly be considered in patients undergoing major intra-abdominal procedures which may preclude oral alimentation for some time (e.g. esophagogastrectomy, pancreatoduodenectomy, total gastrectomy). Early resumption of enteral alimentation with elemental diets in these patients is based on the rapid return of small bowel mobility and absorption in the postoperative period while gastric and colonic adynamic ileus persist. This method allows administration into the upper gastrointestinal tract with maximal absorption in the small intestine.

The desired volume of 100–125 cc/hour is achieved over a three day period at 10% wt/vol concentration with an additional three days to achieve full concentration of 25% wt/vol. The peripheral intravenous support may be discontinued on the second postoperative day, allowing greater patient mobility, with fluid and electrolyte needs being administered via the jejunostomy. The established access to the small bowel allows prolonged enteral support, should this be required. Once full oral alimentation is resumed, the jejunostomy catheter may be left in situ for nutritional support during projected chemotherapy or radiotherapy.

INFECTION AS STRESS: NUTRITIONAL SUPPORT

Any patient who is recovering from major intra-abdominal surgery is a potential candidate for the development of infection and sepsis with associated severe hypermetabolism. This is manifested by a 40% to 60% increase in metabolic rate due to sepsis and the febrile response. An aggressive approach to nutritional support of these patients is strongly encouraged because of the marked proteolysis which occurs as a result of increased substrate and energy needs.

The introduction of a foreign body, the central catheter, has been a "theoretical" hindrance to nutritional support of the septic patient. In reality, this is not a problem when one adheres to rigid protocol in catheter insertion and aftercare. Septicemia with endogenous contamination of the catheter is much less common than the catheter sepsis induced by deviation from strict aseptic technique. The danger of inadequate nutritional support in these septic patients far outweighs the potential hazard of an intravenous foreign body.

Nutritional support of the severely septic patient requires careful monitoring of blood glucose levels with exogenous insulin supplementation as necessary. Prolonged hyperglycemia in a range above 200 mg% appears to increase susceptibility to fungus infection in the debilitated patient, especially if broad spectrum antibiotics have been administered.

Marked hyperglycemia can lead to glucosuria with resultant hyperosmolarity, dehydration and death if unchecked. This may occur because of the unique "insulin resistance" of sepsis with decreased glucose uptake by skeletal muscle, despite the presence of hyperglycemia and hyperinsulinemia. The "insulin resistance" mainly affects skeletal muscle, leading to a localized tissue-energy deficit, which is compensated by direct oxidation of branch-chain amino acids within muscle (Fig. 7.6).

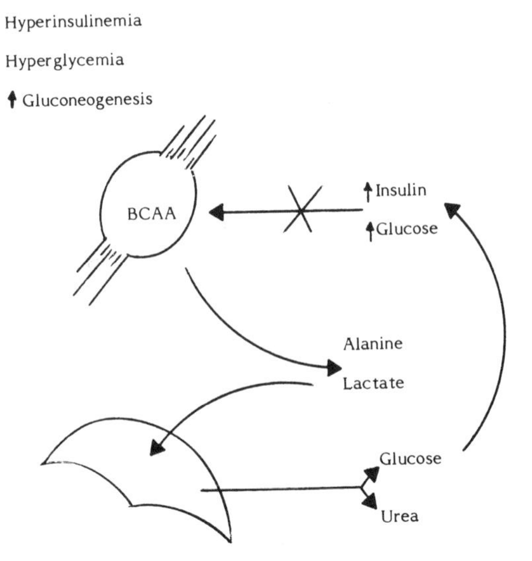

Kaminski et al.

FIG. 7.6. POSTULATED SCHEMATIC REPRESENTATION OF SUBSTRATE CHANGES ASSOCIATED WITH SEPSIS

Transamination results in increased serum levels of alanine, lactate and glycerol which induces increased hepatic gluconeogenesis not suppressed by low levels of glucose infusion (dextrose 5%).[12] Thus, sepsis results in a localized muscle energy deficit, producing hyperglycemia and hyperinsulinemia.[13] This endogenous hyperglycemia in conjunction with glucose in parenteral hyperalimentation solutions can then be compounded by peripheral resistance to the action of insulin. This is the framework which, if not closely monitored and treated, can easily lead to hyperglycemic, hyperosmolar, nonketotic dehydration.[14] The increased insulin requirements of the septic patient should not deter one from the use of parenteral nutrition but rather be accepted as a metabolic derangement in these critically ill patients which needs close monitoring.

Once therapy has been directed against the septic focus (abscess drainage, antibiotic therapy) and the patient has entered a period of convalescence with cessation of the septic hypermetabolic state, the need for nutritional support remains of paramount importance. The protein deficits associated with the hypermetabolic state will persist after fever lysis. With the patient in the recovery phase of illness, an aggressive approach to nutritional repletion is warranted to repair these deficits and restore immune competence. The goal is to return the patient rapidly to an immune competent state whereby he will be capable of handling any further septic insults which may occur during the remainder of hospitalization.

REFERENCES

1. MACFADYEN, B.J. JR., and DUDRICK, S.J.: Management of Gastrointestinal Fistulae With Parenteral Hyperalimentation, Surgery 74:100, 1973.
2. COPELAND, E.M.; MACFADYEN, B.V. JR.; MACCOMB, W.S.; GUILLAMONDEGUI, O.; JESSE, R.H., and DUDRICK, S.J.: Intravenous Hyperalimentation in Patients With Head and Neck Cancer, Cancer 35:606, 1975.
3. HUME, D. M., and EGDAHL, R.H.: Importance of the Brain in the Endocrine Response to Injury, Ann. Surg 150:697, 1959.
4. IVERSON, J.: Adenergic Receptors and the Secretion of Glucagon and Insulin From the Isolated Perfused Canine Pancreas, J. Clin. Invest. 52: 1202, 1973.
5. EGDAHL, R.J.: Pituitary-Adrenal Response Following Trauma to the Isolated Leg, Surgery 46:9, 1959.
6. BAXTER, J.D., and FORSHAM, P.H.: Tissue Effects of Glucocorticoids, Am. J. Med. 53:573, 1972.
7. HARPER, H.A.; RODWELL, V.W., and MAYES, P.A.: The Chemistry and Function of the Hormones, in *Review of Physiological Chemistry*, 16th edition, Lange Medical Publications, Los Alto, Calif.

8. BLACKBURN, G.L.; BISTRAIN, B.R.; MAINI, B.S.; SCHLAMM, H.T., and SMITH, M.F.: Nutritional and Metabolic Assessment of the Hospitalized Patient, JPEN 1:11, 1977.
9. STUDLEY, H.O.: Percentage of Weight Loss—A Basic Indicator of Surgical Risk in Patients with Chronic Peptic Ulcer, JAMA 106:458, 1936.
10. BISTRAIN, B.R., BLACKBURN, G.L.; SHERMAN, M., and SCRIMSHAW, N.S.: Therapeutic Index of Nutritional Depletion in Hospitalized Patients, Surg. Gyn. Obst. 141:512, 1975.
11. PAGE, C.P.; RYAN, J.A., and HOFF, R.C.: Continual Catheter Administration of an Elemental Diet, Surg. Gyn. Obst. 142:184, 1976.
12. LONG, C.L.; KINNEY, J.M., and GEIGER, J.W.: Nonsuppressability of Gluconeogenesis by Glucose in Septic Patients, Metabolism 25:193, 1976.
13. WANNEMACHER, R.W., and BEISEL, W.R.: Metabolic Response of the Host to Infectious Disease, in *Nutritional Aspects of Care in the Critically Ill*, by Richards, J.R., Kinney, J.M. (eds.), pp. 135–159, 1977.
14. KAMINSKI, M.V.: Review of Hyperosmolar Hyperglycemic Nonketotic Dehydration (HHND); Etiology, Pathology and Prevention During Intravenous Hyperalimentation, JPEN 2:5, 1978.

8

DIETARY MANAGEMENT OF GASTROINTESTINAL DISORDERS

Ben J. Dolin, M.D. and H. Worth Boyce, Jr., M.D.

Transit, digestion and absorption of food represent a complex interplay of mechanisms by which the body alters food into suitable form to permit its utilization. Conversely, food may alter the body by its effects on the gastrointestinal tract. In the daily exercise to maintain adequate nutrition and satiation, man constantly is exposing himself to a variety of nutritious and non-nutritious chemical agents. Gastrointestinal dietotherapy is designed to direct the patient to a proper diet to promote health and prevent injury. This may consist of the avoidance of foods that in certain persons may cause illness, or alternatively, dietotherapy may be used as a guide to certain eating habits that likely will improve intestinal function.

For years many foods have enjoyed an almost revered position in the therapy of a variety of bodily dysfunctions. In this discussion we will review the influence of certain dietary factors upon some of the more common gastrointestinal disorders. Appropriate mention will be made of the physiology involved to permit an understanding of the interactions of food and gastrointestinal dysfunction. Lactose intolerance and gluten sensitive enteropathy have been directly linked to factors found in normal diets and will be discussed in more detail. In addition, problems with dietary oxalate, fiber and factors that possibly influence the incidence of gastrointestinal malignancies will be discussed. Finally, sev-

---

Dr. Dolin is in private practice and is Associate Director of Nutritional Support Service, Methodist Hospital, Peoria, Illinois. Dr. Boyce is Director of the Division of Gastroenterology, Department of Internal Medicine, University of South Florida College of Medicine, Tampa, Florida.

eral traditional beliefs concerning effects of diet on peptic ulcer and gallbladder disease will be discredited based on recent clinical research.

LACTOSE INTOLERANCE

One of the most common gastrointestinal disorders related to diet is lactose intolerance. Lactose is a disaccharide composed of glucose and galactose. The sole source of lactose in nature is the milk from the mammary glands of placental mammals. Cow's milk contains about 5 grams and human milk about 7 grams of lactose per 100 ml. One quart of cow's milk, therefore, contains about 50 grams of lactose. Lactose in the American diet totals about 10% of the average daily carbohydrate intake.

In the human, lactase is the enzyme that hydrolyzes each molecule of lactose to one molecule of glucose and one molecule of galactose. Lactase is present in the so-called brush border covering the luminal surfaces of the mucosal cells. In mammals other than man, lactase activity is highest at term and decreases rapidly at the time of weaning. High incidences of lactose malabsorption have been found in the populations of eastern Asia, the Pacific, black Africans, Jews, Italians, Arabs and Blacks in the United States.[1] For example, over 70% of black Americans are lactase deficient. Only about 30% or less of the people from Northern Europe are intolerant of lactose. Besides the genetic predisposition to lactose intolerance, there are a variety of diseases of the gastrointestinal tract which may be accompanied by acquired lactose malabsorption. These include some forms of gastroenteritis, malnutrition, fibrocystic disease of the pancreas, tropical and nontropical sprue and giardiasis.[2] These diseases may lead to a temporary lactase deficiency and improve after the predisposing condition is resolved.

Persons with significant lactose intolerance often will be symptomatic with the ingestion of small amounts of lactose, usually that present in an eight ounce glass of milk (about 12 grams.)[3] They typically complain of abdominal distention, flatulence and diarrhea. These symptoms can be explained wholly by the osmotic effects and bacterial fermentation of undigested lactose remaining in the lower gastrointestinal tract. If no lactase is present, lactose, an osmotically active disaccharide, remains in the gut lumen. The osmotic effect of the unhydrolyzed lactose results in a net fluid accumulation or volume overload in the small intestine. This fluid excess results in osmotic diarrhea.

In addition to the osmotic effect, lactose malabsorption may cause symptoms in two other ways. When the unabsorbed lactose enters the colon, it is fermented by the microflora causing a reduction in the colonic pH and the liberation of hydrogen and carbon dioxide gases. Most of the hydrogen is eliminated as flatus. A similar process is the cause of the increased flatus from beans which contain the sugars raffinose and stachyose. Since the gut of man contains no enzyme capable of hydrolyzing these substances, the resulting fermenting process causes gas production and a reduction in the pH, which leads to an increase in circular muscle activity and rapid propulsion of osmotically derived fluid.

The diagnosis of lactose malabsorption usually can be suspected from the symptoms and knowledge of the patient's ethnic background. Confirmation may be made with a lactose tolerance test. A dose of 50 g/M^2 for children or 50–100 g lactose for adults is ingested and the blood glucose is determined at 0, 15, 30, 60 and 90 minutes. A rise of less than 20 mg/100 ml of serum glucose plus occurrence of symptoms is presumptive evidence of lactase deficiency. The test assumes a normal mechanism for the absorption of glucose and galactose. The demonstration of reduced lactase activity in a small intestinal mucosal biopsy is considered the most reliable test, but this test is presently available only in research laboratories.

The easiest treatment for a patient with symptomatic primary lactose intolerance is complete withdrawal of lactose from the diet, since the symptoms do not seem to correlate well with the amount of lactose consumed. To date, it has not been possible to induce an increase in lactase activity in either lactase deficient or normal individuals. The frequency of lactase deficiency and the value of lactose-free diets have not been appreciated by the medical profession at large, even among populations where lactase deficiency is common. In a recent survey, only 42% of hospitals reported even having lactose restricted diets in their diet manuals.[4] Occasionally the use of chocolate milk may improve symptoms. Chocolate milk has a higher osmolality than plain milk because of its sucrose content, and empties from the stomach at a slower rate. If the use of milk is felt necessary for its nutritional value, such as in school lunch programs, the lactose may be hydrolyzed before ingestion by the addition of lactase. Studies have shown that a commercially available lactase enzyme (Lact-Aid®), derived from yeast, may be used to hydrolyze the lactose in milk before ingestion, and thereby lessen the symptoms and signs of lactase deficiency.[5]

GLUTEN SENSITIVE ENTEROPATHY

Gluten sensitive enteropathy, or celiac sprue, is a well-known but uncommon disease with a direct relationship to the diet. It has an incidence of 1 in 2000–3000 births, with a slight predominance in women. Affected persons are sensitive to dietary gluten, which is found in wheat, barley and rye. The toxic substance in gluten is gliadin. When this substance comes into contact with the small bowel mucosa of a sensitive individual it produces severe mucosal changes. These changes are characterized by atrophy of the mucosal villi, hyperplasia of the cells of the mucosal glands and lymphocytic infiltration in the lamina propria. The mechanism of toxicity is unknown, although there are indications that gliadin activates an endogenous mechanism of toxicity, probably mediated through the immunological system.[6]

Common manifestations include steatorrhea, diarrhea, weight loss and malnutrition. Symptoms also may include vague abdominal pain and distention or bloating. Some persons may not complain of gastrointestinal symptoms but rather present with difficulties arising from consequence of malabsorption. They may have bleeding due to clotting abnormalities, edema related to hypoproteinemia and protein-losing enteropathy, develop severe peripheral neuropathy and anemia due to iron, folic acid or B-12 deficiency, hypocalcemia causing tetany, bone pain associated with osteomalacia or with hypokalemia leading to nephropathy. The clinical picture may be confusing since the classical malabsorption syndrome with multiple manifestations may be absent and steatorrhea may be detectable only by chemical tests. Small intestine mucosal biopsy findings are supportive but are not specific for this entity.

The mucosal atrophy leads to malabsorption of many nutrients. Fat is poorly absorbed because of mucosal atrophy as well as asynchrony between meal transit, gallbladder emptying and pancreatic secretion.[7] Carbohydrate malabsorption is present due to a universal decrease in brush border disaccharidase activity and reduced absorptive surface area. In patients improved by gluten-free diet, lactase deficiency may persist and clinical symptoms may follow milk ingestion. Protein abnormalities occur as a result of both impaired absorption and increased fecal loss. Inadequate protein digestion may result from impaired enzyme release from the pancreas. Brush border proteolytic enzymes (oligopeptidases), responsible for the breakdown of small peptides, are present in decreased concentrations. Increased fecal protein is due partially to undigested dietary protein and the loss of protein secreted into the bowel in the form of enzymes.

Since the causative substance in celiac diseases is the gliadin component of gluten found in wheat, barley and rye, treatment is aimed at totally removing these substances from the diet. Strict adherence to a gluten-free diet should result in improvement in symptoms and gradual return of the histologic pattern to normal. Improvement may be expected in a few weeks but a longer time is required in some. The avoidance of gluten-containing foods may sound simple but is relatively difficult due to the ubiquitous nature of rye, barley and especially wheat flour in the normal American diet. Wheat flour is found in some brands of instant coffee, mustard and candy bars and is used as an extender in many processed foods such as ice cream, salad dressing and canned goods. Even if the patient has a satisfactory response to gluten withdrawal, lactase deficiency and subsequent lactose intolerance may continue. If a patient does not respond to confirmed gluten withdrawal, the diagnosis must be questioned since similar histologic findings may be found in a variety of other diseases.

ENTERIC HYPEROXALURIA

It has been known for some time that patients with several types of bowel disease are prone to develop kidney stones. Recently it has been shown that stones composed primarily of oxalate are characteristic of these intestinal diseases.[8] In the normal state, much of the dietary oxalate combines with calcium in the gut to form insoluble salts which cannot be absorbed. In some patients with terminal ileitis (Crohn's disease), after jejunoileal bypass surgery or following extensive distal small bowel resection, steatorrhea may result from bile acid malabsorption. In this instance the unabsorbed fat combines with dietary calcium to form insoluble soaps and calcium is then not available to form insoluble complexes with dietary oxalate. This situation leaves the oxalate in a soluble form which may readily be absorbed. It has been shown that there is a linear correlation between fat malabsorption, oxalate absorption and urinary oxalate excretion. The increased oxalate absorption leads to an increase in urinary oxalate excretion which predisposes to nephrolithiasis.

Therapy for enteric hyperoxaluria includes the reduction of steatorrhea by restricting dietary fat and/or the administration of calcium to bind oxalate as insoluble calcium oxalate. Hypercalcemia has not been a problem since most of the additional calcium is bound to malabsorbed fatty acids or oxalate and excreted in the stool. Aluminum hydroxide gels also may be given to bind oxalate and decrease its absorption.

The average diet contains about 100 mg of oxalate daily. Most of this comes from vegetable sources and breads because animal products are low in oxalate. The amount of ingested oxalate can be lowered by a low oxalate diet.[9] This includes avoidance of tea, cocoa, leafy green vegetables and products made with unbleached flour. Reduction of fat and oxalate ingestion, plus administration of calcium supplements to bind oxalates in the lumen, provide the only means for controlling oxalate renal stone formation in the previously mentioned gastrointestinal disorders.

THE ROLE OF DIETARY FIBER

Fiber is considered an undigestible material which, to the extent it escapes bacterial digestion, is eliminated unchanged in the stool. Fiber is a combination of several substances, including cellulose, lignin, hemicellulose and pectin. Cellulose is a complex polysaccharide derived from cell walls of plant tissues. It is not digested by any enzyme in the human intestine. In most foods crude fiber content corresponds well with their cellulose content. Lignins make up the principal part of the woody structures of plants but unlike cellulose are not carbohydrates. Lignin acts in the gut like an ion exchange resin combining with bile acids and other substances to form insoluble complexes which are not absorbed. The hemicelluloses are a large group of complex polysaccharides which form mucilages and gums. Pectin also is present and is similar to the hemicelluloses. It is frequently mixed with kaolin for the treatment of diarrhea.[10]

It is known that stool weight is proportional to the amount of fiber in the diet. Most American city dwellers have a formed and relatively hard daily stool weighing about 100–200 grams. Feces of rural Africans, eating native diets, is soft, formless and weighs about 400 grams daily. The addition of increased fiber to the diet will increase fecal weight and stool frequency. Since the increase in fecal weight is greater than the weight of the fiber added, much of the increased weight is the result of water entering the gastrointestinal tract. It has been shown that as fecal weight increases, the intestinal transit time diminishes. The transit time for Europeans is about 80 hours, whereas for African villagers, it is about 35 hours.[11]

Knowledge of the effects of increased dietary fiber has resulted in its use for a variety of conditions. In some patients with ileal disease or distal ileal resection, who are unable to absorb bile salts normally, increased fiber has been shown to bind bile salts and reduce the diarrhea caused by bile salt stimulation of the colon.[12] High dietary fiber intake in persons with an intact and normal ileum may reduce serum cholesterol levels. The dietary fiber-bile salt complexes formed in the small intestine result in reduced bile salt absorption in the terminal ileum. This leads to a reduction in the body's bile salt pool. Since bile salts are made from cholesterol the decreased bile salt pool causes more cholesterol to be converted to bile salts. The result of this response is a lowering of the serum cholesterol in an attempt to increase the bile salt pool.

Several epidemiologic studies and observations by many clinicians have demonstrated the salutary effects of increasing dietary fiber on colon evacuation and symptoms of chronic constipation, irritable colon syndrome and diverticular disease of the colon. A high fiber diet is safe, simple, inexpensive and has a rational basis. Current opinion among gastroenterologists is that a normal diet high in fiber does promote a more regular bowel evacuation and likely reduces the incidence of common lower bowel disorders such as constipation, hemorrhoids and diverticulosis of the colon.[13]

The average American consumes 4–5 grams of crude fiber daily. The easiest way to increase this amount is to add more fruits, vegetables, and especially cereals to the diet. A high fiber diet is most easily accomplished by increased use of unprocessed bran, cereals with high fiber content, whole wheat bread, fresh fruits, nuts and vegetables. The richest source of fiber among ordinary foods is unprocessed wheat bran which contains 11% crude fiber. Several commercially available cereals (Kellogg's All-Bran, All-Bran Buds or Nabisco 100% Bran) provide about 1–2 grams of crude fiber per ounce (one-half cup). Unprocessed or miller's bran is now available in grocery and health food stores. One rounded teaspoon of unprocessed bran contains 2.4 grams of fiber and may be taken with fluids, added to cereals or used in baked goods. The average daily diet should contain 12–15 grams of fiber, i.e. six rounded teaspoons of unprocessed bran or its equivalent in other sources of fiber.

The old belief that low fiber or low residue diets are best for patients with diverticular disease of the colon and irritable bowel syndromes has no current support and in our opinion these diets should no longer be used as therapy for these conditions.

DIET AND GASTROINTESTINAL MALIGNANCIES

In recent years it has been realized that many malignancies of the gastrointestinal tract show marked regional and worldwide variation. These observations have led investigators to speculate that environmental factors may initiate or contribute to a variety of neoplasms. There is now increasing evidence that the diet that man consumes may in some way be related to the pathogenesis of gastrointestinal malignancies. Current evidence relates colon cancer, the most common gastrointestinal malignancy in the United States, to dietary factors. There is also epidemiologic evidence linking diet to cancer of the stomach, liver, pancreas and esophagus.[14]

Burkitt observed that Africans had a high daily intake of fiber and a low incidence of colon cancer.[11] He attempted to correlate the 90% reduction of dietary fiber in the United States and England between 1890 and 1960 with the rise in colon cancer. His observations suggested that the decrease in stool bulk and frequency associated with the diet in developed countries correlated with an increase in cancer of the large bowel.

Several mechanisms of action have been suggested to explain how dietary fiber might have an effect on the incidence of colon cancer.[15] First, fiber shortens the transit time and thus reduces the duration of exposure of the mucosal cells to possible carcinogens in the lumen. Fiber may alter bile salt metabolism in such a way as to decrease the formation of potential carcinogens. This may be done by binding bile salts, cholesterol and its degradation products and augmenting excretion of sterols, which are structurally similar to known carcinogens. Bulking properties of fiber may also dilute potential carcinogens. Animal studies show that the high fiber diet correlates with reduced activity of certain enzymes that can promote the formation of potent carcinogens. Increased dietary fiber causes a change in the intestinal bacterial flora which may result in less degradation products of bile salts that may have potential carcinogenic effects. The studies supporting the postulated relationship between dietary fiber and colon cancer rest on epidemiologic grounds, have no experimental proof and therefore must be regarded as unproven.

Although the relationship between dietary fiber and colon cancer may not be convincing, other dietary influences have stronger scientific support. A positive correlation between daily consumption of meat and colon cancer has been noted in the analysis of statistics from 23 countries. The critical factor appears to be a positive correlation with consumption of animal fat. In studies of Japanese immigrants to Hawaii, the incidence of colon cancer rises as migrants abandon the practice of eating at least one Japanese-style low meat meal each day. The rise in meat consumption parallels the increased incidence of bowel cancer in Japanese immigrants.

Studies have shown that people on a mixed Western-type diet, in which the incidence of colon cancer is high, degraded and excreted acid and neutral sterol metabolites to a greater degree than people with a low rate of colon cancer. Patients with familial polyposis excrete significantly more bile acids and cholesterol in their feces than do controls.

Gastric cancer has a widely varying incidence in mortality depending on the country of residence.[14] In countries where there is a high incidence of gastric cancer, there is usually a low incidence of colon cancer. In Japan and Finland the high rate of gastric cancer is associated with high smoked fish consumption. Additionally, low intake of fat and micronutrients (vitamins and minerals) such as vitamin A have been identified in these high risk populations. The common factor seems to be a high carbohydrate diet and a low consumption of fat, fresh fruit, vegetables and probably micronutrients. Another factor implicated in cancer of the stomach is the ingestion of nitrites. It has been shown that nitrosamines, which are known gastric carcinogens in animals, can be formed in the human stomach from nitrites and suitable substrate amines. Nitrite is used as a food additive in meat and fish to inhibit spores of clostridial bacteria (botulism). Fish preserved by salting may contain nitrites which can form nitrates. In Chile and Columbia, which have high death rates from gastric cancer, there are large nitrate deposits believed related to correspondingly high levels of nitrates in food and drinking water. Nitrate production can be inhibited by proper refrigeration and vitamin C. It has been suggested that the reduction of gastric cancer in the United States is due to widespread introduction of refrigeration and the increased availability of fresh fruits.

To a lesser degree, cancers of other parts of the gastrointestinal tract may correlate with dietary influences. Several studies have shown that extensive use of alcohol significantly increases the risk of cancer of the esophagus in smokers. In the rare Plummer-Vinson syndrome, there is also a strong association of iron deficiency and cancer of the mouth, hypopharynx or upper esophagus. It has been postulated that riboflavin deficiency, which may accompany both alcoholism and iron deficiency, also may be an etiologic factor in this syndrome.

Even though the relationship of diet and gastrointestinal cancer is unproven, it is thought that certain dietary precautions should be followed. The "prudent diet" for a person without specific diet-related disorders calls for a reduction of fat calories in the average American diet from its present 44% to 35% or less, and cholesterol to less than 300 mg per day. Adequate protein should be included and efforts should be made to minimize alcohol intake. Although the exact role of fiber in gastrointestinal malignancies is unknown, it would probably be wise to eat a diet high in fiber content to at least improve intestinal transit and colonic evacuation and thereby probably lessen problems related to constipation, hemorrhoids and diverticulosis of the colon.

PEPTIC ULCER DISEASE

Much confusion remains concerning dietary measures useful in the treatment of peptic ulcer disease. This has in part been fostered by opposing views (neither based on controlled studies) given in major textbooks on internal medicine and gastroenterology. There is no scientific proof that a "strict" Sippy-type or bland diet promotes ulcer healing. Several studies have shown that slightly modified or regular diets produce radiological healing or relief of symptoms as well as bland diets in patients with duodenal or gastric ulcers.[16] In accordance with these studies the American Dietetic Association in 1971 stated that an individualized regular diet with few restrictions should be used for people with duodenal ulcer disease.[17] Despite this modern approach adopted by both gastroenterologists and the ADA, a recent survey showed that some type of bland diet is still used in 77% of hospitals.[16] This practice is indicative of a hesitancy to give up ineffective, traditional treatments that have no proven benefit. Tea, coffee or carbonated beverages have been shown to stimulate gastric acid secretion and it is therefore still recommended that restriction of such caffeine-containing beverages is a reasonable though unproven therapeutic gesture for peptic ulcer disease. Unfortunately, and contrary to popular belief, decaffeinated coffee has been shown to stimulate gastric acid secretion probably as much as regular coffee.[18] A bedtime snack may stimulate gastric acid secretion at night when the patient is not awake to take antacids and therefore should be avoided.

Milk, although frequently recommended to ulcer patients, is a poor acid neutralizer and may result in acid rebound. The protein and calcium content of milk are potent stimulants for gastric acid secretion and probably are responsible for this acid rebound effect after the neutralizing effect of milk wanes.

Alcohol has been shown to alter the gastric mucosal barrier but it does not stimulate acid production by the human stomach. Therefore it is best avoided in a patient with peptic ulcer disease since the alteration in the mucosal barrier may potentiate the ulcer diathesis.

None of the traditional dietary measures used for peptic ulcer disease appear to have any proven effect on ulcer healing. Therefore, we recommend that the bland diet, frequent feedings, bedtime snacks and milk not be used as a treatment for gastric or duodenal ulcer diseases. The best diet therapy appears to be a regular, well-balanced diet containing calories appropriate to maintain or achieve ideal body weight. Physicians also should be aware of recent advances in the drug therapy of peptic ulcer diseases, including proper antacid dosage and a histamine-2 receptor antagonist.

GALLBLADDER DISEASE

Generations of physicians have been taught that obesity is a common accompaniment of gallbladder disease. Recent studies show that the incidence of cholesterol cholelithiasis is increased in obese patients as compared to controls of normal body weight.[19] Despite the fact that most gallstones in this country are believed to result from cholesterol supersaturation of the bile, a diet low in cholesterol does not prevent their formation. In fact, in a group of male patients with coronary artery disease treated with a lipid-lowering low cholesterol diet, the incidence of gallstones was actually greater than in controls.[20]

Other dogma concerning gallbladder disease is that fatty foods will increase symptoms. It is true that when fat reaches the duodenum it causes the release of the hormone cholecystokinin which causes gallbladder contraction. However, except for individual intolerances, there is no justification, based on presently available data, for patients with cholelithiasis to avoid fatty foods. In patients who report fatty food intolerance, the incidence of gastrointestinal complaints will decrease even though they are given fat in a disguised form.[21] It seems wise then in treating patients with gallbladder disease, as in peptic ulcer disease, that one should strive to maintain or attain ideal body weight by eating three balanced meals a day and avoid only those foods that are known by personal experience to be poorly tolerated.

SUMMARY

We have reviewed how a limited number of diseases are related to specific dietary patterns. Only two common disorders, lactose intolerance and gluten sensitive enteropathy, have been directly linked to common dietary components. Popular diet therapy, such as for peptic ulcer disease and gallbladder disease, has little or no scientific basis. Epidemiologic evidence has strongly linked diverticular disease of the colon and large bowel cancer to dietary factors but scientific proof is lacking. At this time it seems wise to follow a balanced diet to achieve and maintain ideal body weight with a reduction in fat intake and an increase in dietary fiber. Future dietary recommendations, when possible, should be made on the basis of scientific evidence and not tradition.

REFERENCES

1. RANSOME-KUTI, O.: Lactose Intolerance—A Review, Postgrad. Med. 53(2): 73, 1977.
2. JOHNSON, J.D.; KRETCHNER, N., and SIMOONS, F.J.: Lactose Malabsorption: Its Biology and History, Adv. Pediat. 21:197, 1974.
3. BEDINE, M.S. and BAYLESS, T.M.: Intolerance of Small Amounts of Lactose by Individuals with Low Lactase Levels, Gastroenterology 65(5):735, 1973.
4. WELSH, J.D.: Diet Therapy in Adult Lactose Malabsorption: Present Practices, Am. J. Clin. Nutr, 31(4):592, 1978.
5. PAIGE, D.M.; BAYLESS, T.M.; HUANG, S.S. and WEXLER, R.: Lactose Hydrolyzed Milk, Am. J. Clin. Nutr, 28(8):818, 1975.
6. STORBER, W.: Gluten-Sensitive Enteropathy, Gastroenterology 5(2):429, 1976.
7. TRIER, J.S.; FALCHUK, Z.M.; CAREY, M.C. and SCHREIBER, D.S.: Clinical Conference: Celiac Sprue and Refractory Sprue, Gastroenterology 75(2):307, 1978.

8. EARNEST, D.L.: Perspectives on Incidence, Etiology and Treatment of Enteric Hyperoxaluria, Am. J. Clin. Nutr. 30(1):72, 1977.
9. PIEPMEYER, J.: Planning Diets Controlled in Oxalic Acid Content, J. Am. Diet Assoc. 65(10):438, 1974.
10. BING, F.C.: Dietary Fiber—In Historical Perspective, J. Am. Diet Assoc. 69(11): 498, 1976.
11. BURKITT, D.P.; WALKER, A.R.P. and PAINTER, N.S.: Dietary Fiber and Disease, JAMA 229(8):1068, 1974.
12. DWYER, J.T., GOLDIN, B.; GORBACH, S., and PATTERSON, J.: Drug Therapy Reviews: Dietary Fiber and Fiber Supplements in the Therapy of Gastrointestinal Disorders, Hosp. Pharm. 35:278, 1978.
13. MENDELOFF, A.I.: Dietary Fiber and Gastrointestinal Diseases, M. Clin. North America 62(1):165, 1978.
14. WYNDER, E.L.; BANDARU, S.R.; McCOY, G.D., and WEISBURGER, J.N.: Diet and Cancer of the Gastrointestinal Tract, Ann. Int. Med. 22:397, 1977.
15. ALCANTARA, E.N. and SPECKMANN, E.W.: Diet, Nutrition and Cancer, Am. J. Clin. Nutr. 29(9):1035, 1976.
16. WELSH, J.D.: Diet Therapy of Peptic Ulcer Disease, Gastroenterology 72:740, 1977.
17. THE AMERICAN DIETETIC ASSOCIATION Position Paper on Bland Diet in the Treatment of Chronic Duodenal Ulcer Disease, J. Am. Diet Assoc. 59:244, 1971.
18. COHEN, S. and BOOTH, G.H.: Gastric Acid Secretion and Lower Esophageal-Sphincter Pressure in Response to Coffee and Caffeine, New England J. M. 293(18):897, 1975.
19. WHEELER, M.; HILLS, L.L., and LABY, B.: Cholelithiasis, A Clinical and Dietary Survey, Gut 11:430, 1970.
20. STUDEVANT, R.A.L.; PEARCE, M.L., and DAYTON, S.: Increased Prevalence of Cholelithiasis in Men Ingesting a Serum-Cholesterol-Lowering Diet, New England J. M. 288(1):24, 1973.
21. DONALDSON, R.M.: Diet and Gastrointestinal Disorders (editorial), Gastroenterology 52(5):897, 1967.

9

TOTAL PARENTERAL NUTRITION

Ralph T. Guild, M.D., and James J. Cerda, M.D.

The need for adequate nutrition is now considered a fundamental tenet in the management of most diseases. In the last decade, total parenteral nutrition has evolved as an important means for accomplishing this goal.

The concept of intravenous alimentation is rooted in antiquity. Sir Christopher Wren described the first intravenous infusion in 1656, utilizing a hollow quill to administer various solutions to dogs. Later, Biedl and Kraus administered intravenous nutrition to man for the first time in 1896. By the time of the first World War, infusions of glucose and water were widely utilized. Studies on the use of intravenous proteins were conducted in the 1930's. The use of intravenous fat emulsions became widespread in the 1950's in the United States but their use was prohibited in 1964 because of several toxic side effects. The advances that have led to our modern techniques of total parenteral nutrition were achieved in the 1960's. Wretlind and his colleagues in Sweden developed a safe fat emulsion which made possible parenteral alimentation which could safely be delivered through a peripheral venous route. In 1968 Dr. Stanley J. Dudrick of the University of Pennsylvania reported that parenteral nutrition utilizing hypertonic glucose and protein hydrolysates achieved positive nitrogen balance in postoperative patients. Because of the hypertonicity of the glucose solutions they required infusion via a central vein. The superior vena cava was utilized, via the subclavian vein. The term, "hyperalimentation," was derived from this description of a "hypertonic intravenous alimentation." More recently, the term,

Dr. Guild is Instructor in Gastroenterology, and Dr. Cerda is Professor of Medicine and Associate Chairman, and also Director of the Nutrition Laboratory, University of Florida College of Medicine, Gainesville.

"hyperalimentation," has been used interchangeably with "total parenteral nutrition" especially with solutions delivered centrally.

The aim of total parenteral nutrition is to provide and maintain adequate nutrition by an intravenous route to patients in whom enteric feedings are inadequate, poorly tolerated, or contraindicated. Enteric feedings should always be utilized when the clinical situation so permits. The goal of therapy is to maintain or achieve the patient's ideal weight or usual weight and to maintain positive nitrogen balance.

The basic principles of total parenteral nutrition (TPN) are: (1) evaluate the individual patient for the advisability of total parenteral nutrition and that individual's particular requirements for parenteral nutrients; (2) establish and maintain an aseptic intravenous route, usually central, using a large-bore catheter for administration of the nutrient solution; (3) infuse nutrient solutions in a concentrated form in order to avoid volume overload; (4) provide sufficient nonprotein calories to insure the utilization of administered amino acids for protein synthesis, and (5) establish a steady-state delivery, i.e., a constant flow rate, in order to minimize fluctuations in the physiological responses to nutrient infusion. One additional principle would appear to be the desirability of a team approach. Several studies have shown that such nutritional support units maximize the benefits of TPN programs and minimize the complications which marred early TPN utilization. Such teams should include a physician with an interest and knowledge of basic nutrition; a pharmacist to aseptically prepare the solutions and provide medical/nutrient interaction information; and a nurse to supervise aseptic technique in placing and maintaining intravenous catheters, monitor infusion of the nutrient solutions and correlate monitoring data for individual patients. Fewer complications in catheter placement appear to result when a select few physicians skilled in this technique regularly provide this service. The involvement of a dietitian provides a valuable input not only from a general nutritional standpoint but also in integrating the transition in diets which occurs when patients do respond to TPN. Additional members of a team are occasionally needed to provide input into the management of individual patients and, sometimes, their complications.

INDICATIONS FOR TOTAL PARENTERAL NUTRITION

Total parenteral nutrition may be indicated in certain patients of the following groups: gastrointestinal tract disorders; massive burns or severe trauma; cancer patients receiving chemotherapy or radiotherapy; postsurgical patients not expected to receive oral intake for seven days; emaciated or obviously debilitated patients prior to undergoing nonemergency surgery; and infants suffering from respiratory difficulties during feeding and longstanding failure to thrive. A variety of studies have demonstrated the efficacy of total parenteral nutrition in these conditions.[2-5]

The gastrointestinal disorders in which TPN may be of benefit can be classified in two groups. The first are those patients unable to ingest nutrients because of an obstructing lesion or a disorder of motility. The second includes patients with impaired digestion or absorption in whom bowel rest may eventually result in marked clinical improvement secondary to adequate nutrition. In particular, patients with fistulas, inflammatory bowel disease, pancreatitis, diverticulitis and complete bowel obstruction seem to benefit.

In most patients with inflammatory bowel disease in whom hospitalization is required, significant malnutrition from a variety of causes is a significant contributing factor. In a recent review article, Driscoll concluded that most studies do not show that TPN alters the unpredictable and recurrent course of Crohn's disease. In patients without associated fistulae, the approach may be useful in the following situations: (1) nutritional repletion during diagnostic investigation; (2) primary therapy for the patient in whom medical management has failed, where surgery is contraindicated or hazardous; and (3) preparation for surgery and maintenance in the postoperative period; (4) immediate or long-term management of the patient with short bowel following intestinal resection. In the above cases, TPN is usually utilized in association with bowel rest. Patients with Crohn's fistulae present special problems and benefits remain controversial. Nutritional repletion can usually be achieved but closure usually requires surgical intervention. The possible exception to this would appear to be the postoperative fistulae in the region of resected bowel which may close spontaneously with hyperalimentation. In the pediatric age group, patients with inflammatory bowel disease with growth retardation may be unable to meet their energy and protein requirements with oral feedings alone. There has been some success in these refractory patients with the use of TPN to meet these needs. Patients with ulcerative colitis do not usually respond to TPN as primary therapy. Even when remissions are achieved they are usually for only a short term. Hyperalimentation does appear useful to replenish the malnourished patient in preparation for surgery and to support patients in the postoperative period.

Patients with massive burns and trauma are frequently unable to ingest nutrients because of involvement of the anatomy in such a way as to prevent oral feeding. Other patients may simply not be able to ingest sufficient nutrients to meet the requirements imposed in this hypermetabolic state. Wound healing in particular seems to be improved by total parenteral nutrition. Dudrick has shown that burn patients on

TPN also evidence less septic complications, enjoy better graft survival and demonstrate accelerated healing.

Although the question of the use of hyperalimentation in the management of terminally ill patients with malignancies remains unanswered, TPN does appear to be an important adjunct to both chemotherapy and radiotherapy. Frequently malnutrition may have resulted in loss of immunocompetence in cancer patients, such immunocompetence actually being required for the efficacy of some chemotherapeutic agents. TPN has also been shown to increase the tolerance of some patients to chemotherapeutic agents such as methotrexate and 5-fluorouracil which have significant gastrointestinal side effects. Radiation therapy, which frequently results in significant gastrointestinal side effects, is also better tolerated by patients on adequate TPN programs. Additionally, it is believed that TPN is of benefit in cancer patients because of the improvement in the quality of life.

Patients who have not been fed for seven days following surgery or who are expected to have a period of intolerance to oral feedings for greater than two weeks should be considered for TPN. It has been shown that such patients enjoy better wound healing and fewer complications than malnourished, debilitated patients. As concerns preoperative patients an effort should be made to delay surgery when anergy or significant protein calorie malnutrition, as evidenced by the patient's nutritional assessment profile, is demonstrated. Meakins and others have demonstrated that such patients are at a higher risk for complications. It should be noted, however, that with sepsis there is poor utilization of nutrients. Surgery should not be withheld in such patients pending nutritional improvement.

Patients in the pediatric age group present additional problems. They require nutrition not only adequate for homeostasis but also to sustain growth. In our hospital, the primary indications in the neonatal age group would include (1) patients with hyaline membrane disease who are ventilator dependent (2) gastrointestinal disease including necrotizing enterocolitis and bowel distention of unknown etiology; and (3) neonates of less than 1500 g body weight. In the general pediatric age group, the most common indication for the use of TPN is in preparation for bowel surgery. Hyperalimentation may be used in malnourished patients to replete them prior to surgery and maintain them postoperatively. Long-term TPN is used to meet maintenance and growth requirements in pediatric patients in whom surgery must be delayed until further growth and development takes place, or in whom staged surgical procedures are required.

In general one should consider total parenteral nutrition for patients in the high risk categories mentioned. Any patient who has been, or might be, deprived of adequate oral nutrition for seven or more days or who has had a recent loss of 10% or more of body weight due to inadequate nutrition should also be considered.

NUTRITIONAL STATUS EVALUATION

Prior to implementation of total parenteral nutrition in any patient, a thorough evaluation of that individual's nutritional status should be made. Such evaluations are helpful in assessing the degree of nutritional impairment, need for nutritional support in an appropriate form and the data base against which the results of therapy may be evaluated. Blackburn, Bistrian and colleagues have suggested an extensive protocol which utilizes anthropometric data, laboratory studies and measures of a patient's immunocompetence.[6] They have emphasized the inadequacies of any single test to define any patient's nutritional deficiencies.

Initial assessment should include height and weight which are important indicators of the patient's somatic status. The patient's weight should be compared to his usual weight as well as to his ideal weight for height. The usual reference table for ideal body weight-for-height is presented in the Recommended Dietary Allowances published by the NAS/NRC (See Appendix F.). A simple rule for estimating ideal body weights for adults is: (1) for women, allow 100 lb for the first 5 feet and 5 lb for each additional inch; (2) for men, allow 110 lb for the first 5 feet and 6 lb for each additional inch; (3) allow 10% variation above or below the calculated weight for individual differences. A more definitive measure of lean body mass is the Creatinine/Height Index which is calculated by comparing the patient's actual urinary creatinine (mg/24 hr) to an ideal urinary creatinine calculated from ideal body weight. For men of ideal weight for their height, the value is 23 mg/kg²4 hr; for women, the value is 18 mg/kg/24 hr. A greater than 20% deficit indicates nutritional depletion. Other anthropometric measurements which are useful in evaluating the patient's nutritional status include the triceps skinfold, mid-arm circumference and mid-arm muscle circumference. Triceps skinfold allows an estimation of the body's fat reserves. A fold of skin on the posterior aspect of the arm midway between the shoulder and elbow is grasped and pulled gently away from the underlying muscle. Special calipers are then applied to measure the skinfold. For adult males, the standard is 12.5 mm and for females 16.5 mm. The mid-arm circumference is measured on the nondominant arm halfway between the acromial process of the scapula and the olecranon process of the ulna. The usual values for adults are 29.3 cm for males and 28.5 for females. The third anthropometric indicator is calculated from the triceps skinfold and the mid-arm circumference. This is the arm muscle circumference which is an indicator of the level of somatic protein deficit. The relationship is: arm muscle circumference (in cm) equals mid-arm circumference minus (0.314 × triceps skinfold in cm). The usual standards are 25.3 cm for males and 23.2 cm for females. The values obtained from these anthropometric measures are usually presented as percentages of the ideal or standard. These standards are based on World Health Organization figures compiled by Jelliffe. It has recently been suggested that these figures may underestimate malnutrition in the general U.S. population; however, widespread use of the WHO figures provides a benchmark by which results can be compared between centers.

The degree of visceral protein depletion in the malnourished patient may be determined by the depression of secretory proteins and of the cellular immune system. Blackburn and Bistrian have demonstrated that albumin and transferrin are good parameters of visceral protein compartment status. For albumin, a value of 3.5 g/dl is considered normal. A mild impairment is considered to be between 3.5 and 3.0 g/dl; moderate between 3.0 and 2.5, and severe less than 2.5 g/dl. Utilization of this parameter is not valid if albumin has been provided to the patient prior to assessment. Serum transferrin may be estimated from the total iron binding capacity by the formula: transferrin = (0.8 × TIBC) – 43. A result between 200 and 180 mg/dl is considered a mild impairment; between 180 and 160 moderate; and less than 160 severe.

The cellular immune system is evaluated by the total lymphocyte count and delayed hypersensitivity reactions to antigens. A lymphocyte count between 1800 and 1500 per mm^3 indicates a mild deficiency; between 1500 and 900 moderate, and less than 900 severe. The usual skin test antigens utilized are PPD, Tricophyton, Candida, Mumps and Streptokinase/Streptodornase. The delayed cutaneous hypersensitivity is evaluated at 48 hours. Normal response is a wheal at least 15 mm in diameter for any one of the skin tests. A result between 10 and 15 mm represents a mild deficiency; between 5 and 10 mm moderate, and less than 5 mm severe immunodeficiency or anergy. Recently, anergy has been correlated with increased morbidity and infection in chemotherapy. Prognosis seems to be improved if the patient retains or achieves immune competence as measured by skin test and poor if an initially immune competent patient becomes anergic or remains anergic.

It is sometimes helpful to classify nutritional deficiencies as marasmus, kwashiorkor or a combined deficiency state. These estimations of protein calorie malnutrition are readily identified by International Classification of Diseases, Adapted numbers. Nutritional marasmus (268.0) is characterized by depression of anthropometric measurements and kwashiorkor (267.0) by decreased visceral protein stores even though anthropometric measures may appear normal. The combined state (269.9) is a life-threatening form of malnutrition in which both anthropometric and laboratory studies are abnormal.

An additional test which should be utilized in evaluation of the patient's nutritional status is determination of nitrogen balance. Nitrogen intake is estimated by dividing grams of protein consumed by 6.25. The nitrogen output is estimated by a formula based on urea nitrogen excreted during a 24-hour period. A constant of 3 to 4 g of nitrogen is added to cover the excretion of non-urea nitrogen lost through the skin, in the feces or as non-urea urinary nitrogen. This estimation of nitrogen balance is easily carried out and provides a good estimation of the sufficiency of nutritional support.

Additional baseline laboratory studies should include a complete blood count, differential, platelets and clotting studies. Frequently, abnormalities in these studies may be the first indication of a patient's inadequate vitamin status. Other important laboratory tests would include electrolytes, calcium, phosphate, magnesium and serum iron.

NUTRITIONAL REQUIREMENTS

The next step in instituting total parenteral nutrition is to establish the nutritional requirements of the individual patient. The caloric requirement for the resting adult patient is 27–30 kcal/kg/day for men and 23–26 kcal/kg/day for women (Recommended Dietary Allowances, 1974). Infants and young children will require approximately 100–150 kcal/kg/day to maintain body weight. Many centers have adopted the recommendation of Blackburn *et al.* regarding basal energy expenditures (BEE) which are based on experimental data (Harris-Benedict equations).

$$\text{Men's BEE} = 66 + (13.7 \times W) + (5 \times H) - (6.8 \times A)$$
$$\text{Women's BEE} = 655 + (9.6 \times W) - (1.7 \times H) - (4.7 \times A)$$
where W = actual weight in kg; H = height in cm; A = age in years.

However, these values approximate the requirements for a nonstressed hospital patient at bed rest. Ambulation will increase metabolic expenditures by about 20%. Fever will increase metabolic requirements by 11–13% for each degree centigrade body temperature elevation. Major stress will increase requirements by up to 20%; peritonitis by 50%; and significant burns by 100%. Jeejeebhoy and colleagues have suggested that the provision of 40 kcal/kg/day will permit positive caloric balance and weight gain in most patients with gastrointestinal problems. Blackburn's recommended energy requirements for anabolism in patients on TPN are 1.75 × BEE. In the calculation of nutrients to supply the patient's caloric needs, protein calories are not included by convention. Consideration for the calorie:nitrogen ratio in the diet must be given. In the normal diet, the ratio is in the range of 200–300 kcal/gram of nitrogen consumed. For resting metabolic expenditure, the ratio of nitrogen:calories falls in the range of 1:100–200. Acute injury and infection may increase nitrogen loss compared to energy expenditure. Thus, the appropriate nitrogen:calorie ratio is in the range of 1:75–150. Conversely, in disease states such as renal failure where nitrogen accumulation occurs, the optimum nitrogen:calorie ratio is increased to 1:450–700 to suppress ureagenesis and catabolism.

In determining the protein requirement of a patient receiving total parenteral nutrition, both the amount of the protein infused and its composition are important. The recommended dietary allowance of protein for an average adult is approximately 0.9 g/kg of body weight of an "ideal" protein. The present state of the art is such that amino acid solutions containing both essential as well as sufficient nonessential amino acids to balance the mixture (approximating an ideal protein) are now utilized as a protein source. With a daily infusion of protein in the range of 1–1.5 g/kg (body weight), most patients will achieve a positive nitrogen balance. This represents a minimum of 12–15 g of nitrogen (75–95 g protein) daily. Because of the availability of the readily utilizable clinical tool of nitrogen balance, adjustments to achieve a positive nitrogen balance can be made in the individual patient.

Most of the caloric requirements for a patient receiving total parental nutrition are supplied by carbohydrates. The standard intravenous carbohydrate source in the United States is monohydrate dextrose which supplies 3.4 kcal/g. Eighty to 90% of caloric requirements are generally supplied as carbohydrate. Solutions of 5–50% dextrose are available to supply these requirements. Fructose, maltose and sorbitol have also been utilized as carbohydrate sources but are not readily available for general clinical use.

Fats in the normal diet may constitute up to 40% of total calories. In the United States, the utilization of intravenous lipids is generally restricted to 10–20% of the caloric requirements. This will supply 4% of calories as essential fatty acids. Only two lipid products are currently available in the United States. The older of the two is Intralipid® (Cutter), which is based on soybean oil. Liposyn® (Abbott) has a safflower oil base. Both utilize egg phosphatides as emulsifying agents. They are generally utilized as 10% or 20% solutions of the basic lipids. Lipids are desirable for several reasons. First, they supply a concentrated source of calories, approximately 9 kcal/g. They are not hypertonic and may be used peripherally if necessary. Because they do not promote insulin release, lipids may improve nitrogen retention in catabolic patients. As an alternative to I.V. fat emulsions in patients able to tolerate oral feedings, safflower or corn oil may be given in dosages of 25–50 ml/day to treat symptoms of fatty acid deficiency.

Requirements for vitamins in total parenteral nutrition have not been established. Several factors such as disease states and even the amount of nutrients infused may significantly alter the requirements in individual patients. Generally, one to two ml of any of several commercially available water-soluble B-complex vitamins will fulfill the daily requirements for this important group. Vitamin B_{12} may be administered I.M. in doses of 100–200 micrograms monthly or added (usually with folacin) in dosage of 100 micrograms weekly to bottles of nutrients containing no other vitamins. The usual weekly dosage of folacin is 2.5 mg. Vitamin C requirements are 300–500 mg daily. This water-soluble vitamin is available as a mixture with B-complex vitamins. Presently, the only commercially available emulsion of the fat-soluble vitamins A, D and E is M.V.I.® (Multi-Vitamin Infusion, USV Laboratories). Generally, 5 ml of M.V.I. concentrate is administered twice weekly for fat soluble vitamin maintenance. As M.V.I. also contains water-soluble B-complex vitamins and vitamin D, the requirements for those vitamins are also met on the days in which it is infused. Vitamin K preparations are compatible with TPN solutions, but are often administered I.M. Weekly doses should be adjusted to the patient's prothrombin time and are usually in the range of 10–15 mg weekly. These are essentially maintenance requirements for vitamin additives. For patients with specific deficiencies, greater amounts of specific vitamins may be required.

Electrolyte requirements in total parenteral nutrition vary widely in individual patients. In general, they parallel the requirements of standard I.V. feeding. Alterations may be required for patients with cardiac or renal disease as well as for disease states which lead to significant losses of electrolytes. Additional amounts of potassium, phosphate, calcium and magnesium are introduced by total parenteral nutrition. Potassium is required for the intracellular movement of glucose and amino acids. It is required for the deposition of protoplasm and lean mass at a rate of 3 mEq for each gram of nitrogen retained. In addition, potassium is necessary to replace obligatory losses, usually 40–60 mEq/day in patients with normal renal function. Usual adult phosphate requirements are 10–12 mM phosphorus (20–24 mEq of dibasic phosphorus) per liter of TPN solution. The amount infused should be about 1.5 times the calcium infusion. The usual calcium requirement is 15–20 mEq/day. Therefore, about 30 mEq/day of phosphate will also be required due to reciprocal relationships between serum calcium and phosphate levels. Magnesium is retained at a rate of 0.5 mEq for each gram of nitrogen. The recommended daily requirement for magnesium is approximately 24 mEq for adults. Additional requirements for magnesium occur in several disease states because of significant losses. These include prolonged diarrhea, short bowel syndromes, cirrhosis, alcoholism and thermal burns. Patients with renal disease should be monitored closely to prevent hypermagnesemia.

Attention must also be given to the addition of minerals and other micronutrients which may be required only in trace amounts on a monthly basis. Particularly, in patients on prolonged total parenteral nutrition, deficiencies of trace elements may be expected. Currently, no standard recommendation or preparation including these minerals is available. Iron is required at levels of 1 to 15 mg/day. This may be administered I.M. or I.V. as iron salts or iron dextran preparations. Zinc may be required at levels of 2 to 4 mg or more per day, particularly in patients with significant trauma or small bowel fistulae. Other trace elements for which requirements have been suggested include iodine, copper, manganese, chromium and selenium. Transfusions of whole blood and fresh frozen plasma have been utilized in the past to provide micronutrients. However, the use of blood products is not without significant risk and little uniformity in replacement can be guaranteed. Most of these trace elements are available in a soluble form compatible with other TPN nutrients. These may be administered to correct specific deficiencies and it is anticipated that a commercial preparation of trace elements will soon be available to fill this nutritional gap.

Finally, in administration of nutrients, fluid requirements must be considered. The basic fluid input should be 1.2–1.5 ml/kcal. In the theoretical 70 kg man with a caloric requirement of 40 kcal/kg, amounts to 40–60 ml/kg or 3.5–4.2 l would be required daily and patients with impaired renal function should be limited to approximately one liter/day. Jeejeebhoy and colleagues have suggested that, in patients with congestive heart failure, infusions of 40 ml/kg is tolerated in most patients provided sodium input is restricted to about 20–30 mEq/day.

In actual practice, with a specialized physician order form for TPN, a typical order need not be unduly complicated. To illustrate, Figure 9.1 is a reproduction of the order form utilized at the University of Florida Teaching Hospitals. The solutions ordered represent what might be termed a standard formulation for a mythical 70-kg adult without complicating metabolic problems. For such an individual, an equal mixture of amino acid 5.5% with electrolytes and D50W would be utilized to provide a final concentration of 2.75% amino acids and 25% glucose. At the maintenance rate shown of 125 ml/hr (3 L per day) the patient will receive 82.5 g of protein (approximately 1.2 g per kg body weight) and 2,550 kcal of non-protein calories in the form of glucose. This represents an energy intake of approximately 35 kcal per kg body weight. Use of

University of Florida
Shands Teaching Hospital and Clinics
Gainesville, Florida 32610

ADULT

DOE, JOHN
40-01-01

Patient Addressograph

TOTAL PARENTERAL NUTRITION (TPN)
PHYSICIAN ORDER FORM

*Please complete sections I, IA, IB, &II
SIGN & forward to Pharmacy by 9:00 a.m.

Sec. I. AMINO ACID/CARBOHYDRATE ORDER (A.A./C.H.O.)

NO CHANGE	CENTRAL LINE	PERIPHERAL LINE	OTHER
from Previous Day's Order	Amino Acid 5.5% with Electrolytes ______ 500 ml. $D_{50}W$ ______ 500 ml. Sterile H_2O ______ 0 ml.	Amino Acid 5.5% with Electrolytes ______ 500 ml. $D_{10}W$ ______ 500 ml. Sterile H_2O ______ 0 ml.	"CIRCLE" Amino Acid ___ % with/without electrolytes ______ ml. D ___ W ______ ml. Sterile H_2O ______ ml.
[ ] "X"	[X] "X"	[ ] "X"	[ ] "X"

Sec. IA ADDITIVES

Electrolytes in Standard Solution (Amino acids 8.5% or 5.5% with electrolytes) "CROSS OUT STANDARD CONCENTRATIONS IF DIFFERENT"		FINAL Concentration of Formulation
Sodium Chloride	35mEq/L	mEq/L
Potassium Phosphate	30m Eq/L	mEq/L
Magnesium	~~5mEq/L~~	10 mEq/L
Calcium Gluconate		10 mEq/L
Will be added to only liter 1 unless otherwise designated		
Vitamin K_1		mg/L
Will be added to only liter 1 unless otherwise designated		
Insulin (Reg.)		u/L
Iron Dextran		mg/L
		/L
		/L
		/L
		/L

Sec. IB PHARMACY STANDING ORDERS

START	D/C	
X		MVI Conc 5 ml/L on Monday
X		Vitamin B with C 5 ml/L on Tuesday through Sunday
TO BE PLACED IN FIRST LITER ONLY		
X		Folic acid 5 mg on Monday
X		Vitamin B_{12} 500 mcg on 1st and 15th days of the month
X		Trace Element Solution 1 ml. Daily *SEE STHC TPN HANDBOOK
		Elemental Zinc ______ mg Daily
		Elemental Copper ______ mg Daily
NOTE:		Charges in Standing Orders should be indicated in Additive Sec. IA.

ANTICIPATED D/C SOLUTION
DATE/TIME: 1-1-80
OTHER COMMUNICATION:

Room 439 Weight (kg) 70 Date to be infused 12-15-79 Infusion Rate (A.A./C.H.O.) 125 ml/hr

Sec. II FAT ORDERS

Infuse ______ ml. at ______ ml./hr. for ______ hours.

12-14-79 Date Ralph Guild, M.D. M.D. (Sign)

Orig.—CHART COPY NCR—PHARMACY Copy immediately after signing. REV. 5/79

FIGURE 9.1. A SPECIALIZED PHYSICIAN ORDER FORM FOR TPN UTILIZED AT THE UNIVERSITY OF FLORIDA TEACHING HOSPITALS

the standard solution also lessens the number of additives that are required to meet the patient's nutritional needs—thus, also reducing the possibility for potential contamination or error. As noted, additional magnesium must be added to the solution to produce a final concentration of 10 mEq/L (30 mEq/day). Calcium gluconate need only be added to 1 L daily in the amount of 10 mEq. Routine standing orders for vitamins and trace elements are utilized as detailed in Section IB to simplify ordering these routine additions. As noted previously, B and C vitamins are added daily with fat-soluble vitamins added on one day each week. Folacin is added on one day each week and vitamin B_{12} is given twice monthly. Trace elements are added as a solution in the amount of one ml/day. Although not ordered on this example, Section II allows the physician to order Intralipid® in amounts necessary to avoid essential fatty acid deficiency in patients on total parenteral nutrition. As discussed previously, the usual requirement is approximately 4% of total calories per week. The standard unit for both Intralipid and Liposyn is a 500-ml container. Typically, two units (1000 ml) are required per week. This may be given via the central line or by a peripheral catheter. Infusion of the glucose amino acid mixture is usually continued during infusion of Intralipid® by the central line.

The use of a standardized order sheet provides several benefits for both the physician and the pharmacist in meeting the needs of patients. The physician is reminded of the standard solutions which are available which lower the cost of hyperalimentation per unit as well as providing greater safety because of the fewer number of additions required. After the patient has been stabilized on total parenteral nutrition, only a few minutes are required to complete Sections I and IA of this form. At the same time, most changes in solutions involve electrolytes, thus affecting easy accessibility to such changes. In our hospital, these forms are in duplicate with a non-carbon copy being made at the same time as the original. This pharmacy copy is then utilized as the worksheet for the pharmacist, providing a form which is printed and thus less likely to lead to potential errors in formulation. A separate form (not shown) is used to order TPN solutions for pediatric and neonatal patients.

ADMINISTERING TOTAL PARENTERAL SOLUTIONS

The technical aspects of administering total parenteral solutions involve the catheter and associated infusion equipment, preparation of solutions, and monitoring of administration. As noted earlier, to reduce complications, a team approach is best. Individuals knowledgeable and skilled in applying known techniques generate optimal outcomes.

A plastic cannula introduced into the superior vena cava via a percutaneous cannulation of the subclavian vein continues to be the preferred route of administration for adult patients. The technique is relatively safe and the area lends itself to good antiseptic technique both in the placement of the catheter and its maintenance. Dressings over the catheter are changed daily or every other day. Infusion tubing is replaced daily. The line established for total parenteral nutrition is used solely for that purpose. No blood or pressure measurements are taken from the TPN catheter. Additionally, no medications are given via this catheter. To prevent infusion of contaminants, a 0.22 micron disposable millipore filter is generally utilized in the infusion line as close to the catheter as possible. Although a gravity drip may be utilized in infusing TPN solutions, current practice is to utilize a controlled infusion pump. Monitoring features and warning alarms associated with the use of such equipment provide visual and auditory cues to both patient and personnel when complications arise. The use of this equipment does restrict the mobility of the patient somewhat. As many become more sophisticated in the management of their own nutrition, gravity drip monitored by such patients can be employed. Because of the cost of such equipment, gravity may be utilized in home TPN administration.

While TPN solutions are ordered on individual patients by a physician, the storage, inspection and preparation of such solutions are generally under the purview of a pharmacist. Indeed, the use of laminar flow hoods, aseptic technique and careful monitoring of mixtures by a knowledgeable pharmacist have done much to minimize potential complications. While individuals require a TPN solution tailored to their needs, the use of basic formulations with individual additives has increased the safety factor and lowered the costs of total parenteral nutrition. In general, TPN solutions are composed of a concentrated protein source (usually a mixture of crystalline amino acids) with or without a standard electrolyte solution added, a concentrated carbohydrate source, vitamins and trace elements. Sterile transfer and administration sets are used in preparing the final solution.

In initiating total parenteral nutrition, care must be taken to allow time for the body to respond appropriately to the increased nutrient load. During the first 24 hours of therapy, only a single liter of TPN solution is infused. This will allow time for the pancreas to respond to the hypertonic glucose load with increased insulin. Electrolyte solutions with 5–10% glucose may be given peripherally to meet fluid requirements. On the second day, two liters are infused and the patient is advanced to three liters by the third day if the blood glucose stays within acceptable limits. Glucose-amino acid solutions and the currently available lipid infusion (Intralipid) are not compatible when mixed. The lipid emulsion is not compatible with additives such as vitamins and minerals. Intralipid may be infused through the central catheter when connected by a "y" connector or given peripherally.

Monitoring and careful record keeping are essential to the success of a program of total parenteral nutrition. Baseline studies have been outlined previously. After initiating infusion of the TPN solution, fractional urines should be tested four times daily for glucose and acetone. Accurate fluid balances should be recorded daily. Weights and temperatures should be recorded daily. Nutritional assessment should be made on a regular basis: nitrogen balances twice weekly, skin tests for anergy every one to two weeks until the patient is nutritionally repleted; lymphocyte counts and TIBC's weekly until the patient is nutritionally repleted; anthropometrics every three weeks. In general, serum electrolytes and blood glucose should be obtained daily until the patient is stabilized. They are then followed thrice weekly. Other laboratory tests including CBC, liver function studies, lipid profiles, minerals and renal function studies are obtained twice weekly until the patient is stabilized and, thereafter, weekly. If Intralipid is infused, the patient's ability to clear lipids should be assessed by checking the triglyceride level. It should be normal within 12 hours of infusing the emulsion. Platelet count should be checked weekly if Intralipid is being infused regularly.

POSSIBLE COMPLICATIONS

Total parenteral alimentation is, by its very nature, a complicated process. To say that complications may arise represents profound understatement. These complications fall into two categories; first, those involving the mechanical aspects of the process especially the intravenous catheter and, secondly, metabolic complications which may arise particularly during prolonged administration. One of the principal advantages of an experienced knowledgeable hyperalimentation team is the reduction of complications by careful attention to detail and procedure.

The intravenous alimentation catheter is the most vulnerable component of the system. As discussed previously, meticulous care must be utilized in placing and maintaining the catheter in order to avoid complications. Pneumothorax, hemothorax, visceral trauma, emboli and misplacement are the most commonly reported complications of catheter placement. Other complications involving the catheters include phlebitis and thrombosis of the superior vena cava or subclavian veins. Patients should be placed in a Trendelenberg position during placement and redressing of the catheter to avoid the introduction of air embolus.

The most common and serious complication involving the mechanical aspects of TPN is sepsis. Reported series would suggest a rate of septic complications ranging from 4–7% even in the best of hands. Also of pertinence is the extremely high incidence of fungal infections which comprise more than 50% of infections in most series. The usual organism is Candida although Torulopsis has also been reported. A patient receiving total parenteral nutrition should have his body temperature monitored frequently. When a significant fever elevation is noted, the hyperalimentation solutions should be discontinued and the solutions cultured. Blood should be withdrawn from the catheter and cultured, following which an isotonic dextrose solution should be infused through the catheter to prevent hypoglycemia. A standard fever workup including the taking of a careful history, physical examination and appropriate cultures should be carried out. If a source for the temperature elevation can be determined, appropriate therapy should be instituted and TPN resumed. If the source is not identified within the first 12 hours and fever persists, the I.V. catheter should be replaced and the tip of the withdrawn catheter should be cultured.

Perhaps the most frequent metabolic complications are those involving the infusion of glucose. As mentioned previously, the initiation of infusion should be in a stepwise fashion to allow the patient's insulin secretion to adjust to the increasing glucose load. Hyperglycemia and glycosuria may produce an osmotic diuresis leading to hyperosmolar, hyperglycemic, nonketotic dehydration. Exogenous insulin may be required in some patients—particularly patients with carbohydrate intolerance, sepsis or stress as well as patients receiving steroid therapy. Inadequate potassium may lead to significant glycosuria and this factor should be reviewed before insulin is administered. Hypoglycemia may occur with blockage of the catheter or other interruption of infusion. Should it be necessary to discontinue the hyperalimentation solution, infusion of isotonic 5–10% dextrose solution will prevent significant hypoglycemia. Another recently recognized complication of hyperalimentation has been fatty metamorphosis of the liver in patients receiving an exceptionally high calorie: nitrogen ratio. This complication may be managed by lowering this ratio to 50:1 or less or by cyclic hyperalimentation omitting hypertonic glucose solutions for short periods of time during the day.

Relatively few other complications are associated with infusion of protein. Patients may develop prerenal azotemia if excessive amino acids are infused. This may be corrected by decreasing the total dose of amino acids or by increasing the calorie:nitrogen ratio. Occasionally, in primary hepatic disorders or with the infusion of some crystalline amino acid solutions, hyperammonemia may result. The specific amino acids which may be deficient include arginine, ornithine, aspartic acid and glutamic acid. Hyperammonemia was more commonly associated with the no-longer utilized hydrolysate solution.

After several weeks of total parenteral nutrition, patients may develop deficiency states involving minerals, vitamins or essential fatty acids. It may be very difficult to distinguish between these several deficiency states and, indeed, multiple deficiencies may coexist. A careful review of the composition of the solutions infused will usually suggest the deficient component(s). Utilization of standard solutions has helped to minimize these difficulties. The potential for electrolyte and acid base imbalances is great; however, with frequent monitoring and careful record keeping such complications can usually be avoided.

Compatibility of additives and stability of alimentation solutions may also be significant problems. These are perhaps less well appreciated by clinicians and the participation of a cautious well-trained pharmacist is essential if these complications are to be avoided. Fortunately, the use of in-line filters will usually prevent serious complications, should precipitation of a solution occur during infusion. Indeed, perhaps the most serious complication is the inactivation of some vitamins and other additives should they be mixed in the same solution. Because of the relative paucity of published data regarding some of these complications, careful testing and monitoring by the pharmacist are necessary.

CONCLUSION

Despite the potential for complications, total parenteral hyperalimentation represents one of the most significant developments of our modern health care system. Under the direction of a knowledgeable, experienced team, the nutritional status and demands of individual patients may be evaluated and total parenteral nutrition instituted where indicated. With the utilization of modern techniques and careful monitoring, the risks are slight compared to the potential benefits. In addition, careful study of patients maintained on total parenteral nutrition have generated much additional knowledge and insight into general nutritional requirements as well as specialized requirements in certain disease states. With the increased use of total parenteral nutrition have come refinements in techniques, solutions and equipment which suggest an even greater promise in the future.

SELECTED REFERENCES

1. DUDRICK, S.J., WILMORE, D.W., VARS, H.M. and RHOADS, J.E.: Long-term Total Parenteral Nutrition with Growth, Development and Positive Nitrogen Balance. Surgery 64:134–143, 1968.
2. JEEJEEBHOY, K.N., ANDERSEN, J.H., SANDERSEN, I. and BRYAN, M.H.: Total Parenteral Nutrition: Nutrient Needs and Technical Tips. Modern Med. of Canada 29:21, No. 9-10, Sept.-Oct., 1974.
3. FLEMING, C.R., McGILL, D.B., HOFFMAN II, H.N., and NELSON, R.A.: Total Parenteral Nutrition. Mayo Clin. Proc. 51:187–199, 1976.
4. LAW, D.H.: Total Parenteral Nutrition. N. Engl. J. Med. 297:1104–1107, 1977.
5. ODA, D.M., IMBEMBO, A.L. and ZUIDEMA, T.D.: Total Parenteral Nutrition. Surgery 83:503–520, 1978.

6. BLACKBURN, G.L., BISTRIAN, B.R., MAINI, B.S., SCHLAMM, H.T., and SMITH, M.F.: Nutritional and Metabolic Assessment of the Hospitalized Patient. J. Parenteral and Enteral Nutr. 1:11–22, 1977.
7. DRISCOLL, R.H. and ROSENBERG, I.H.: Total Parenteral Nutrition in Inflammatory Bowel Disease. Medical Clinics of North America 62(1):185–202, 1978.

10

NUTRITION AND ORAL HEALTH

Thomas E. Grow, Ph.D.

Of the many diseases that affect man, certain disorders of the oral cavity are the most prevalent. These diseases are, of course, dental caries and periodontal disease (gum disease). Like many diseases, these have complex etiologies and may be mediated by a variety of factors, nutrition being among the most important. What is presented here is a brief summary of current thinking of the cause of these two diseases and a somewhat more detailed description of the nutritional aspects that may play important roles in the cause and prevention of these disorders.

Dental caries (tooth decay) typically begins with the dissolution of the mineral components of the enamel portion of the tooth. If allowed to progress, this process may lead to involvement of the dentin, infection of the pulp, and ultimately to the loss of tooth viability requiring endodontic therapy or extraction. The initiating process is the formation of a complex bacterial colony, called plaque, on the surfaces of the tooth. The normal metabolic reactions of certain plaque organisms, notably *Streptococcus mutans*, result in production of organic acids, e.g. lactic acid, which in turn lowers the pH of the plaque colony. The localized increased concentration of acid at the surface of the tooth is such that a pH as low as 4.5 may be reached. At this low pH hydroxyapatite, the major tooth mineral, dissolves resulting in the formation of an incipient carious lesion. If the plaque is removed these early lesions may remineralize. However, if the plaque is not removed or if the lesion is repeatedly exposed to new plaque formation, dental caries result. During the discussion of the nutritional aspects of the process, keep in mind the following points: (1) the bacteria must be present in the oral cavity and they must adhere to the

Dr. T.E. Grow, Department of Basic Dental Sciences, University of Florida College of Dentistry, Gainesville.

tooth surface; (2) these organisms must produce the organic acids necessary to lower the pH of the plaque colony; (3) the plaque colony is constantly bathed in saliva whose chemical composition may mediate adherence and acid formation; and (4) the chemical composition of the enamel may alter its susceptibility to dissolution by acid. Each of these factors can be modified by the nutritional status of the individual.

Both dental caries and periodontal diseases are conditions in which essentially 100% of the population are "at risk." It has been estimated that 94 million Americans have some form of periodontal disease while 32 million have advanced disease. In excess of 80% of tooth loss after the age of 35 has been attributed to this chronic, destructive disease process. Although there is still some disagreement, the consensus of opinion is that the major etiologic agent in periodontal diseases appears to be a variety of anaerobic microorganisms that exist in the subgingival plaque that develops between the teeth and gums. Species of the genera *Actinomyces, Bacteroides,* and *Fusobacterium*, among others, have been implicated in this disease. Other local irritants such as faulty restorations and traumatic tooth contact may also contribute significantly to the problem. The ultimate loss of the tooth in severe periodontal disease results from the loss of the supporting structures around the tooth, most notably the alveolar bone. Although the end products of the metabolism of the microorganisms may contribute to direct tissue damage, i.e. loss of epithelial attachment of the tooth, the major factor contributing to the destruction of both soft and hard tissue seems to be the host's own defense mechanisms. One explanation of bone loss is that the antigenic components on the surface of the invading bacteria stimulate previously sensitized lymphocytes to release proteins called lymphokines. One such lymphokine is osteoclast activating factor (OAF) which will, if present, activate the osteoclasts to resorb the alveolar bone. This is a localized phenomenon which may occur at a very specific site. It should be remembered that periodontal disease manifests itself in a variety of inflammatory responses. Destruction of tissues certainly occurs by other mechanisms such as release of collagenase enzymes by macrophages. The example of OAF is used to point out that host defensive mechanisms appear to play a vital role in this disease. Again during the discussion of the nutritional aspects of periodontal disease keep the following in mind: (1) bacterial plaque must form and remain in contact with the tissues; (2) the integrity of the epithelial attachment is important in maintaining periodontal health; (3) systemic factors may play a significant part in the severity of the disease process by affecting host defense and repair mechanisms; and (4) loss of alveolar bone and other supporting structures is the basis for the irreversible damage caused by periodontal disease.

For more detailed explanations of the problems of dental caries and periodontal disease, see Gibbons and van Houte,[1] Socransky,[2] and Nisengard.[3]

With this information as a basis for discussion, some current concepts on nutrition and oral health will be presented. The discussion will be divided into three major areas: nutrition and growth and development of the oral cavity; nutritional aspects of dental caries, and nutritional aspects of periodontal disease.

GROWTH AND DEVELOPMENT

The process of growth and development of the oral cavity is similar to that of any other organ. Winick and Noble have defined distinct growth phases based upon biochemical events taking place during each phase.[4] These are: (1) hyperplastic growth—a period in which the number of cells is increasing by the process of cell division; (2) hyperplastic and hypertrophic growth—a period in which both cell number and cell size are increasing; and (3) hypertrophic growth—a period in which net cell numbers remain constant while there is an increase in cell size. Stages 1 and 2 are characterized by net increases in the DNA content of the organ while stages 2 and 3 are periods in which a dramatic increase in the rate of protein synthesis is observed. It is apparent that the nutritional requirements of the organism will vary depending upon the stage of growth of the specific organ. Requirements for higher levels of folic acid (important in DNA and RNA precursor synthesis) might certainly be characteristic of phases 1 and 2 while excess essential amino acids would be required during growth phases 2 and 3.

It has been suggested that each developing structure undergoes certain "critical periods" during which nutritional stress or other stimuli may lead to irreversible changes or damage.[5] Nutritional deficiencies during stages of intense hyperplastic growth often lead to irreversible damage to the developing tissue. Nutritional stress after hyperplastic growth normally results in reversible change unless the deficiency state is very extreme or is maintained for long periods of time. In the oral cavity, the development of the teeth is especially characterized by these critical periods. Other oral structures such as alveolar bone, salivary glands, and oral epithelium also have critical periods during development and, as we will see, the normal growth of these tissues is vitally important in the maintenance of oral health in later life.

MATERNAL AND INFANT NUTRITION AND DEVELOPMENT OF TEETH

The development of the teeth takes place both in utero as well as after birth up until about age 18. Since much of the development takes place before birth the nutritional status of the mother is quite important. During development, two processes occur. First is the formation of a protein matrix model of the tooth or bone and, second, the mineralization of this matrix. In teeth, these processes are accomplished by the ameloblasts. The enamel mineral is deposited in stages such that temporary deficiencies or problems during mineralization may result in localized defects in the enamel. This is best illustrated by the fluorescent staining patterns found on teeth of children who were given tetracycline therapy during tooth formation. It is important to remember that once the teeth have erupted, changes in the nutritional status of the individual have very little effect upon the composition of the enamel. Most of the information we have at this time comes from animal studies since human experimentation in this area is not feasible.

Menaker and Navia have shown that if female rats are fed low protein diets during fetal development the offspring develop a variety of oral manifestations.[6] When compared to controls, the deficient offspring have smaller molars, delayed eruption of 1st and 2nd molars, and impaired salivary gland function. The offspring also have significantly increased susceptibility to caries. The authors attribute the changes to amino acid deficiencies during the critical periods of development of these structures. When young rats are fed fatty acid deficient diets during periods of tooth development, significant alterations in tooth morphology and ameloblast structure are also noted.[7,8]

Since tooth enamel is essentially hydroxyapatite ($Ca_{10} (PO_4)_6 (OH)_2$) it is not surprising that severe calcium or phosphate deficiency during critical periods of development has an effect on both tooth structure and caries resistance after eruption. Early studies by Gaunt and Irving indicate that calcium and phosphate deprivation leads to much greater effects on bone than on the incisors of rats.[9] The ratio of calcium and phosphate in the diet was also shown to be of importance. The ash content of incisors of deficient rats was only slightly lower (95% of controls) and was only mildly affected by the Ca:P ratio of the diet. Bone ash was significantly reduced in deficient animals (40% of controls) but bone appeared better able to adapt to a relative calcium deficiency (low Ca:P ratio). Further studies of Sobel *et al.*, and Stanton have suggested that variations in the Ca:P ratio in the diet of both test animals and humans may be of extreme importance in determining the caries resistance of teeth.[10,12] Sobel *et al.*, reported that animals raised on diets with high Ca:P ratios develop teeth with increased susceptibility to caries.[11] These authors suggest that the increased carbonate content of the teeth of the experimental animals leads to increased crystal defects which, in turn, render the enamel more labile to dissolution by acid. This effect is opposite to that of fluoride which is believed to increase the "crystallinity" of enamel apatite. Although the extreme Ca:P ratios used in animal studies are greater than those likely to be found in human diets, support for this idea comes from the studies of Stanton and Kreitzman who have shown that caries levels may be directly correlated to Ca:P ratios in the diet.[12,13] Interestingly, the correlation is much greater than that obtained when caries and carbohydrate intake are compared.

Although the mineral portion of teeth is composed mainly of compounds of calcium and phosphate, a number of other inorganic components have been identified and recent research has suggested that these minor components may play a major role in governing the caries resistance of teeth. It can be shown that the composition of the minor components of enamel reflects the mineral content of the intracellular fluid at the time of calcification. Once the tooth has erupted the trace mineral composition of the tooth may change depending upon the solubility of the particular component and its concentration in the diet. Many of these components affect the caries susceptibility of enamel by altering the organization and composition of the hydroxyapatite crystals within the enamel structure. Navia suggests that the following grouping of the minor mineral components of enamel can be made: (1) Cariostatic—F, P; (2) Mildly cariostatic—Mo, V, Cu, Sr, B, Li, Au; (3) Doubtful—Be, Co, Mn, Sn, Zn, Br, I; (4) No effect—Ba, Al, Ni, Fe, Pd, Ti; and (5) Caries promoting—Se, Mg, Cd, Pt, Pb, Si.[14] In later work Curzon and Losee, studying the caries rate in humans as compared with the trace element composition of extracted teeth, suggest the following: (1) F and Sr were found associated with low levels of caries; (2) Mg and Cu could be statistically correlated to high caries incidence; (3) Li, Be, Al, S, Ti, V, Cr, Fe, Co, Zn, Se, No, Mo, Zr, Sn, I, and Pb could not be correlated with either high or low caries incidence.[15] It is pointed out that these results do not preclude possible effects on caries by these elements in surface enamel, plaque, or bacterial metabolism.

Certainly, no trace element has received as much attention as has fluoride. Although a detailed discussion of fluoride is beyond the scope of this paper, a few basic facts regarding this important and often controversial element are presented for consideration. As early as the 1940's, it was evident from epidemiological data that there was a significant correlation between the fluoride content of drinking water and the incidence of dental caries in humans consuming that water. It was also known at that time that concentrations of fluoride greater than 2 or 3 ppm could be associated with randomly distributed, irregular white specks in the enamel, a condition known as mottling. In order to maximize the caries-protective nature of fluoride and to minimize the mottling problem, it was suggested that fluoride be either added or removed from the drinking water to attain a final concentration of 1 ppm. In 1945 residents of Grand Rapids, Michigan began to add fluoride to their drinking water. By the 1970's over 130 million people were drinking artificially fluoridated water where the fluoride content of drinking water is low. The American Dental Association recommends fluoride supplements for children at the following level: Up to two years of age—no specific recommendation, age two to three years—1.1 mg of NaF daily (0.5 mg F^-), over three years of age—2.2 mg NaF daily (1.0 mg F^-). Other groups have recommended 0.25 M.q.F^-supplements daily for the first two years and Glenn recommends 2.2 m.g.NaF once daily for the pregnant woman during the last two trimesters.[16]

Fluoride appears to be most effective in reducing dental caries if two conditions are met. First, fluoride must be present in the tissue fluids of children whose teeth are in the process of mineralization. Second, after eruption, fluoride must be present in the diet to prevent the loss of fluoride from the surface enamel. When fluoride is present during mineralization, some of the mineral crystals formed are fluoroapatite ($Ca_{10}(PO_4)_6F_2$). For reasons not yet fully understood fluoroapatite is resistant to dissolution by the acids of the plaque organisms.[17] Because the surface enamel is the region first exposed to caries producing conditions, the maintenance of high concentrations of fluoride in the surface enamel is important. The continual exposure of the tooth surface to fluoride in drinking water, fluoride containing toothpastes and mouthrinses, or topically applied fluoride is necessary to maintain the high fluoride content of the surface enamel.

The fluoridation of water has been opposed on three major grounds, namely, that it is not sufficiently effective to justify the cost, that there are doubts about its safety and effects of long term exposure, and that it interferes with the liberty of the public. The suggestions that there may be damaging effects is not made without grounds since fluoride has been known for years to be a potent inhibitor of many enzymes, especially those enzymes whose action depends upon metal cations such as magnesium.[18] As little as 10 ppm fluoride will inhibit the enzyme enolase by 45% and it has been suggested that the inhibition of bacterial metabolism is one mechanism by which fluoride may reduce caries. However, the concentration of fluoride in human tissue normally does not reach inhibitory levels of even most sensitive enzymes and studies of the overall health of individuals in communities consuming high levels of naturally occurring fluoride have shown no differences when compared to populations where fluoride is not present.[19] A small number of individuals, however, do seem to have an immediate unfavorable reaction to fluoridated water that resembles an allergic reaction by hypersensitivity.[20] The symptoms include rashes, tremors, diarrhea, stomatitis, visual disturbances, tinnitis, and mental depression. Whatever the minor risks are, the fact that fluoridation of water can reduce the caries rate by an average of 50% probably ranks water fluoridation as one of the more effective public health measures ever attempted.

Trace elements may play important roles other than protecting the tooth mineral itself. Recent studies by Iqbal *et al.* have shown that salivary gland activity in the developing rat was inhibited when the animals were given zinc deficient diets.[21] Alkaline phosphatase, an enzyme that may play an important role in the mineralization process, was inhibited and the gland weight was reduced to 70% of controls.

Because of the difficulties in raising offspring from vitamin deficient mothers, few animal experiments involving vitamin deficiency during growth and development have been done. Most experiments have involved vitamin deprivation after birth and observation of the structure of teeth that develop after a deficient state is achieved. No changes in the growth or structure of the teeth have been observed in developing animals maintained on diets deficient in vitamin K and apparently studies have not been reported involving vitamins other than A, C, D and E. Lady Mellanby demonstrated that both animals and humans that developed with vitamin D deficiency displayed a condition known as hypoplasia (thin, irregular enamel).[22,23] Although attempts to correlate enamel hypoplasia, rickets, and dental caries have been made, no conclusive evidence has been presented. When vitamin E is given in excess to developing rats it can be shown that the teeth developing during the exposure period are more susceptible to caries than in control animals.[24] Most studies involving vitamin C deficiency have been concerned with the collagen containing structures of the adult oral cavity. The only human observation reported was made by Boyle who examined the tooth germs in two fatal cases of infantile scurvy.[25] He found little changes in developing teeth and noted that the size, arrangement, and development of the various parts appeared quite normal. This is in contrast to changes in the soft tissues that occur during clinical scurvy.

Vitamin A deficiency in developing rats caused significant alteration in the structure of the third molars.[26] These teeth were poorly mineralized, had irregular dentine, showed irregular root formation, and degeneration of some of the odontoblasts (cells found within the tooth). These changes are similar to changes reported in the incisors of deficient adults (rat incisors are continually growing). Bloch described the macroscopic structure of the teeth of 64 human patients aged between eight and 12 who were severely vitamin A deficient.[27] Although some changes were noted, many could be attributed to vitamin D deficiency and it was concluded that no gross disturbance of the enamel organ had occurred in spite of the severe vitamin A deficiency.

In terms of growth and development, I believe it can be concluded that although animal experiments have clearly shown the importance of vitamins A, D, and C and minerals in the developmental process, the teeth appear to be less sensitive to changes that significantly affect other tissues. However, the minor changes that do occur may play an important role in oral health in later life.

DIET AND DENTAL CARIES

With the exception of the concentration of certain ions such as fluoride at the enamel surface, once teeth have erupted, the basic chemical composition does not significantly change. In the previous section, fluoride and other trace minerals were discussed and it was indicated that their continued presence in the diet may govern their actual concentration in different parts of the tooth. Aside from those considerations, the major effect of dietary components on the formation of dental caries probably involves the accumulation, maintenance, and metabolism of the acid producing organisms in the plaque. The one dietary substance most often associated with caries is sucrose. Sugar intake has been clearly implicated as the major dietary factor contributing to this disease in modern man.[28] Probably the most noted report was the Vipeholm study in which the sucrose intake and caries incidence of an institutional population were compared.[29] This study concluded that the total sucrose intake and the frequency of intake along with the retentive nature of the food were all factors associated with the caries incidence of these individuals. High caries rates could be correlated with "sticky," high sucrose containing, "between meal" snacks. Many animal studies have also supported this contention. When rats are fed diets with high levels of sucrose (30–70%) a high caries rate is observed when compared to controls.[30] However, recent studies by Huxley suggest that much lower levels of sucrose were equally as cariogenic and that raising the sucrose level above 15% did not increase caries.[31] Studies using *Streptococcus mutans* infected gnotobiotic rats have suggested even lower sucrose levels are still cariogenic.[32] In this study, maximal caries rates were obtained with 3% sucrose and even concentrations as low as 0.1% provided sufficient substrate for the accumulation of *S. mutans* plaque in monoinfected rats. It should be pointed out that the strain of *S. mutans* used was a highly cariogenic one.

Beside the clinical and animal studies, sucrose has been singled out for two reasons. First, in the presence of sucrose but not other sugars, *S. mutans* in vitro manufactures extracellular polysaccharides that allow the organism to accumulate on the tooth surface. Second, of a variety of sugars tested, sucrose is one of the most acidogenic. This is not to suggest that many other sugars do not lead to the production of acid by plaque of *S. mutans*, but the combination of accumulation and acid production fits well with the clinical and animal experimental data. Based on this type of information, the dental profession has eagerly embraced the idea that refined sugar is "the enemy" and has accepted the premise that a reduction in sucrose intake would lead to a reduction in dental caries. A number of investigators have been skeptical of this simplistic approach to what certainly is a complex problem. We have already seen that the trace mineral content of teeth may play a role in caries. Other factors appear equally important. Harris has shown that the caries challenge of high sucrose diets in rats can be completely overwhelmed by additions of sodium trimetaphosphate to the diet.[33] Stanton made the interesting observation that caries could be correlated to the Ca:P ratio in the diet regardless of the sucrose intake.[12] It has been suggested that sucrose may be important in caries only in diets deficient in phosphorous or with Ca:P ratio significantly different from 0.55.[13] Curiously, few clinical studies have been done to test whether or not a reduction in sucrose intake will lead to a reduction in the rate of formation of dental caries. Dental caries appears to be a problem of a complex nature with many factors of equal importance. One should consider all these factors before recommending anything as far reaching as a significant reduction in dietary carbohydrate.

As mentioned earlier, the physical consistency of the diet may play a role in dental caries formation. A variety of studies have been done and most have shown that the longer the food is retained, the more cariogenic it is. Stookey fed rats a diet which included presweetened cereal.[34] One group received the diet premoistened while the other group ate it dry. The caries incidence was measured after 104 days and the conclusion made that because the dry diet was retained longer it was more caries promoting.

Little work has been done to relate caries to vitamin intake. Studies have been done using vitamin B_6 supplements and suggest a reduced caries rate in both animals and humans receiving vitamin B_6.[35-37]

Whether dental caries is a problem that can be controlled by simply altering sucrose intake or whether it is a highly complex problem only aggravated by dietary sucrose remains to be seen. There are other factors not considered in this paper, i.e. the composition of saliva as it related to diet. These may be of greater importance than those mentioned. Under the circumstances, I would suggest careful consideration of the facts before specific recommendations are made.

DIET AND PERIODONTAL DISEASE

Probably the most controversial topic in the subject of oral health is the relationship of nutrition and periodontal disease. Although most investigators believe in a microbiological etiology for periodontal disease some researchers have suggested that it is essentially a nutritional problem with microbiologic involvement acting as a secondary factor. Rather than try to support one side or the other evidence is presented supporting both views; comment is included.

The effect of the consistency of food has been studied in relation to periodontal health. In some animal model systems, a firm, fibrous diet apparently helped prevent the accumulation of plaque and gingivitis when compared to a nutritionally equivalent soft diet.[38-40] Although this was true for dogs, ferrets, and cats, rodents developed more periodontal lesions on a hard granular diet.[41] Attempts to relate plaque removal by fibrous diets in man mave proven unsuccessful.[42] Although it has been suggested that hard diets promote keratinization of gingival tissues this has not been demonstrated in man. One possible beneficial effect is to promote salivary function which is known to play a role in both periodontal disease as well as caries.

Since the periodontium contains a number of important protein-based structures, it is not surprising that protein deficiency can lead to changes in periodontal health. Teeth are held in place by the collagenous periodontal ligament and the gingiva contains both collagen and keratin. When a variety of animals are subjected to protein or protein-calorie deficient diets, the effects on the periodontium are similar. In the presence of plaque, typical symptoms include gingival inflammation, loss of alveolar bone density, degeneration of the periodontal ligament, and increased periodontal pocket depth.[43-45] Studies of protein deficient human populations have also suggested the importance of protein in periodontal health. Indian children with severe protein deficiency showed more periodontal problems than did healthy children.[46] Cheraskin and Ringsdorf examined the effects of protein supplementation, local therapy, and a combination of both on periodontal health and reported that although each provided benefits, a combination of the two gave best results.[47-49]

Several vitamins have been examined for the possible effects of supplementation or deficiency on periodontal health. Although studies using rats have suggested significant alterations in epithelial integrity, bone structure, and periodontal pocket depth if the animals were fed vitamin A deficient diets,[50-52] human studies show little or no correlation between vitamin A deficiency or serum levels and the subject's periodontal status.[53,54] Deficiency of B complex vitamins has been studied and data similar to that for vitamin A have been obtained. Animal studies have demonstrated that deficiency of vitamin B complex causes changes in the gingiva, periodontal fibers, and alveolar bone.[55-57] Although in one survey urinary levels of thiamine and riboflavin could not be correlated to periodontal health,[53] in another, persons with clinical signs of B complex deficiency showed increased periodontal disease scores.[58] Vogel *et al.* have recently shown that folic acid supplementation reduces the flow of gingival exudate, an observation that suggests improvement in gingival health.[59]

Certainly no vitamins have received as much attention in recent years as have C and E. Their role in periodontal health has been a subject of controversy for a number of years with no solution in sight. In the case of vitamin C, deficient animal models have shown that even in the absence of local irritants certain clinical symptoms of periodontal disease develop.[60-62] The symptoms include tooth mobility, hemorrhage, and loss of periodontal fibers, symptoms not unexpected considering the alterations in collagen metabolism known to accompany vitamin C deficiency. Again, as in the case of vitamins A and B complex, human investigations have not been in agreement. Although attempts to correlate serum levels of vitamin C with the presence or severity of periodontal disease have generally failed,[53,63] supplementation of excess vitamin C may be beneficial to the maintenance of periodontal health.[64-67] However, this suggestion has been disputed by other studies.[68-70] Careful clinical studies are needed to better define this complex problem.

Vitamin E supplementation of human diets has shown some beneficial effect in patients with periodontal disease. When patients were given 800 mg of vitamin E daily for 21 days, there was an apparent reduction in the production of gingival exudate possibly due to a reduction in the prostaglandin-mediated inflammatory response.[71] However, using another group of subjects, when the serum vitamin E levels of both diseased and healthy individuals were measured significant differences between groups could not be determined.[72]

Aside from a recent report that iron deficiency increases the severity of periodontosis in rats,[73] most work concerning the minerals has been centered around the controversy involving calcium deficiency, osteoporosis, and periodontal disease. The observation that one effect of calcium deficiency is to create osteoporosis and that in periodontal disease the changes in alveolar bone in some resembled osteoporosis has led to the suggestion that alveolar osteoporosis induced by calcium defiency is the primary event in the development of the periodontal disease. This idea has been supported in experiments by Henrickson, Krook *et al.*, and Ericsson and Ekberg who have all shown that calcium deficiency in animals and humans leads to osteoporosis of alveolar bone and the development of certain symptoms characteristic of periodontal disease.[74-76] However, evidence that disputes this hypothesis has been reported. It has been shown that although calcium deficiency created osteoporosis in animals, no tooth loosening or gingivitis was observed in the absence of plaque.[77-79] This supports the evidence which points to local factors as the main cause of most periodontal disease.

The main body of evidence indicates that nutrition plays a modifying rather than an initiating role in periodontal diseases and that the maintenance of good nutritional status may alter both the susceptibility to, or severity of, periodontal disease.

CONCLUSIONS

The complexity of the relationship between oral health and nutrition is apparent from the data presented. Unfortunately until more research is carried out and some of the more controversial questions answered, only general statements regarding recommendations can be made. Based on the current state of understanding it can be suggested that nutrition plays a major modifying role in the etiologies of both dental caries and periodontal disease. Although apparently neither disease can be prevented nor cured by only dietary restrictions or supplementation, to ignore the nutritional considerations of these disease processes is a serious mistake. The role of nutrition in oral health is becoming increasingly evident and nutritional counseling should become part of the responsibility of the practicing dentist, as well as the practicing physician.

REFERENCES

1. GIBBONS, R.J. and VAN HOUTE, J. 1975. Ann. Rev. Med. *26*:121–136.
2. SOCRANSKY, S. 1977. J. Periodontol. *48*:497–504.
3. NISENGARD, R.J. 1977. J. Periodontol. *48*:505–516.
4. WINICK, M., and NOBLE, A. 1965. Develop. Biol. *12*:451–466.
5. MILLER, S.A. 1969. In Mammalian Protein Metabolism, Vol. III. (Munro, H.N., ed.) pp. 183–233, New York, Academic Press.
6. MENAKER, L., and NAVIA, J.M. 1973a. J. Dent. Res. *52*:680–687.
6. MENAKER, L., and NAVIA, J.M. 1973b. J. Dent. Res. *52*:688–691.
6. MENAKER, L., and NAVIA, J.M. 1973c. J. Dent. Res. *52*:692–697.
7. PROUT, R.E.S., and TRING, F.C. 1971. J. Dent. Res. *50*:1559.
8. PROUT, R.E.S., and TRING, F.C. 1973. J. Dent. Res. *52*:462.
9. GAUNT, W.E., and IRVING, J.T. 1940. J. Physiol. *99*:18.
10. SOBEL, A.E. and HANOK, A. 1958. J. Dent. Res. *37*:631.
11. SOBEL, A.E. and HANOK, A. 1960. J. Dent. Res. *39*:462.
12. STANTON, G. 1969. N.Y. State Dent. J. *35*:399–407.
13. KRITZMAN, S.N. 1976. Dent. Clin. of N.A., *20*:491–505.
14. NAVIA, J.M. 1972. Int. Dent. J. *22*:427–437.
15. CURZON, M.E.J. and LOSEE, F.L. 1978. FADA, *96*:819–822.
16. GLENN, F.B. 1977. J. Dent. Child. *44*:391–395.
17. BROWN, W.E., KÖNIG, K.G. (Eds) 1977. Caries Res., *11*:Suppl. I.

18. WISEMAN, A. 1970. In *Handbuch der experimentallen Pharmakolgie*, Springer-Verlag, Berlin.
19. McCLURE, F.J. 1970. In Water Fluoridation. The Search and the Victory. National Inst. of Dent. Res., Bethesda, Maryland.
20. GRIMBERGEN, G.W. 1974. Fluoride 7:146.
21. IQBAL, M., MEYER, J. and GERSON, S.J. 1977. J. Dent. Res. 56:Abstr. 243.
22. MELLANBY, M. 1929. Spec. Rep. Ser. Med. Res. Coun., London 140.
23. MELLANBY, M. 1936. Spec. Rep. Ser. Med. Res. Coun., London 140.
24. ALAM, S.W., ALAM, B.S., and ALVEREX, C.J. 1978. J. Dent. Res., *57*:244.
25. BOYLE, P.E. 1933. J. Dent. Res., *14*:172.
26. JENKINS, G.N. 1978. In the Physiology and Biochemistry of the Mouth, 4th ed., Blackwell Scientific Publications, Oxford.
27. BLOCH, C.E. 1930. Amer. J. Dis. Child., *42*:263.
28. ANDLAW, R.J. 1977. J. Hum. Nutr., *31*:45–52.
29. GUSTAFSSON, B.E., QUENSEL, C.E., LANKE, L.S., LUNDQVIST, C., GRAHNEN, H., BONON, B.E., and KRASSE, B. 1954. Acta Odont. Scand. *11*:232–364.
30. HUXLEY, H.G. 1971. N.Z. Dent. J. *67*:85–98.
31. HUXLEY, H.G. 1977. Caries Res. *11*:237–242.
32. MICHALEK, S.M., McGHEE, J.R., SHIOTA, T., and DENENYNS, D. 1977. Infect. Immun. *16*:712.
33. HARRIS, R.S., NIZEL, A.E., and WALSH, N.E. 1969. J. Dent. Res. *40*:290–294.
34. STOOKEY, G.K. 1978. J. Dent. Res. *57*:730.
35. HILLMAN, R.W., *et al.* 1962. Amer. J. Clin. Nutr. *10*:512.
36. STREAN, L.P., *et al.* 1958. N.Y. State Dent. J. *24*:133.
37. RINEHART, J.F. and GREENBERG, L.D. 1956. Amer. J. Clin. Nutr. *4*:318.
38. KRASSE, B. and BRILL, N. 1960. Odontol. Revy *11*:152.
39. KING, J.D. and GLOVER, R.E. 1945. J. Pathol. Bac. *57*:353.
40. EGELBERG, J.E. 1965. Odontol. Revy *16*:31–41.
41. PERSON, P. 1961. J. Periodontol. *32*:308.
42. SREENBY, L.M. 1972. Int. Dent. J. *22*:394–401.
43. RUBEN, M.P., McCOY, J., PERSON, P., and COHEN, D.W. 1962. Oral Surg. *15*:1061.
44. FRANDSEN, A.M., BECKS, H., NELSON, M.M., and EVANS, H.M. 1953. J. Periodontol. *24*:135.
45. BAVETTA, L.A., and BERNICK, S. 1956. Oral Surg., *9*:906.
46. PINDBORG, M.B. 1967. J. Periodontol. *38*:40/218.
47. CHERASKIN, E., and RINGSDORF, W.M.J. 1965. J. Oral Ther. Pharmacol., *1*:497.
48. CHERASKIN, E., and RINGSDORF, W.M.J. 1967. J. Periodontol., *38*: 227.
49. CHERASKIN, E., and RINGSDORF, W.M.J. 1969. J. Periodontol., *39*: 316.

50. FRANDSEN, A.M. 1963. Acta Odontol. Scand. *21*:19–34.
51. MELLANBY, H. 1941. J. Dent. Res. *20*:489–509.
52. GLICKMAN, I. and STOLLER, M. 1948. J. Dent. Res. *27*:758.
53. RUSSELL, A.L. 1963. J. Dent. Res. *42*:233.
54. RUSSELL, A.L., CONSOLAZIO, C.F. and WHITE, C.C. 1961. J. Dent. Res. *40*:604.
55. CHAPMAN, O.D. and HARRIS, A.E. 1941. J. Infect. Dis., *69*:7–17.
56. SHAW, J.H. and GRIFFITH 1962. J. Dent. Res. *41*:264.
57. TOPPING, N.H. and FRASER, H.F. 1939. Public Health Reports *54*: 416–443.
58. WAERHAUG, J.A. 1966. In World Workshop in Periodontics, p. 197.
59. VOGEL, R.I., FINK, R.A., SCHNEIDER, L.C., FRANK, O., and BAKER, H. 1976. J. Periodontol. *47*:667.
60. DREIZEN, S., LEVY, B.M., and BERNICK, S. 1969. J. Periodont. Res. *4*:274.
61. WAERHAUG, J.A. 1958. J. Periodontol. *29*:87.
62. MACKENZIE, I.C., KOLAR, G., KASHANI, H. and DAHLBERG, S. 1977. J. Dent. Res. *56*:Abstr. 237.
63. PARFITT, G.J. 1963. J. Periodontol. *34*:347.
64. EL-ASHRY, G.M., RINGSDORF, W.M., and CHERASKIN, E. 1964. Int. J. Vitamin Nutr. Res., *34*:202.
65. EL-ASHRY, G.M., RINGSDORF, W.M. and CHERASKIN, E. 1964. J. Periodontol. *35*:250.
66. CARVEL, R.L. and HALPERIN, V. 1961. Oral Surg., *14*:847.
67. CHERASKIN, E. 1975. In Diet, Nutrition and Periodontal Disease, American Society for Preventive Dentistry, Chicago.
68. COVEN, E.M. 1965. J. Periodontol., *36*:494.
69. KUSTNER, A.H. 1953. N.Y. State Dent. J. *19*:422.
70. O'LEARY, T.J. 1969. J. Periodontol. *40*:284.
71. GOODSON, J.M. and BOWLES, D. 1973. J. Dent. Res. *52*:217.
72. SLADE, E.W., BARTUSKA, D., ROSE, L.F. and COHEN, D.W. 1976. J. Periodontol. *47*:352.
73. MURPHY, N.C., SWEDLOW, D.B., and BISSADA, N.F. 1977. J. Dent. Res. *56*:Abst. 247.
74. HENRIKSON, P. 1968. Acta Odontol. Scand., Suppl. No. 50.
75. KROOK, L., WHALEN, J.P., LESSER, G.V., and LUTWAK, L. 1972. Cornell Vet. *62*:371–391.
76. ERICSSON, T., and EKBERG, O. 1975. J. Periodont. Res. *10*:256–260.
77. RASSMUSSEN, P. 1977. J. Periodont. Res. *12*:491–499.
78. SVANBERG, G., LINDHE, J., HUGOSON, A. and GRÖNDAHL, H.G. 1973. Scand. J. Dent. Res. *81*:155–162.
79. GLICKMAN, I. 1972. Clinical Periodontology. 4th ed. W.B. Saunders Co., Philadelphia.

11

NUTRITION AND CHILDHOOD DIABETES

John I. Malone, M.D.

The role of diet in the management of diabetes in children is usually presented in rather simplistic terms. The concept of balancing caloric intake against energy expenditure is presented in a manner suggesting that careful observation plus a pocket calculator will lead to success in this adventure.

This approach has been reasonably effective in the management of diabetes in adults.[1] A standard goal for this type of dietary management is maintaining "consistency in food intake from day to day." Implicit in this statement is maintenance of constant energy expenditure from day to day. Although something approaching consistency of energy expenditure may be approached in certain healthy compulsive young adults, this goal is physiologically impossible for vigorously growing, physically maturing children (see also Chapter 26).

The nutritional problems of childhood differ from those of adults. The nutrients must provide energy for physical activity. This varies on a daily basis that depends on school and social activities, TV programs and the weather. Energy expenditure varies with age during the first years of life as the child increases physical abilities and decreases the proportion of time spent sleeping.

Energy and nutritional requirements are also directly related to physical growth. Growth rate is not constant throughout childhood. The highest rate of increase occurs during the first two years of life with another spurt in adolescence. The age at which increased energy is required for

Dr. Malone is Professor, Department of Pediatrics, University of South Florida College of Medicine, Tampa, and Director, Suncoast Regional Diabetes Program.

the adolescent growth spurt is variable and occurs between 10 and 18 years of age. An indicator of sufficient caloric intake and utilization in a healthy child is the rate of growth and weight gain. However, at insufficient levels of energy intake a child may maintain normal growth rates by a reduction of physical activity as an adaptive mechanism. This dysfunction is more difficult to assess than growth failure.

Casual observations of normal nondiabetic children suggest that quantity and quality of intake vary widely from day to day. More objective quantitation of the dietary consumption of children confirms that impression.[2] Children provided the opportunity to self-select their diet demonstrated variable daily intake. Certain foods were consumed in excessive quantities while others were refused. The long term quality and quantity of food ingested, however, were appropriate. This suggests that constant day to day caloric intake may not be optimal for normal growth. It is more likely, however, that the individual child has an effective innate indicator of the quantity and quality of required calories. This indicator, by definition, is more physiologic than external calculated regulation of calories. The more compulsive meal planner would have to abandon his calculator and resort to a computer to consider all of the important variables regulating caloric need in children.

This is not to suggest that the growing child should not have his diet planned. The great attachment of children to television viewing and the coincident exposure to the highly desirable claims for high-calorie, low-quality food demands counter education and regulation of the eating habits of children. A problem of equal importance is the present practice of continual snacking which is encouraged by and while watching television. In short, food ingestion is a major activity unrelated to nutritional need in many families. The physiologic directors of eating habits are being overridden by social and commercial influences.

Coronary heart disease is a major cause of death in both the diabetic and nondiabetic population. Two factors firmly established as leading to an increased risk of coronary heart disease are hypertension and hypercholesterolemia.[3] There is much recent interest in the influence of childhood diets upon these factors.

Communities that have a high salt intake tend to have high average blood pressure.[4] Experimental evidence in rats indicates that animals have more hypertension in adult life if subjected to high sodium intake during infancy.[5] Although there is yet no direct evidence in humans that high salt intake predisposes to later hypertension, it seems logical to limit the use of salt in children at risk for hypertension. Children with diabetes are at an increased risk for both hypertension and coronary heart disease. Accordingly, these families are advised to avoid excess salt in their diet.

Hypercholesterolemia is also associated with increased risk for myocardial infarction. Hypercholesterolemia occurs in association with diabetes mellitus. A low cholesterol diet is the first step in correcting hypercholesterolemia.[6] This diet features avoidance of egg yolk, fatty meats and the use of skimmed milk (1% fat) and low cholesterol margarine. Early reports of using low cholesterol feedings to prevent hypercholesterolemia in infants with familial hypercholesterolemia suggest that it is beneficial.[7]

Long term benefits from such a diet have not been determined. Dietary planning to avoid hypercholesterolemia in children with diabetes, however, seems judicious at this time. Thus, dietary and nutritional counseling is appropriate for the well being of all children. It is of particular importance for children who have diabetes, a dysfunction in normal energy metabolism that prevents physiologic compensation for poor eating habits.

Since children with diabetes have the same energy requirements for normal growth and development as nondiabetic children, the preceding discussion should serve as a model for action. When calorie intake must be varied from day to day the best regulator is the child's appetite center. No defect has been demonstrated in this function in children with diabetes. Meal planning and supervision must be employed, however, to allow this center to function optimally without interference from the continuous external advice to consume food products for reasons other than physiologic need.

Specific guidelines helpful for families and their children with diabetes have been offered by Schmitt in the form of an "unmeasured diet" for children and adolescents with diabetes.[8]

A modified version of this plan is used in our clinic.

AN UNMEASURED DIET

Meals

Main Course

1. Meals should contain a variety of foods necessary to provide the nutritional requirements for normal growth and development. Information required for this can be provided by a nutritionist who may use the Exchange Lists for Meal Planning[9] as a guide. Major goals during the educational process are the utilization of a large variety of foods and avoiding the concept of "safe" and "bad" foods. It is possible to consume too much of any food. All food items

may be taken at appropriate times. Those foods with high sugar content while deficient in other nutritional value are only appropriate at times of high energy needs. Thus, they should only be used at times of unusual energy expenditure (physical exertion) or in the treatment of hypoglycemia.

2. The child should be allowed to decide the amount of food he eats. He should not be forced to finish a meal if he doesn't want all of it. However, skipping meals should not be allowed. One must also understand that some children manifest hypoglycemia by refusing to eat. Thus, some degree of food consumption during at least three meals and a bedtime snack is mandatory.
3. The food should be served or selected in standard restaurant size portions. When this has been consumed, seconds of similar size of any or all of the meal constituents may be taken. If the child continues to be hungry following seconds, a time delay of approximately 15 minutes should be employed before allowing thirds, etc. Food consumption beyond this, even in growing adolescents, is a bit unusual and should serve as an indicator of hypoglycemia and possible excessive insulin dosage.
4. The meals should be planned for approximately the same time each day and be the same for the entire family. The child with diabetes should not be served different foods at mealtime than other family members.

Snacks

1. Snacks are light meals taken between the three major meals of the day to prevent hypoglycemia. Routinely they should contain fewer calories than the major meals and be selected from one or two food groups.
2. Mid-afternoon snacks (4:00 p.m.) are common for most children and are usually required for children with diabetes. Bedtime snacks are important for most children, but many adolescents taking a single dose of intermediate acting insulin may not desire or need a bedtime snack.

   Mid-morning snacks are helpful for most preschool children but older children rarely need them.
3. Good snack foods are one or two of the following: low-fat milk, crackers, cheese, peanut butter, sandwich, fruit.
4. A snack is especially important before or directly after vigorous exercise. This may be an appropriate time for a concentrated sweet (i.e. sugar sweetened beverage, candy bar, etc.).

Sweets

1. Dessert foods are frequently the sweetest foods in the diet. If they are part of the family diet plan, they should be limited to one meal each day.
2. The helping size again should be conservative and no seconds are allowed.
3. Good dessert foods are: pudding, jello, fruit, ice milk.
4. Concentrated sugar, sweetened beverage, honey, candy and sugar should routinely be avoided. These are appropriate for treating hypoglycemia and during vigorous athletic events.

"Insulin Reactions"—Hypoglycemia

1. Children with diabetes should always have a quick source of glucose with them. Individually wrapped sugar cubes are ideal since they are less tempting for unrequired treats and less likely to become so gooey in the wrapper that they cannot be used in time of emergency.
2. If doubt exists about the occurrence of an insulin reaction—treat. Food is harmless, untreated insulin reactions are not.

Salt

1. The salt shaker should not be on the dining table.
2. Salt may be used in moderation for cooking, but extra salt is not to be added at the table.

Avoid Cholesterol

1. Use margarine instead of butter.
2. Use skim milk (1% Fat) instead of whole milk.
3. Trim your meat before eating it.
4. Three eggs per week maximum.

Obesity

1. The above rules apply only to young, growing, maturing individuals. When growth is complete, then limitations on amounts of food are appropriate.
2. The Exchange System of Meal Planning with greater emphasis upon calorie restriction is then appropriate.

Nutritional management is an important aspect in the care of children with diabetes. It should not be ignored or left up to the nondiscretion of the families involved. A greater degree of hypoglycemia occurs with unmanaged diets.[10] Undesirable and potentially dangerous hypoglycemia also occurs when unplanned nutrition results in inadequate calories. However, one must keep in mind while directing such activities that the appropriate quality and quantity of nutrients for growing, physically maturing individuals is quite variable. Both individual and daily changes make specific diet prescriptions too inflexible to be appropriate for the child with diabetes. The great importance of appropriate nutrition for the child with diabetes is a compelling reason for the medical management of these individuals to be controlled by those most knowledgeable of the normal growth, development and energy requirements of children—their pediatricians.

REFERENCES

1. DAVIDSON, J.K.: Controlling Diabetes Mellitus With Diet Therapy, Postgrad. Med. 59:114–112, 1976.
2. DAVIS, C.: Feeding After the First Year; in J. Brennemann (Ed): Practice of Pediatrics. Hagerstown, Md., W.F. Prior Co., Inc. 1957, Vol. 1, Chapter 30.
3. LEVY, R.I. and RIFKIND, B.M.: Diagnosis and Management of Hyperlipoproteinemia in Infants and Children, Am. J. Cardiol. 31:547, 1973.
4. BURMAN, D.: Nutrition in Early Childhood *in* Textbook of Pediatric Nutrition, Churchill Livingstone, London and New York, 1976, p. 46.
5. DAHL, L.K.: Salt and Hypertension, Am. J. Clin. Nutrition 25:231, 1972.
6. LEVY, R.I.; BONNELL, M., and ERNST, N.D.: Dietary Management of Hyperlipoproteinemia, J. Am. Diet. Asso. 58:406, 1971.
7. GLUECK, C.J.; HECKMAN, F.; SCHOENFELD, M., *et al.*: Neonatal Familial Type II Hyperlipoproteinemia: Cord Blood Cholesterol in 1,800 Births, Metabolism 20:597, 1971.
8. SCHMITT, B.D.: An Argument for the Unmeasured Diet in Juvenile Diabetes Mellitus, Clin. Ped. 14:68–73, 1975.
9. EXCHANGE LISTS FOR MEAL PLANNING: New York and Chicago: American Diabetes Association and American Dietetic Association, 1977.
10. KNOWLES, H.C. JR.; GUEST, G.M.; LAMPE, J., *et al.*: Course of Juvenile Diabetes Treated with Unmeasured Diet, Diabetes 14:239–273, 1965.

12

NUTRITION: JOINT RESPONSIBILITY OF AGRICULTURE AND MEDICINE

George K. Davis, Ph.D.

The need for good nutrition is given "lip service" by almost every lay or professional person but the ultimate responsibility for adequate nutrition and its role in maintaining human health can be said to rest squarely on the sister disciplines of agriculture and medicine.

The charge is often made that agriculturalists are too concerned with quantity production of food products with little concern for the effects of their products on health. Physicians, on the other hand, are often charged with ignoring the importance of nutrition, concentrating on treatment of disease conditions without concern for either the preventive or supportive roles of good nutrition practice.

As is often the case, the actual situation is quite different, for food producers are concerned about nutritional quality and physicians recognize the need for good nutrition, but there is great need for improved concern on the part of both agriculture and medicine. This discussion will suggest that agriculture and medicine are sister disciplines in maintaining human health. There are many ways in which they can and should support each other. Since nutrition is a discipline of great common interest, it is natural to examine areas where research and practice in agriculture and in medicine are jointly supportive.

Dr. Davis is Professor of Nutrition, I.F.A.S., University of Florida, Gainesville.

INTERACTION BETWEEN AGRICULTURE AND MEDICINE

Production of adequate food to meet energy and nutrient requirements of humans and animals has always been a basic responsibility of agriculture. We too often forget that famine is still the lot of many humans and it has only been in comparatively recent times that, at least in more developed countries, adequate food supplies could be assured. In a country such as the United States the availability of adequate food and a wide variety of foodstuffs in all seasons of the year has made it possible for physicians to take for granted that the nutritional needs of patients will be met, whether to prevent disease or to aid in the treatment of disease conditions.

The ethical considerations of research have inevitably meant the need for animal models in investigations that can contribute to knowledge applicable to humans. In turn, agriculturalists concerned with the nutrition of animals have uncovered information that has resulted in improved nutrition for humans.

Looking back it is easy to point out that solutions to many of the deficiency diseases have resulted from research carried out by agricultural scientists whose primary interest was in solving problems of animal nutrition. It can be demonstrated that knowledge of many of the vitamins, trace elements, amino acids and lipids and their functions resulted from research in agricultural research centers. But it is also true that transfer of this information to humans became and remains the responsibility of investigators and practitioners in the field of medicine.

Illustration is always better than generality and two recent examples can demonstrate the importance of the interaction between agriculture and medicine.

Agriculturalists and physicians have realized for years that vitamin D is necessary for good metabolism of calcium and phosphorus. This vitamin, which results from ultraviolet radiation of ergosterol or 7-dehydrocholesterol, has been regularly included in the diet of humans and animals or developed internally by exposure to sunlight or a source of ultraviolet light. Prior to 1968, the mechanism of vitamin D function was a matter of constant discussion among investigators. Conditions in humans and animals that did not respond to vitamin D were recognized and often given the appellation "idiopathic." Perhaps, in this way, we used a big word as a means of covering our ignorance.

But, since 1968, as a result of work at the experiment stations, especially Cornell and Wisconsin, a whole new explosion of knowledge about vitamin D, its biochemistry and its metabolism in the body has taken place. A team of workers at Wisconsin, under the direction of Dr. Hector F. DeLuca, demonstrated that vitamin D had to be modified within the body before it could function in its role in the absorption of calcium and phosphorus from the intestinal tract. Actually, it has been demonstrated that vitamin D, when it is absorbed, goes to the liver where an OH group is added in the 25 position. This product is then transported to the kidney where a second OH group is added in the 1-α position. It is this product, 1-α,25$(OH)_2D_3$, that is transported to the cells of the intestinal mucosa where a compound known as calcium binding protein (CaBP) is formed. The metabolite of vitamin D functions as a hormone to stimulate this formation. The CaBP then serves as a mechanism for the transport of the calcium across the membranes of the intestinal cell walls.

It should be pointed out that Dr. Robert H. Wasserman at Cornell and his colleagues had been actively investigating the formation of CaBP and had demonstrated its role in a number of species of animals. Consequently it was very convenient and natural that the investigations of these two groups of investigators at agricultural experiment stations should be correlated and confirmed by investigators at other agricultural experiment stations.

With the discovery that vitamin D functioned as a hormone after the formation of metabolites, it was but one step further to have this compound, the metabolite, synthesized and prepared for use in special medical problems. This is particularly true inasmuch as people with kidney failure often suffer from an inability to form the 1-α,25$(OH)_2D_3$ and, therefore, to form the CaBP needed for the absorption of calcium and phosphorus from the intestinal tract. It had been known that some individuals on dialysis for long periods of time suffered from a loss of calcium in the bones and were unable to replete this calcium. With the development of the information about the role of the kidney in the formation of the vitamin D metabolite it now is within the realm of possibility to correct this deficiency and, in fact, this has been carried out with good success experimentally. A quote from a statement released from the University of Wisconsin is pertinent: "The drug [1,25$(OH_2)D_3$] similar to a hormone has been tested on about ten patients in the United States and Canada and has succeeded in eliminating the crippling effects and severe pain that bone deterioration may bring in kidney patients.

"The drug will probably be useful to some extent to everyone who must use kidney machines to replace failed kidneys. It is estimated that there are about 100,000 such patients in the U.S. Only a few of them suffer from severe and sometimes fatal bone disease. Dr. DeLuca feels that it will be at least two years before all the safety testing will be done on the drug and it becomes available to physicians. Various forms of the drug are manufactured by Hoffman-LaRoche Company and the Upjohn Company."

While interest in the application to humans is, of course, primary for the physician, the agriculturalist also has an interest since the drug is strikingly effective in the prevention of milk fever disease in dairy cattle, reducing milk fever incidence from as high as 80% in a susceptible herd to less than 10%. Of special importance is the fact that the repeated doses can be given without danger to the animals.

The end of this research is far from apparent. Investigations in Argentina and collaborative work in the United States have demonstrated that a plant, *Solanum malacoxyln*, contains a compound which Dr. Wasserman at Cornell has shown to be 1-α,25(OH)D_3 glycoside. It had been known for many years that cattle and sheep and horses grazing in a large part of South America developed excess calcification of the cardiovascular system. With the investigations carried on by agricultural investigators it was possible to demonstrate that this calcification resulted from the animals consuming some of the plant which caused a rapid elevation of calcium and phosphorus in the blood. It has now been demonstrated that at least three genera of plants contain a compound that is either the same as the vitamin D metabolite or is easily converted to the metabilite in the digestive tract, with the result that abnormal amounts of calcium and phosphorus are absorbed. This results in metastatic calcification of the elastic tissues, especially those in the cardiovascular system. The question is raised as to whether or not there are other plants which may contain this substance or a similar substance that influences the absorption of calcium and phosphorus. It is apparent that, by avoiding the normal metabolism of vitamin D through introduction of the hormone form of vitamin D directly into the intestine, the homeostatic controls that are functioning within the normal individuals are bypassed and the absorption of calcium and phosphorus can be excessive with resulting development of disease.

There are good reasons to suspect that many plants, as yet to be investigated, may contain small amounts of the compounds that are now recognized as derivatives of vitamin D and, consequently, can influence the metabolism of calcium and phosphorus in animals and in humans. As long ago as 1947–1948, investigators at the Florida Agricultural Experiment Station were able to show that Florida milk naturally contains more vitamin D than milk from areas in Wisconsin and Minnesota. Since homeostatic controls would rule out the possibility that the additional sunshine to which dairy cattle are exposed in Florida might be the factor which caused this higher vitamin D in the milk, it was necessary to examine the forage that the cattle were consuming. It was shown that this forage did have unexpected vitamin D activity. Consequently, it was assumed that animals consuming this forage, therefore consuming excess vitamin D, were excreting some of this vitamin D in the milk. Now

30 years later, it would appear that much more fundamental differences may exist between the types of forage growing in subtropical areas such as Florida and those commonly produced in more northern latitudes.

The study of the nutrient requirements for trace elements has been a particularly effective one for interaction between agriculture and medicine. The role of iodine in thyroid function, the need for iron and the interaction of iron and copper in hemoglobin formation, the role of cobalt as a part of vitamin B_{12} and its relationship to pernicious anemia are just a few examples of human health benefits from the research and interaction between agriculture and medicine.

When Dr. W.D. Salmon and his colleagues at Auburn, Alabama reported in 1955 that zinc was a key to prevention and cure of parakeratosis in swine, it came as a shock to investigators in animal nutrition who had been convinced that a zinc deficiency was a remote possibility in animal feeding. Once it was demonstrated that zinc played such an important role, numerous investigators found that zinc deficiency was a frequent problem in other classes of livestock as well as swine. It was not long before zinc and its role in human nutrition was attracting the interest of physicians and research investigators concerned with human health. In 1961 zinc deficiency was suspected in humans and by 1963 it had been demonstrated.

The close resemblance between zinc deficiency in animals and in humans suggested that many of the same biochemical reactions occur in both animals and humans and this encouraged application of information developed with animal models to human problems.

When a conference on zinc metabolism was held at Wayne State University (proceedings published in 1966), zinc was being examined as a factor in human endocrine abnormalities, in bone metabolism and in myocardial metabolism, with strong indications that zinc influenced biochemical reactions in all of these areas.

The reports and discussions taking place at the Western Hemisphere Nutrition Congress V in 1977 emphasized that zinc is a factor in taste acuity and, therefore, appetite, in normal development of children, in wound healing, in skin dermatoses and, perhaps, in many other metabolic functions. Truly the agriculture research into a problem affecting livestock has provided another step forward in our knowledge of the role of proper nutrition in the prevention of disease and maintenance of health.

JOINT RESPONSIBILITY

Perhaps these two examples emphasize the joint responsibility that rests on agricultural scientists and the medical profession. They may also emphasize the need for better communication and collaboration between the disciplines of agriculture and medicine and between the scientists and the general public.

The close working relationship existing between agriculture and the health professions at the University of Florida, located on the same campus, provides an unusually valuable situation where interchange of ideas and research results and collaborative research stimulates and accelerates the development of answers to problems of both areas. In the areas of nutrition, physiology, neurology, biochemistry and gastroenterology to name a few, major advances are being made through collaboration between the disciplines in agriculture and the health sciences.

Investigators and practitioners in agriculture and medicine have one great principle in common which is that we still have many unknowns influencing production and human health. Fortunately, the basic investigations carried on by interdisciplinary teams can go a long way toward obtaining solutions to each other's problems.

It is good for all of us to examine the relationship between agriculture and medicine for not only is agriculture concerned with the production of adequate amounts of nutritious food but there is a tremendous research effort being expended to solve the basic problems that may eventually enable the practicing physician to better perform his task of keeping people healthy. The research also enables the practicing agriculturalist to provide the products that meet human and animal nutrition needs. Hopefully, good nutrition can be provided to all of our people and not only prevent many health problems from developing but assist in the treatment of diseases that arise from other causes.

REFERENCES

1. DeLUCA, H.F.; CHAN, J.C.M., OLDHAM, S.B., and HOLLICK, M.F.: 1-α-hydroxy Vitamin D_3 in Chronic Renal Failure. A Potent Analogue of the Kidney Hormone, 1,25-dihydroxycholecalciferol, JAMA 234: 47–52, 1975.
2. NUTRITION IN TRANSITION. Proceedings, Western Hemisphere Nutrition Congress V. AMA. Monroe, Wisconsin, 1978.
3. TUCKER, H.F., and SALMON, W.D.: Parakeratosis of Zinc Deficiency Disease in the Pig. Proc. Soc. Exptl. Biol. Med. 88:613, 1955.
4. WASSERMAN, R.H., and TAYLOR, A.N.: Evidence for a Vitamin D_3-Induced Calcium-Binding Protein in New World Primates, Proc. Soc. Exptl. Biol. Med. 136:25–28, 1971.
5. WASSERMAN, R.H.; HENION, J.D.; HAUSSLER, M.R., and McCAIN, T.A.: Evidence That a Calcinogenic Factor in Solanum malacoxylon is 1,25-dihydroxy Vitamin D^3 Glycoside, Science 194:853–855, 1976.
6. ZINC METABOLISM, Anada S. Prasad, ed., Charles G. Thomas, Springfield, Illinois, 1966.

13

MEETING RECOMMENDED DIETARY ALLOWANCES

Alfred E. Harper, Ph.D.

Recommended Dietary Allowances (RDA) are the best known and most widely used nutrition standards in the United States. They are established by the Food and Nutrition Board (FNB) of the National Academy of Sciences/National Research Council (NAS/NRC) as guidelines for assessing the adequacy of intakes of essential nutrients. Such standards are needed for evaluating the nutritional adequacy of diets both for maintenance of health and for treatment of disease. They are needed as guides for recommendations for modification of the diets of persons who may be at risk of nutritional inadequacy owing to inappropriate food selection. They serve as the basis for recommendations for modification of the national food supply when some type of nutritional inadequacy is identified as a public health problem.

WHAT ARE RECOMMENDED DIETARY ALLOWANCES?

Recommended dietary allowances are defined as amounts of essential nutrients that will meet the known physiological needs of essentially all healthy persons. They are amounts that, if consumed daily by each person in a population, should meet the needs of all, or at least almost all. They are recommendations for population groups, and are, therefore, set high enough to cover the needs of those with the highest requirements.

Dr. Harper is E.V. McCollum Professor of Nutritional Sciences, Departments of Nutritional Sciences and Biochemistry, University of Wisconsin-Madison, Madison, Wisconsin.

The RDA are not "recommended" intakes in the sense that they are guidelines for the most appropriate intake of each essential nutrient. They are not "ideal" intakes of nutrients. The most appropriate intake of a nutrient depends on many factors; it can vary with the individual and can differ from time to time. The concept of an "ideal" nutrient intake or diet is a theoretical concept; it can be defined only by those who profess to have absolute knowledge. The RDA are recommendations for desirable lower limits of intake for population groups. They represent adequate or satisfactory intakes of essential nutrients for healthy people. They are not recommendations for therapeutic management of those who are ill.

The RDA are based on the available scientific knowledge of human requirements for nutrients, on information about the way requirements change with age and physiological state, upon knowledge of factors that influence the utilization of nutrients after they have been consumed, and upon information about variability among individuals in their requirements for nutrients. Since the RDA are designed to meet the needs of those with the highest requirements, they cannot be equated with average requirements. They exceed the needs of most people. The RDA do not take into account losses of nutrients that may occur during food preparation. They are not amounts of nutrients that should be present in the food supply but, rather, are the amounts that should be consumed.

RDA FOR ENERGY

It is important in discussing RDA to recognize at the outset that allowances for energy, i.e. for calories, are based on a different concept than that used for establishing allowances for the various essential nutrients. The RDA for energy are estimates of the requirements of persons with average energy expenditure in each age-sex group for which recommendations are made. If energy allowances were designed to cover needs of those with the highest requirements, they would be recommendations for obesity for most people. Energy requirements of individuals vary widely, depending upon body size, age and physical activity. However, since the amount of food a person consumes is ordinarily controlled well by the body to balance energy expenditure, there is little need to be concerned about meeting these needs in a population with an adequate supply of palatable food. Of much greater concern is the tendency for a substantial number of people to consume more calories than they need. The energy allowances are based on the average requirement for resting metabolism plus an additional allowance for the average amount of physical activity for each age group. They are, thus, reasonable guides for the energy needs of large groups of people, since about half will have energy requirements above the average and about half below.

There are conditions in which meeting energy needs deserves special consideration. The energy needs of the elderly are low because both basal metabolic rate and physical activity decline with age. Energy expenditure is also low whenever physical activity is restricted as the result of chronic illness or physical disability. When energy needs are low, probably on the order of 1500 kcal/day, it becomes increasingly difficult to meet the needs for essential nutrients from the amounts of foods needed to meet caloric needs. It is important for those with low energy requirements to select foods that are rich in essential nutrients and to limit the amounts of those that provide mainly calories, such as highly refined starches, sugars, oils, fats and alcohol. This is also important for those who are restricting food intake in an effort to lose weight.

RDA AND FOOD LABELS

Before discussing the RDA for essential nutrients, it is necessary to distinguish clearly between the NAS/NRC RDA, which are used as nutritional standards, and the U.S. RDA which have been established by the Food and Drug Administration (FDA) for regulatory purposes and for nutritional labeling. The NAS/NRC RDA, with which we are concerned here, are established for a wide range of age groups from infancy through adulthood. They take into account differences in body weight, sex and physiological state. They can be used as guides for the amounts of nutrients needed by groups who differ greatly in age or size. The U.S. RDA of the FDA, on the other hand, are a single set of values based usually on the highest NAS/NRC RDA, that for adult man. These serve as guides for comparing the nutrient content of different food products. They are not adjusted for differences in age and physiologic state so cannot be used as guides to nutritional needs, except for physically mature men. They greatly exceed the needs for the younger and smaller members of a family or population.

PROCEDURE FOR ESTABLISHING RDA

The starting point for establishing RDA is the available information about human requirements for essential nutrients. There have been relatively few studies in which human subjects have been fed diets that contain inadequate quantities of specific nutrients for long enough periods of time to establish the amount that will just prevent the development of deficiency signs. There have, however, been a larger number of studies in which the amount of a nutrient that is required to prevent a fall in the concentration of the nutrient in blood or losses from the body has been determined.

The balance procedure has been used extensively for estimating the requirements of adults for protein and for minerals. All of the nitrogen from dietary protein is excreted, primarily in urine and feces. This is also true of mineral elements that are essential nutrients. Measurements of the minimum amount of such nutrients that must be consumed to just balance the amounts lost from the body while body weight remains constant provide estimates of the minimum requirements of these nutrients for maintenance. Some additional amount over the urine and fecal losses must be added to this to compensate for the amounts lost in sweat, sloughed skin, hair and other body excretions and secretions. This procedure has been used to estimate the average protein requirement of adults of about half a gram of high quality protein/kg body weight/day.

Most of the vitamins are degraded to end products that are not readily measurable, therefore, techniques other than the balance procedure must be used to estimate requirements for this group of nutrients. For several of the vitamins, human volunteers have consumed diets containing inadequate amounts of the vitamin until signs of a specific deficiency disease began to develop. The amount of vitamin A and of several of the B-vitamins required to prevent such specific diseases has been determined in this way. For some of the B-vitamins, a readily identifiable metabolic end product or the vitamin itself is excreted in the urine. The concentration of the vitamin or its metabolites in the urine usually remains low until the requirement has been met. When the requirement is exceeded, urinary excretion then rises sharply. This method has been used to establish requirements for thiamin, riboflavin and niacin.

For some nutrients, it is possible to estimate the requirement from measurement in human subjects of changes in the blood concentration or in a metabolic function for which the nutrient is required. Vitamin E, for example, is required to maintain the integrity of the membrane of the erythrocyte. In fact, vitamin E status can be assessed by examining the resistance of erythrocytes to hemolysis in standard laboratory tests. In a study in which men consumed a diet almost devoid of vitamin E for many months, a clear-cut deficiency disease did not develop but eventually the red blood cells showed increased susceptibility to hemolysis and the blood concentration of the vitamin fell. It was difficult to establish the requirement for the vitamin accurately in this study. However, from the information obtained and from knowledge that the requirement cannot exceed the lowest amount of the vitamin found in diets that will prevent such changes an average requirement for vitamin E could be estimated. It would appear not to exceed 7–9 mg/day for adults.

For vitamin C, it has been possible, through studies in which a small amount of isotopically-labelled vitamin C has been consumed by human volunteers, to determine with a high degree of confidence the rate at which the vitamin is lost from the body. In such experiments, it has also been possible to determine how much of the vitamin is retained in the body in relation to the amount consumed. In studies of this type, it was established that only 10 mg of vitamin C was required to prevent signs of scurvy from developing. It was also established that with an intake of just over 30 mg of vitamin C per day, adult men would retain the vitamin until their bodies contained about a gram of ascorbic acid. This was enough to ensure maintenance of health for at least 40 days even if they consumed diets that provided no ascorbic acid. Where the requirement lies in this case between 10 mg and 30 mg/day is a matter of judgment as to how large the body pool of ascorbic acid should be to ensure maintenance of health.

ADDITIONAL FACTORS THAT MUST BE CONSIDERED IN ESTABLISHING REQUIREMENTS

Infants and children who are growing rapidly require more food and more nutrients per unit of body weight than adults. As experiments of the type that have been done on adults might impair development of the child, estimates of requirements for growth must be made using indirect methods. Guidelines for requirements for infants can be obtained from measurements of the amount of milk or formula consumed by infants who are growing satisfactorily and from knowledge of the composition of the milk or formula. The amounts of specific nutrients they are consuming can then be calculated. Although this procedure does not provide values for minimum nutrient requirements, it does set an upper limit for requirements.

For intermediate age groups, for the most part, there have been so few experiments that it is necessary to calculate, from knowledge of growth rates and body composition, how much of a nutrient accumulates in the body during growth and to estimate from such calculations the requirements at different ages. This type of approach is also used to estimate the additional requirements for reproduction and lactation. The amounts of nutrients accumulating in the fetus and in the mother's tissues can be estimated from knowledge of weight gain and body composition. The amounts of nutrient secreted in milk can also be calculated to estimate the additional requirements during lactation. When this procedure is used, the value obtained is adjusted for inefficient utilization of the ingested nutrients on the basis of measurements made on adults.

Nutrient requirements for men and women are essentially the same if they are expressed per unit of body weight. The one exception is the requirement for iron which is higher for women of child-bearing age because of the extra amount of iron they lose during menstruation.

Several factors influence requirements. For some nutrients, mainly the mineral elements, the efficiency with which they are absorbed from the intestine must be considered. Average values for iron absorption are estimated to be only about 10%, therefore, even though body losses of iron by men are only about 1 mg/day, their requirement for iron is about 10 mg/day.

There are precursors of some nutrients in foods. Tryptophan, for example, is a precursor of niacin in the body. The amount of niacin needed thus depends on the amount of tryptophan consumed as about 1 mg of niacin is formed for each 60 mg of tryptophan ingested. The contribution of precursors must also be considered in estimating vitamin A requirements since several carotenoids, the orange pigments in many vegetables and fruits, are precursors of vitamin A. For vitamin E, for which there are several naturally occurring forms that differ in their biological activity, the requirement will depend upon the relative proportions of each in the diet.

Finally, the efficiency of utilization of proteins depends upon their amino acid composition. The requirement for protein thus depends upon how efficiently the dietary protein is utilized by the body. In the United States, the quantity of protein consumed is high and the mixture of proteins in the diet is usually of good quality so low efficiency of utilization is not a serious concern. However, if much of the dietary protein is derived from cereal grains, the quantity of protein required to meet the requirement is much greater than it is with diets that contain a large proportion of animal protein.

CONVERTING REQUIREMENTS TO ALLOWANCES

The requirements of about half the people in a population would be expected to exceed the average. As those who have low requirements cannot be distinguished from those who have high requirements without elaborate metabolic studies, a statistical approach is used in order to convert average requirements to RDA, intakes of nutrients that should cover the needs of those with the highest requirements. To do this, it is necessary to know how much requirements vary from individual to individual.

Although there is not enough information to permit calculations of individual variability to be done for all nutrient requirements, enough values have been obtained for several of the requirements to permit calculation of the standard deviation of the average. Since nutrient requirements that have been studied most extensively appear to follow a statistically normal distribution, the average plus twice the standard deviation should include the requirements of all but the 2.5% of the population who have the highest requirements. As estimates of average requirements and adjustments for factors that influence requirements, such as efficiency of utilization of the nutrient, efficiency of absorption and the presence in the diet of precursors of the nutrient, tend to be on the generous side, it is unlikely that many people have requirements higher than two standard deviations above the average. In establishing the RDA, then, the average requirement is increased by an amount equivalent to twice the standard deviation. For nutrients for which enough information about individual requirements is not available, it is assumed that the degree of variability does not differ greatly from nutrient to nutrient. The standard deviation expressed as a percent of the average is the coefficient of variability. This does not usually exceed 15% for requirements for which an adequate number of individual values are available. Therefore, for nutrients for which insufficient information is available, the average requirement is increased by 30% or twice the coefficient of variation in estimating the RDA.

Table 13.1 gives figures for the RDA for young children and for adults. After the various adjustments have been made, the average requirement of 0.5 gm of protein/kg of body weight/day for adults has been increased to 0.8 gm/kg of body weight/day for the RDA. The average requirement for vitamin C falls between 10 and 30 mg/day for adults but the RDA has been set at 60 mg/day in order to assure that there will be enough of this vitamin in the body to provide a store that will last about 60 days even if no ascorbic acid is consumed. For vitamin E, although the average requirement was estimated to be less than 8 mg/day, the RDA is set at 10 mg/day in order to provide an adequate margin of safety. The relationships between the average requirements and the RDA for other nutrients are similar to these.

APPROPRIATE USES OF THE RDA

The two major uses of the RDA are as nutrition standards for: (1) planning food supplies for population groups such as the inmates of institutions or patients in hospitals, and (2) assessing the nutritional adequacy of diets from knowledge of food composition and food intake.

The original use of the RDA was as guides for the planning and procurement of food supplies by the armed services. They are now used by a variety of public and private organizations concerned with the feeding of

TABLE 13.1. RECOMMENDED DIETARY ALLOWANCES (1980)

	Children (1–3 years) (13 kg)	Adults (23–50 years) Male (70 kg)	Female (56 kg)
Energy (kcal)	1300	2400	2000
Protein (gm)	23	56	44
Vitamin A (μgRE)	400	1000	800
Vitamin D (μg)	10	5	5
Vitamin E (mgα-TE)	5	10	8
Vitamin C (mg)	45	60	60
Thiamin (mg)	0.7	1.4	1.0
Riboflavin (mg)	0.8	1.6	1.2
Niacin (mgNE)	9	18	13
Vitamin B_6 (mg)	0.9	2.2	2.0
Folacin (μg)	100	400	400
Vitamin B_{12} (μg)	2	3	3
Calcium (mg)	800	800	800
Phosphorus (mg)	800	800	800
Magnesium (mg)	150	350	300
Iron (mg)	15	10	18
Zinc (mg)	10	15	15
Iodine (μg)	70	150	150
Vitamin K (μg)	20	100	100
Biotin (μg)	65	150	150
Pantothenic acid (mg)	3	5	5
Sodium (mg)	600	2000	2000
Potassium (mg)	1000	3000	3000
Chloride (mg)	1000	3500	3500
Copper (mg)	1.5	2.5	2.5
Manganese (mg)	1.2	3.5	3.5
Fluoride (mg)	1	3	3
Chromium (mg)	0.05	0.1	0.1
Selenium (mg)	0.05	0.1	0.1
Molybdenum (mg)	0.07	0.3	0.3

large groups of people. When the RDA are used as guidelines for planning diets, it is important to recognize that diets are composed of foods, not nutrients. A diet will not be consumed in an amount sufficient to provide the required amounts of essential nutrients unless it is composed of a selection of palatable and acceptable foods that provide psychological and social satisfaction. Only after an acceptable diet has been planned should the RDA be used as a yardstick to assess the nutritional value of the diet and to serve as a guide for making adjustments to ensure that it is of high nutritional quality.

Also, it should be emphasized that, although the dietary standards are termed "recommended" allowances, this term should be equated with "acceptable intakes of nutrients" rather than with the idea of recommended intakes. The RDA are guidelines to the lower limit of adequacy. They should not be used to justify restricting intakes of nutrients to this limit. The objective in diet planning should not be to provide amounts of nutrients that just meet the RDA. Nutrients are not distributed evenly among foods and in order to ensure nutritional adequacy, the diet should be composed of as wide a variety of foods as is possible. When this is done, and the diet has been selected to ensure palatability, some nutrients are bound to be in excess of the RDA. It is well nigh impossible to devise a palatable diet that meets the needs of several of the essential nutrients without exceeding the RDA for protein.

The other major use of the RDA is as a standard for evaluating food consumption records in an effort to assess the probability of nutritional inadequacy occurring in a population. This is an appropriate use of the RDA but great caution must be exercised in drawing conclusions about nutritional status from comparisons of nutrient intakes with the RDA.

One conclusion that can be drawn with confidence from such comparisons is that the probability of nutritional inadequacy is negligible in persons who consume amounts of nutrients equal to or in excess of the RDA. Since the RDA exceed the requirements of most people, consumption of a diet that provides less than the RDA for an essential nutrient cannot be taken as evidence that the diet is nutritionally inadequate. All that can be concluded is that the farther the intake falls below the RDA, the greater is the probability of nutritional inadequacy. Reliable information about the nutritional status of persons whose nutrient intakes are less than the RDA can be obtained only through clinical and biochemical evaluations.

The most serious misuse of the RDA as dietary standards is to assume that the nutritional status of an individual can be evaluated from food intake records alone. They can, nevertheless, help to identify potential dietary problems and to identify problems that have been detected during clinical and biochemical evaluations. This points up a major limitation of dietary standards, such as the RDA; they do not provide guidelines for establishing the point at which a diet becomes inadequate. However, this should not be considered an inadequacy of the RDA. It is not possible to do this with any type of dietary standard. It could be done only if the nutritional requirements of all people were the same.

In evaluating nutrient intakes of populations, similar problems are encountered. If the average intake of a population exceeds the RDA, this does not provide assurance that all members of the population have adequate nutrient intakes. This is the situation in the United States, for example, where the national food supply provides quantities of nutrients other than iron well in excess of the RDA. Despite this, some people have inadequate diets as the result of illness, alcoholism, neglect, ignorance, poverty, or social disintegration within the family. Since only a small percentage of people are found to show evidence of even marginal nutritional inadequacy, mainly as the result of low iron intake, it is evident that nutritional inadequacy is not the result of an inadequate food supply.

The only appropriate conclusions that can be drawn from comparisions of nutrient intakes of populations with the RDA are: (1) the farther the average intake is above the RDA, the less likelihood there is of nutritional inadequacy within the population; and (2) the farther the average intake falls below the RDA, the greater is the likelihood of nutritional inadequacy within the population.

Most of the other uses of the RDA are outgrowths of one or the other of these two primary uses. All of the precautions that must be kept in mind when the RDA are used for planning food supplies or evaluating diets must also be considered when the RDA are used as standards for nutritional labelling, as guides for establishing standards for public assistance or as the basis for regulatory standards for the nutritional quality of foods. The RDA have limitations as nutritional standards. They do not provide guidelines for establishing accurately the point at which diets become inadequate. They do not enable us to make definitive statements about nutritional status of individuals who consume less than the RDA. Nevertheless, they do provide guidelines for ensuring that diets are nutritionally adequate and they do make it possible to identify potential nutritional problems through comparisons between food supplies and the standards. The limitations of the RDA should not be exaggerated. They are the limitations of any nutritional standard.

BIBLIOGRAPHY

BEATON, G.H.: The Use of Nutritional Requirements and Allowances, West Hemis. Nutr. Congress III, pp. 356–363, 1972.

CALLOWAY, D.H.: Human Nutrient Requirements-An Update, Proc. West. Hemis. Nutr. Congress IV, pp. 195–203, 1975.

FOOD AND NUTRITION BOARD. Recommended Dietary Allowances: Revised, 9th Edition. Washington, D.C.: NAS/NRC, 1980.

HARPER, A.E.: Those Pesky RDAs, Nutrition Today 9:15–28, 1974.

HARPER, A.E.: Recommended Dietary Allowances: Are They What We Think They Are? J. Am. Diet. Assoc. 64:151–156, 1974.

HEGSTED, D.M.: Dietary Standards, J. Am. Diet. Assoc. 66:13–21, 1975.

14

DRUG–DIET INTERACTIONS

Myron Brin, Ph.D., and Daphne Roe, M.D.

We live in a chemical world. From the beginning of time this chemical environment was either the source or result of life itself. Therefore our environment contained ozone, carbon monoxide, nitrosamines, etc., long before the industrial era.

Since living matter is composed of carbon, hydrogen, oxygen and mineral elements in organic as well as inorganic forms, these also define the nature of the nutrients. Foods must be digested into their basic components in order for an organism to utilize them metabolically for the building and repair of tissue and to reproduce its kind.

But man does not eat chemical elements, he eats food. However, not only are there nutrients in that food but also other components which comprise exposure to a non-nutritive chemical environment. Among these are safrole, pesticides, herbicides, indoles, organic peroxides, flavones, etc. Although non-nutritive, these materials affect drug metabolism, but since they are food they might also be considered nutritional influences on drug metabolism. How confusing!

More recently, as the industrial era developed there accumulated in the environment certain residues of chemical development such as DDT and other halogenated hydrocarbon insecticides, urea herbicides, polychlorinated biphenols, heavy metals, etc., to which we are exposed inadvertently in our physical as well as in our food environment. Accordingly, it may be somewhat difficult to differentiate between the nutritive and the non-nutritive influences which are carried by foods on drug metabolism.

What we propose to do in this paper is to describe the effects of various nutrients in our diet on drug metabolism, and then to describe the effects

Dr. M. Brin is in the Department of Clinical Nutrition, Roche Research Center, Hoffmann-La Roche Inc., Nutley, N.J.; Dr. D. Roe is Professor, Division of Nutritional Sciences, Savage Hall, Cornell University, Ithaca, N.Y.

of drug use on nutrient needs. The material presented here should be considered a compressed overview of the available information in view of the fact that the study of drug metabolism is in itself a young discipline and, therefore, is an active field of investigation.

NUTRITIONAL STATUS IN THE UNITED STATES

While it is generally believed that the United States populations are adequately, if not overly, nourished, this may not in fact be universal. Contrary to most assumptions, the largest incidence of obesity is in the lower socioeconomic group.[1] Little protein or calorie deficiency has been revealed. On the other hand, the U.S. Department of Agriculture Market Basket Survey revealed extensive inadequacies in certain portions of our populations for iron, calcium, and vitamins A, C, B_1, B_2, B_6 and folate.[2] It was shown too that a large portion of our population consumes approximately ½ of the United States Recommended Daily Allowance (USRDA) of 2 milligrams per day for vitamin B_6. (It should be noted that an average consumption of ½ an RDA means that 50% of the population consumes less than that). These findings were confirmed and extended by HEW's Ten State Nutrition Survey and further confirmation has been obtained from the HANES (Health and Nutrition Examination Survey) in which approximately 50% of the population was less than adequate in two nutrients.[3]

As will be noted later, the composition of the diet and nutritional status both influence the rate of metabolism of drugs.

A complete and properly varied diet will deliver to us a full quota of macronutrients (carbohydrates, protein and fat) and micronutrients (vitamins and minerals). Dietary guidelines have been established by the appropriate use of the four food groups and it is assumed that by the use of these guidelines an adequate diet will result. As it happens the Type A school lunch program uses the food groups to describe a specific distribution of food to be included in every federally paid lunch and must be delivered by all participating school boards. However, the United States Department of Agriculture analyzed the school lunches served to 301 schools for vitamins and minerals only to find that the diet was grossly inadequate in both.[4] Another study was done in 21 schools in North Carolina and a summary of data is shown in Table 14.1.[5] Whole trays of food were collected as served and submitted for vitamin and mineral analysis. It was clearly evident that over 50% of lunches did not meet even ⅓ of an RDA for iron, calcium, vitamins B_1 and C (and probably vitamins B_6 and folic acid which were not assayed for). Accordingly, the following of guidelines does not necessarily assure getting adequate nutrition, nor does simply telling a patient to eat a balanced diet (without careful instruction). Yet nutritional status influences drug metabolism.

TABLE 14.1. NUTRIENT ADEQUACY OF TYPE A SCHOOL LUNCH

Nutrient	Percent of meals less than 1/3 RDA
Calories	100
Protein	0*
Vitamin C	56
Vitamin B_1	77
Vitamin B_2	0*
Vitamin A	28
Iron	87
Calcium	72*

*These numbers would be higher if milk were not consumed.

THE MARGINAL DEFICIENCY STATE

In Table 14.2 we present five stages in the development of vitamin deficiency.[6] In the first stage there is inadequate availability of vitamin due to diet, malabsorption or abnormal metabolism. This is the preliminary stage in which there is a depletion of body stores of nutrient. The second stage is called the biochemical one because depletion has progressed sufficiently to interfere with coenzyme formation, thereby resulting in depressed enzyme activity. Urinary excretion of vitamins is reduced to negligible levels. In the physiological or third stage there begin to appear some clinical signs of illness, or malaise. Although these signs are not specific for vitamin deficiency per se, there is loss of weight concurrent with loss of appetite, general malaise, insomnia, increased irritability, somnolence, other behavioral changes, and modified drug metabolism. As the deficiency becomes more severe there appear specific clinical syndromes of vitamin deficiency such as beriberi, pellagra, rickets, etc. The fifth state, which is referred to as the anatomical one, is a situation of extremely severe depletion in which there is specific tissue pathology and in which, unless the situation is reversed by the administration of the missing nutrients, death results.

We refer to the first three stages as the stage of marginal (or preclinical) deficiency because one can reveal specific biochemical and metabolic modifications which result from vitamin depletion but without any specific clinical signs of deficiency. The clinical findings in stage three are behavioral effects (except for drug metabolism) which would not by themselves direct one toward a diagnosis of nutritional deficiency because they are so nonspecific. Nutritional researchers, however, recognize that these findings have been routinely observed where specific deficiencies have been studied under controlled laboratory conditions and often during drug therapy.

It should be borne in mind therefore that a patient who appears clinically normal may not be adequate in all nutrients. As will now be

TABLE 14.2. DEVELOPMENT OF VITAMIN DEFICIENCY

Sequence	Deficiency State	Demonstrable Symptoms and Comments
1	Preliminary	Inadequate availability of vitamin due to diet, malabsorption, and abnormal metabolism
2	Biochemical	Enzyme-coenzyme activity depressed. Urinary vitamin reduced to negligible levels
3	Physiological	Loss of body weight concurrent with appetite loss, general malaise, insomnia, and increased irritability
4	Clinical	Increased malaise, loss of body weight with the appearance of deficiency syndromes
5	Anatomical	Establishment of specific deficiency disease with specific tissue pathology. Unless reversed by repletion, death results

described, this state of marginal deficiency can influence the metabolism of and therefore the action of administered drugs.

SOME INTERRELATIONSHIPS BETWEEN DRUGS AND VITAMINS

Effects of Marginal Vitamin Deficiency on Drug Metabolism

A summary of the effects of vitamin inadequacy on drug metabolism is shown in Table 14.3. These studies were largely done in experimental animals although there is a very high correlation to such findings in man.[7] It is noted that vitamin E deficiency shows markedly reduced hydroxylation and demethylation of drug substrates.[8,10] This is noted also with deficiencies of vitamin A and vitamin C.[11-15] In the case of riboflavin there is decreased metabolism of benzopyrene (a potent carcinogen found in tobacco smoke, etc.) but increased oxidative metabolism of aminopyrene, hexobarbital and aniline.[16,17] It is noted that thiamin deficiency, unlike the others, results in increased metabolism of heptachlor and aniline while large doses of thiamin decrease the rate of metabolism of zoxazolamine.[18,19] As a matter of fact, excessive amounts of vitamin C also have a reverse effect.[15]

It was noted that for vitamins A, E and C reduced drug metabolism resulted from marginal deficiencies before there were any clinical signs of vitamin deficiency. And a recent report has demonstrated that a vitamin deficiency results in an enhanced intestinal transport of passively absorbed drugs.[20] These two effects of vitamin inadequacy on increased absorption and on the reduction in the rate of drug degradation may individually or both result in an increased residence time of the drug in the body and, therefore, may possibly potentiate the action of the drug. This possible potentiation of drug action may not have been accorded adequate attention to this point.

TABLE 14.3. EFFECTS OF VITAMIN STATUS UPON DRUG METABOLISM

Vitamin	Status	Cytochrome P-450	Microsomal Metabolism
E	D	0	–
A	D	–	–
B_1	D		+
	E		–
B_2	D		–
C	D	0	–
	E	+	+

Key to abbreviations: D Deficiency; E Level of administration in excess of ANRC recommendations; 0 No effect; + Increased; – Decreased. All data obtained from experimental animals.

Effects of Drug Use on Vitamin Needs

Some of these findings are summarized in Table 14.4. It is noted that needs for both fat- and water-soluble vitamins are increased as a consequence of drug therapy. Anticonvulsants such as diphenylhydantoin and phenobarbital can cause vitamin D and folic acid deficiencies.[21] In other situations such as with oral contraceptive steroids or aspirin, only marginal deficiency states may result as reflected by reduced blood or urine levels of large numbers of vitamins and/or reduced enzyme activity. In the case of oral contraceptive steroid administration, the activity of certain enzymes may be specifically induced so that the vitamin B_6 requirement is increased to levels in excess of what may possibly be obtainable from diet.[22,23] It is more generally recognized that in the case of certain drugs such as isoniazid and penicillamine, the therapeutic agents combine directly with the vitamin B_6 and/or compete for vitamin B_6 at the enzyme binding sites, thereby again markedly increasing the requirement to levels far beyond what could be obtained from diet. For general interest the effects of certain environmental pollutants such as nitrosamines are also included in the Table. In this case the adverse effects can sometimes be reversed by vitamin C and by vitamin E.[24,25]

While clinical signs of deficiency as described can result from drug administration, in most cases drug administration results in a pre-clinical or marginal deficiency state. This state has been defined by biochemical criteria for the measurement of vitamin adequacy.[26,27] While in most cases simply consuming an additional USRDA of the nutrient per day will correct the abnormal finding, this is not the case for vitamin B_6 upon taking oral contraceptive steroids, where it may be necessary to consume up to four times the USRDA for this vitamin.[22]

Effects of Macronutrient Consumption on Drug Metabolism

Dietary protein and carbohydrate can also have an influence on the rate of drug metabolism. In an interesting series of studies[28] healthy

TABLE 14.4. INCREASED VITAMIN NEEDS AS A CONSEQUENCE OF DRUG AND/OR ENVIRONMENTAL CHEMICAL EXPOSURE

Nutrient	Exposures resulting in increased vitamin needs or reduced bood levels
Vitamin A	Polychlorobiphenyls, benzopyrene, spironolactone, DDT.
Folacin	Oral contraceptives, anticonvulsants, methotrexate, pyrimethamine, alcohol
Vitamin B_{12}	Biguanides, anticonvulsants, oral contraceptive steroids
Vitamin B_6	Isonicotinic hydrazide, thiosemicarbazide, penicillamine, L-dopa, hydralazine, oral contraceptive steroids, alcohol
Niacin	Polychlorobiphenyls, isonicotinic hydrazide, phenylbutazone
Riboflavin	Boric acid
Vitamin D	Anticonvulsants
Vitamin K	Anticonvulsants, antibiotics
Vitamin C	Smoking, aspirin, oral contraceptive steroids, nitrosamines
Vitamin E	Oxygen, ozone

volunteers who did not smoke or drink, who did not use any drugs for three weeks prior to the study, and who were limited to consuming no smoked foods, brussels sprouts, cabbage, or other known inducers or inhibitors of the drug metabolizing enzymes were studied during 14 day periods. The first period comprised the customary home diet. The second period comprised a high protein (44%) low carbohydrate (35%) and the third period a high carbohydrate (70%) and low protein (10%) diet. Following this they returned to their home diets. The special diets were prepared by a metabolic kitchen at a major university hospital. For each subject there was determined the plasma half-life of antipyrine after an oral dose of 18 milligrams per kilogram on day 10 of each of the four periods, and similarly for theophylline at a dose level of 5 milligrams per kilogram on the last day of each of the four periods. It was observed that the half-life of antipyrine was markedly reduced under conditions of high protein intake and that a similar finding was made for theophylline. The difference due to a high carbohydrate diet was less significant than for protein.

The increased rate of drug metabolism (reduced half-life) presented here in human subjects is in accord with studies in experimental animals.[29,30] Furthermore, similar findings obtained from feeding charcoal broiled beef (and which are independent of the protein content of the beef) were probably caused by the presence of polycyclic aromatic hydrocarbons as a consequence of the charcoal broiling.[31] The hydrocarbons in question have been previously shown to be potent inducers of the drug metabolizing enzymes.[32,33] Although the specific studies have indicated that there is considerable individual variation in the responsiveness of humans to dietary change, the findings are of considerable clinical and pharmacological importance since they probably contribute to the large variation in the blood levels and blood action observed in different individuals or in the same individuals on different occasions. Increased rates of metabolism (or reduced life span) mean a lower residence time of the drug in the body, generally associated with lower blood levels and, therefore, potentially a reduced pharmacological effect.

Special Groups at Risk

1. Elderly.—Adverse reactions to drugs are particularly liable to occur in the elderly. Reasons are that they are the chief drug users,[34,35] and the aging process may slow drug metabolism.[36] In the current context, it is important to understand that those who take the most drugs are likely to have the most precarious nutritional status both due to the effect of dietary restriction and the results of acute or chronic disease.[37-39]

Vitamin deficiencies often found in the elderly are those which may affect drug metabolism. Marginal deficiencies of vitamins A, E and C may occur as well as impairment in riboflavin status.[40-47]

Drugs used by the elderly may affect their vitamin needs and contribute to the presence of one or more vitamin deficiencies. Haghschenass and Rao studied serum folacin (folate) levels in 27 elderly patients receiving anticonvulsant therapy with diphenylhydantoin.[44] Although none of their patients showed evidence of overt megaloblastic anemia, serum folacin levels were extremely low in the patient group as contrasted with values for 25 control subjects. Authors comment that the lower serum folacin values were found in people on diphenylhydantoin over 60 years of age.

Osteomalacia is common in elderly people in whom it frequently coexists with osteoporosis. Osteomalacia may be due to abuse of certain laxatives including mineral oil and phenolphthalein.[45-47]

2. Alcoholics.—Whereas acute ingestion of alcoholic beverages with drugs such as central nervous system depressants will tend to cause additive and depressant effects, alcoholics show an increased tolerance for certain drugs. On the other hand, increased sensitivity of alcoholics to certain drugs such as anticoagulants may be on the basis of vitamin K deficiency induced by or associated with alcoholic liver disease.[48]

Deficiencies of fat- and water-soluble vitamins which are common in chronic alcoholics may be exacerbated by intake of therapeutic drugs.[49] In circumstances in which ethanol increases the metabolism of other drugs, it may exert a sparing effect on potential drug-induced vitamin depletion.[50]

3. Epileptics.—Children as well as adults with seizure disorders take anti-convulsant drugs on a long-term basis. Since these drugs have the potential for causing folacin and vitamin D deficiencies, dietary requirements for these nutrients in epileptic children are increased. Chronic anticonvulsant therapy can produce folacin deficiency both in children and in adults. However, an effect of folic acid replacement (high dose) therapy is a reduction in the serum concentration of diphenylhydantoin or phenobarbital which can lead to increased frequency and severity of seizures.[51,52]

Anticonvulsant rickets and osteomalacia may be the result of induction of the hepatic metabolism of vitamin D. At risk are those on chronic high dosage anticonvulsant therapy who are not exposed to sunlight and whose intake of vitamin D is negligible.[53]

Infants born to women on anticonvulsant drugs may develop vitamin K deficiency manifested as hemorrhagic disease of the newborn.[54]

4. Dieters.—In developed countries many individuals frequently modify their diets for the purpose of gaining or losing weight, or as self-imposed or physician-advised treatment of disease. Change in diet often means an alteration in the level of protein consumed. If the dietary change is during drug therapy, rate of drug metabolism may be enhanced, thus reducing therapeutic drug levels and drug efficacy (with high protein intake) or conversely can lead to slowed rate of drug metabolism with prolonged high blood levels of the drug and risks of adverse drug reaction (high carbohydrate intake).

5. Malnourished Children.—Drugs at usual therapeutic dosages may be highly toxic or lethal to malnourished children. Identified causes are: reduction in body weight, slowed drug clearance, and impaired drug metabolism. The attending physician must decide whether to reduce the dosage of the drug (and perhaps not accomplish the therapeutic effects) or realiment the young patient with protein, vitamins, and minerals before the drug treatment, and run the risk of the child succumbing to the disease before the infection is treated.[55]

SUMMARY

It is now recognized that marginal vitamin deficiency will largely result in reduced rates of drug metabolism and that the administration of drugs will often increase the need for vitamin intake. Also, the consumption of high protein diets will increase the rate of drug metabolism and reduce the residence time of the drug in the body thereby reducing its pharmacological effectiveness.

In United States populations there may be extensive marginal deficiency for vitamins as shown by a variety of government and nutritional surveys. Considering this general marginal deficiency state as well as the high variation in protein intake as a consequence of reduced calorie and/or therapeutic dieting, one might expect a large variation in the pharmacological response to drugs depending upon the nutritional state of the patient.

REFERENCES

1. TEN STATE NUTRITION SURVEY (1970) Publ. No. 72-8130 to 72-8134, U.S. Dept. of Health, Education and Welfare, Washington, D.C.
2. U.S. DEPARTMENT OF AGRICULTURE (1965) Household Food Consumption Survey. USDA/ARS, Washington, D.C.
3. HEALTH AND NUTRITION EXAMINATION SURVEY (1974) Publ. No. (HRA)74-1219-1. U.S.D.H.E.W., Rockville, Maryland.
4. MURPHY, E.W., KOONS, P.C., and PAGE, L. (1969) Vitamin content of Type A school lunches. J. Amer. Diet. Assoc. 55:372–378.
5. HEAD, M.K. (1974) A nutrition education program at three grade levels. J. Nutr. Educ. 6:56–59.
6. BRIN, M. (1964) Erythrocyte as a biopsy tissue in the functional evaluation of nutritional status. J. Amer. Med. Assoc. 187:762–766.
7. KAPPAS, A., ANDERSON, K.E., CONNEY, A.H., and ALVARES, A.P. (1976) Influence of dietary protein and carbohydrate on antipyrine and theophylline metabolism in man. Clin. Pharm. Therap. 20:643–653.
8. HORN, L.R., MACHLIN, L.J., BARKER, M.O., and BRIN, M. (1976) Drug metabolism and hepatic heme proteins in the vitamin E deficient rat. Arch. Biochem. Biophys. 172:270–277.
9. GIASUDDIN, A.S.M., CAYGILL, C.P.J., DIPLOCK, A.T., and JEFFREY, E. (1975) The dependence on vitamin E and selenium of drug demethylation in rat liver microsomes. Biochem. J. 146:339–350.
10. CARPENTER, M. (1972) Vitamin E and microsomal drug hydroxylation. Ann. N.Y. Acad. Sci. 203:81–92.
11. BECKING, G.C. (1972) Vitamin A status and drug metabolism in the rat. Can. J. Physiol. Pharmacol. 51:6–11.
12. AXELROD, J., UDENFRIEND, S., and BRODIE, B.B. (1954) Ascorbic acid in aromatic hydroxylation. III. Effect of ascorbic acid on hydroxylation of acetanilids, aniline, and antipyrine in vivo. J. Pharmacol. Exp. Ther. 111:176–181.
13. DEGKWITZ, E., WALSCH, S., DUBBERSTEIN, M., and WINTER, J. (1975) Ascorbic acid and cytochromes. Ann. N.Y. Acad. Sci. 258:201–208.
14. KATO, R., TAKANAKA, A., and OSHIMA, T. (1969) Effect of vitamin C deficiency on the metabolism of drugs and NADPH-linked electron transport system in liver microsomes. Jpn. J. Pharmacol. 19:25–33.
15. SATO, P., and ZANNONI, V.G. (1974) Stimulation of drug metabolism by ascorbic acid in weanling guinea pigs. Biochem. Pharmacol. 23:3121–3128.
16. WILLIAMS, J.R., JR., GRANTHAM, P.H., YAMAMOTO, R.S., and WEISBURGER, J.H. (1970) Effect of dietary riboflavin on azo die reductase in liver and in bacteria of cecal contents of rats. Biochem. Pharmacol. 19:2523–2525.
17. CATZ, C.S., JUCHAU, M.R., and YAFFE, S.J. (1970) Effects of iron, riboflavin and iodine deficiencies on hepatic drug metabolizing systems. J. Pharmacol. Exp. Ther. 174:197–205.
18. WADE, A.E., GREEN, F.E., CIORDIA, R.H., and CASTER, W.O. (1969) Effects of dietary thiamine intake on hepatic drug metabolism in the male rat. Biochem. Pharmacol. 18:2288–2292.

19. GROSSE, W., III, and WADE, A.E. (1971) The effect of thiamine consumption on liver microsomal drug metabolism. J. Pharmacol. Exp. Ther. 176:758–765.
20. MESHALI, M.M., and NIGHTINGALE, C.H. (1976) Effect of α-tocopherol (vitamin E) deficiency on intestinal transport of passively absorbed drugs. J. Pharm. Sci. 65:344–349.
21. RICHENS, A., and ROWE, D.J.F. (1970) Interaction between anticonvulsant drugs and vitamin D. Br. J. Pharmacol. 40:593–595.
22. LUHBY, A.L., BRIN, M., GORDON, M., DAVIS, P., MURPHY, M., and SPIEGEL, H. (1971) Vitamin B_6 metabolism in users of oral contraceptive agents. I. Abnormal urinary xanthurenic acid excretion and its correction by pyridoxine. Am J. Clin. Nutr. 24:684–693.
23. BRIN, M. (1971) Abnormal tryptophan metabolism in pregnancy and with oral contraceptive pill. I. Specific effects of an oral contraceptive steroid on the tryptophan oxygenase and two aminotransferase activities in livers of ovariectomized-adrenalectomized rat. Am. J. Clin. Nutr. 24:699–703.
24. MIRVISH, S.S. (1975) Blocking the formation of N-nitroso compounds with ascorbic acid *in vitro* and *in vivo*. Ann. N.Y. Acad. Sci. 258:175:180.
25. KAMM, J.J., DASHMAN, T., CONNEY, A.H., and BURNS, J.J. (1975) Effect of ascorbic acid on amine-nitrite toxicity. Ann. N.Y. Acad. Sci. 258:169–174.
26. ANONYMOUS (1973) Nutritional assessment in health programs. Am. J. Public Health 63, Suppl.
27. SAUBERLICH, H.E., SKALA, J.H., and DOWDY, R.P. (1974) Laboratory Tests for the Assessment of Nutritional Status. CRC Press, Cleveland, Ohio.
28. CONNEY, A.H., MILLER, E.C., and MILLER, J.A. (1956) Substrate induced synthesis and other properties of benzypyrene hydroxylase in rat liver. J. Biol. Chem. 228:753–766.
29. CAMPBELL, T.C. (1977) Nutrition and drug metabolizing enzymes. Clin. Pharm. Therap. 22:699–706.
30. CAMPBELL, T.C., and HAYES, J.R. (1974) Role of nutrition in drug metabolizing enzyme systems. Pharmacol. Rev. 26:171–197.
31. LIJINSKY, W., and SHUBIK, P. (1964) Benzo(a)pyrene and other polynuclear hydrocarbons in charcoal broiled meat. Science 145:53–55.
32. CONNEY, A.H. (1967) Pharmacological implications of microsomal enzyme induction. Pharmacol. Rev. 19:317:366.
33. CONNEY, A.H., PANTUCK, E.J., KUNTZMAN, R., KAPPAS, A., ANDERSON, A.E., and ALVARES, A.P. (1977) Clin. Pharm. Therap. 22:707–719.
34. MELMON, K.L. (1971) Preventable drug reactions—causes and cures. New Eng. J. Med. 284:1361–1368.
35. THE DRUG USERS. (1968) U.S. Task Force on Prescription Drugs. USDHEW, Washington, D.C., pp. 126–129.
36. O'MALLEY, K., CROOKS, J., DUKE, E. and STEVENSON, I.H. (1971) Effect of age and sex on human drug metabolism. Brit. Med. J. 3:607.

37. EXTON-SMITH, A.N. (1973) Nutritional deficiencies in the elderly. *In* Nutritional Deficiencies in Modern Society. Eds. Howard, A.N. and McLean-Baird, I. Newman Books Ltd., London.
38. BALAKI, J.A., and DOBBINS, W.O. (1974) Maldigestion and malabsorption: Making up for lost nutrients. Geriatrics 29:157–166.
39. EXTON-SMITH, A.N. (1968) The problem of subclinical malnutrition in the elderly. *In* Vitamins and the Elderly. Eds. Scott, B.L. and Exton-Smith, A.N. John Wright and Sons Ltd., London, pp. 12–18.
40. GRANERUS, A., PHILIP, I., and SVANBORG, A. (1972) Intake of calories and nutrients in hospitalized geriatric patients. *In* Nutrition in Old Age. Symp. Swedish Nutr. Founda. Ed. Carlson, L.A. Almquist and Wiksell, Upsalla, Sweden, pp. 134–139.
41. KATARIA, M.S., RAO, D.B. and CURTIS, R.C. (1956) Vitamin C levels in the elderly. Gerontol. Clin. 7:189.
42. ANDREWS, J., BROOK, M., and ALLEN, M.A. (1966) Influence of abode and season on the vitamin C status of the elderly. Gerontol. Clin. 8:257.
43. HAGHSHENASS, M., and RAO, D.B. (1973) Serum folate levels during anticonvulsant therapy with diphenylhydantoin. J. Amer. Geriat. Soc. 21:275–277.
44. MORGAN, J.W. (1941) The harmful effects of mineral oils (liquid petrolatum) purgatives. JAMA 117:1335–1336.
45. FRAME, B., GUIANG, H.L., FROST, H.M. and REYNOLDS, W.A. (1971) Osteomalacia induced by laxative (phenolphthalein) ingestion. Arch. Intern. Med. 128:794–796.
46. HAHN, T.J., HENDIN, B.A., SCHARP, C.R., and HADDAD, J.G. (1972) Effect of chronic anticonvulsant therapy on serum 25-hydroxycalciferol levels in adults. New Eng. J. Med. 287:900–909.
47. KISSIN, B. (1974) Interactions of ethyl alcohol and other drugs. *In* The Biology of Alcoholism, Vol. 3. Clinical Pathology. Eds. Kissin, B. and Begleiter, H. Plenum Press, New York, pp. 109–161.
48. ROE, D.A. (1976) Alcohol and alcoholism. In Drug-Induced Nutritional Deficiencies. AVI Publ. Co., Westport, Conn., pp. 202–210.
49. KATER, R.M.H., ROGGIN, G., TOBORN, F. *et al.* (1969) Increased rate of clearance of drugs from the circulation of alcoholics. Amer. J. Med. Sci. 258:35–39.
50. KLIPSTEIN, F.A. (1964) Subnormal serum folate and macrocytosis associated with anticonvulsant drug therapy. Blood 23:68–86.
51. MATTSON, R.H., GALLAGHER, B.B., REYNOLDS, E.H., and GLOSS, D. (1973) Folate therapy in epilepsy. A controlled study. Arch. Neurol. 29:78–81.
52. RICHENS, A. (1976) Drug Treatment of Epilepsy. H. Kimpton Publ., London, pp. 135–138.
53. MOUNTAIN, K.R., HIRSCH, J., and GALLUS, A.S. (1970) Neonatal coagulation defect due to anticonvulsant drug treatment in pregnancy. Lancet 1:265–268.
54. MONKEBERG, F., BRAVO, M., and GONZALEZ, O. (1978) Drug metabolism and infantile undernutrition. In Nutrition and Drug Interrelation-

ships. Eds. Hathcock, J.N. and Coon, J. Academic Press, New York, pp. 399–408.

55. MEHTA, S., KALSI, H.K., JAYARAMAN, S., and MATHUR, V.S. (1975) Chloramphenical metabolism in children with protein-calorie malnutrition. Amer. J. Clin. Nutr. 28:977–981.

15

DIETETIC SUPPORT OF MEDICAL PRACTICE

Penelope S. Easton, Ph.D., R.D.

The importance of the nutritional status of the patient in acute and chronic disease states is well documented.[1] Actual assessment of the nutriture of an individual patient is difficult[2] and motivating a permanent change in food intake for health reasons is equally if not more difficult to achieve.[3] Physicians have the right to expect professional dietetic personnel to help them design appropriate dietary regimens, as well as to help patients achieve the desired behavior changes.

Specifically, physicians have the right to expect that registered dietitians (R.D.s) will provide the following patient information and services:

1. Assessment of current dietary patterns and self-prescribed supplements with attention to energy intake and use, actual foods eaten, and the possibility of nutrient excesses and/or deficiencies.
2. Summary of economic and/or lifestyle factors which influence food behavior change and affect the translation of the dietary prescription.
3. Comments and data useful for total nutritional assessment, possibly actual determination of assessment components such as skin fold, height and weight.[4]
4. Food composition data which would help the patient to follow the desired dietary regimen or render it inappropriate.
5. Information on current diet fads and faddists as well as accurate data about additives, preservatives and food preparation methods.
6. Preparation of educational materials and methods adapted to the patient's ethnic, religious and educational background.

Dr. Easton is Chairman, Dietetics and Nutrition, Florida International University, Miami.

7. Provide information on feeding modalities, i.e. supplements and tube feeding.
8. Provide a follow-through system for the patient to receive dietetic support and additional information as there is a change in needs, attitude or disease condition.
9. Monitoring of food intake and energy used in both in-hospital and outpatient settings.
10. Information about the patient's comfort and wishes for foods which may be desirable and possible when total food intake and/or the prognosis is considered.

PROFESSIONAL DIETETIC PERSONNEL

The title registered dietitian (R.D.) may be used only by a person with approved academic qualifications, clinical experiences and a passing score on the registration examination (see Definition Table). There are several areas of emphasis in dietetics: clinical, community and administration. However, the R.D. is expected to have entry level competencies in all of these areas. For the rest of this chapter, the term dietitian or R.D. will be used to describe the dietitian who is most often directly related to patient care (general or clinical or therapeutic) and the role expectations will be described for dietitians with these competencies.

The dietetic technician is a new member category of the American Dietetic Association. The technician functions as supportive personnel under the registered dietitian in a subspecialty such as nutritional care. This is an Associate Degree level training. The dietetic assistant training program (usually less than one year at a vocational school level) is also an American Dietetic Association approved program.[5]

DEFINITION TABLE[5]

REGISTERED DIETITIAN (R.D.)

A specialist educated for a profession responsible for the nutritional care of individuals and groups. This care includes the application of the science and art of human nutrition in helping people select and obtain food for the primary purpose of nourishing their bodies in health or disease throughout the life cycle.

CLINICAL DIETITIAN (R.D.)

The clinical dietitian, R.D., is a member of the health care team and affects the nutritional care of individuals and groups for health maintenance. The clinical dietitian assesses nutritional needs, develops and implements nutritional care plans, and evaluates and reports these results appropriately.

DIETETIC TECHNICIAN

A technically skilled person who has successfully completed an associate degree program which meets the educational standards established by The American Dietetic Association. The dietetic technician, working under guidance of an R.D. or an A.D.A. dietitian, has responsibilities in assigned areas in foodservice management; in teaching foods and nutrition principles; and in dietary counseling.

There is much confusion in the use of the title "nutritionist" because it has no legal definition as registered dietitian does. The description of Galbraith summarized the confusion this way.[6]

Nutritionist (non-medical) is not as precisely defined; indeed, that title may be (and is) assumed by individuals with a wide variety of credentials (some of which are authentic, recognized, and prestigious, and some of which are obscure or even non-existent). A small cadre of highly qualified physicians have passed boards in human nutrition as established by the American Board of Nutrition; accreditation of nutrition as a medical subspecialty is advocated.

Physicians have the right to expect that dietetic professionals will have the appropriate credentials, fulfill their continuing education requirements and be paid wages commensurate with their training and experience. Adequate dietetic services cannot be provided by even the most competent dietitians unless sufficient numbers of them and supportive personnel are hired.

DIETARY HISTORIES

For many if not most patients, adequate medical treatment requires information about the patient which is difficult to obtain and assess. Food intake falls within this realm. Food patterns are highly personal and often are a very private part of a patient's life. They involve feelings of guilt, for no one in today's world has escaped information about what he or she should or should not eat. Food habits involve feelings of pride, self image, social behavior, success, "protection" of the food provider and accomplishment in food preparation or hospitality. Food habits are economically and socially influenced and are subjected constantly to change, although these changes may not be because of a diet prescription.

Aging, marriage, children, change of locale, health circumstances and new products on the market must all be considered in food habit changes. A dietary history can determine the direction and extent of change possible as well as provide an estimate of present and usual nutrient intakes.

The data from diet histories should be considered in both in-hospital and outpatient care. The frustration of a patient who follows a strict religious regimen and yet receives "forbidden" foods with the weak excuse "you're allowed it for medical reasons" may be great and probably unnecessary. This stress and anguish could be lessened with personalized dietary care.

A good dietary/activity history takes from one to two hours to determine and may take an additional hour or adequate computer time to calculate. Dietary histories may be "contaminated" with a variety of medical personnel asking questions such as "Do you eat well?" "What do you eat?" "Do you follow your food plan?" Casual questions may make the patient hostile or defensive. It takes a skillful interviewer to provide the supportive climate that allows the patient to give accurate information concerning food habits.

Food habits are indeed a very personal subject, perhaps more personal than sex habits. Certainly in comparison, food habits involve far more time and money!

Discussion of food intake usually involves the answering of many questions concerning the adequacy of the diet and evaluation and correction of the dietary information the patient already has. Although answering these questions when asked during the dietary history interview may render the history useless as "pure" research, it makes the interview become a powerful tool for the dietitian and a good learning situation for the patient.

The use of a dietary record or diary brought in by the patient prevents much of this interchange of information and may include more "expected" behavior than "actual." The assignment of dietary histories to a non-dietetic professional also may produce expected rather than actual food patterns. The sheer number of histories necessary may make it imperative that the dietetic technician take some diet histories. The assessment of these, however, and the supervision of the technician are an integral part of the registered dietitian's responsibilities.

DIETARY MODIFICATIONS

The physician has the right to communicate directly with the R.D. about a patient's food intake and dietary needs—he/she should not have to talk about dietary prescriptions to a "girl from the kitchen" or a nurse's aide. So-called routine diet orders are often ill-advised and may put unnecessary and even life threatening restrictions on patients. For example, the postsurgical diet (called clear liquid or some similar term) even if eaten or drunk, which it rarely is, may cause severe deprivation of all nutrients, even energy. A "high energy, high protein" liquid diet is theoretically possible, but in actuality the energy intake is so low that the protein component will all be used for energy, not for tissue repair.

Patients improve at very different rates and therefore changes in diet orders should reflect this rather than follow a standard number of days. The use of formulated diets is advisable in treatment of debilitated patients, but the numbers and degree of debilitation could be greatly reduced with proper dietary monitoring of all patients.

The diet "as ordered" and even "as delivered" is far different from the diet as eaten. In many instances, even the diet as eaten differs from the diet as absorbed! Vomiting and diarrhea are rarely noted as requiring replacement of food to prevent debilitation. Many hospital trays are delivered to patient's bedside and then no one sees that the food is transferred from the tray to the patient's mouth. The milk carton may be impossible for a weak patient to open. Patients, roommates and visitors may have all eaten from the tray and, therefore, chart notations about food eaten may be inaccurate. The food as well may have been put in the waste basket, down the drain or in a drawer.

The feelings about food are profoundly important, especially in a hospital. Food represents pleasure, punishment, threat or even a waste of money. Food intake should be ascertained in a nonthreatening way if the assessment is to be accurate and useful to the physician in decision making.

The use of a diet order "as tolerated" or "selective" is a reasonable one for the physician concerned with the individualized care of the patient. However, the "as tolerated" diet may become someone else's idea of "as tolerated," not the patient's, or, if the patient is consulted, the same foods may be ordered for days with no rechecking to see if the toleration has changed. "Selective" menus usually are chosen far in advance of the meal being considered. They may be chosen by a family member, who also wishes to eat, or who understandably thinks the patient might eat a little bit of several items by the time the meal arrives. They may be checked by the patient who feels ill at the moment but might feel very different later on. They may be chosen by hospital personnel who wish to help but do not know the patient's likes and dislikes, nor can they predict what the patient's appetite will be four meals hence. The admitting personnel by observing a person without teeth or with ill-fitting dentures may order a "Soft Diet" or what is even worse a "Soft Bland Diet." This convinces the patient who eats well without teeth that he or she is being punished or is really more critically ill than has been told. Such orders may so severely restrict food intake that malnutrition occurs.

Difficult as it is, actual food intake must be determined as accurately as possible in order to monitor the prescribed changes. For example, a person on a restricted sodium diet who eats almost nothing might appropriately be given even a higher sodium food if the total amount of food consumed is actually considered, not the sodium content of the food as served. Multiple restrictions and recommendations may cancel each other out or so restrict intake that actual starvation may occur, such as a high protein, low fat and sodium restricted diet which may be impossible to translate into ordinary foods.

Dietary prescriptions are difficult to determine and even more difficult to follow. Food has a variety of components and food preparation may alter the nutrient contribution significantly. Physicians have the right to expect the dietitians to notify them if the diet prescription is inappropriate for the patient or unreasonable in terms of food composition. Sixty grams of carbohydrates may be unreasonable for a person needing 3000 Kcalories of energy a day, but may be possible for a person using 1200 Kcalories of energy.

The use of formulated diets may make prescriptions easier but they are expensive, unpalatable and unpleasant for the patient and may not produce the nutritional benefits expected even if consumed.

The physician should expect to have persistent problems of food intake pointed out and to have continuing quantitative data recorded in the patient's chart. A notation, "ate approx. 540 Kcal, 20 g Pro, 10 M.Eq. Na" is useful data, but a notation that "patient ate well"—or "half his meal" is not.

DIET COUNSELING

Effective diet counseling is influenced by many social and medical factors. Few if any patients have been untouched by nutrition as a political issue. The dramatic presentations of the dangers of additives, preservatives and colorings, food preparation techniques such as barbecuing and effects of high sucrose diets, bombard the consumer. The physician has the right to expect the registered dietitian to give him or be able to find current information about food components and food chemistry.

The treatment of disease by diet is as much determined by myth and tradition as it is by actual research and physiological fact. The dietitian can help the physician weigh the possible benefits and dangers of food restrictions and regimens. Some restrictions may have been made many years ago for conditions no longer of importance or by professionals no longer in attendance, but the taboos remain. If all professionally given taboos are included along with the admonitions of relatives and friends, the mass of restrictions may become health threatening.

Handing the patient a printed diet pattern or even a book cannot deal with all these questions and uncover necessary information. A "one shot" diet instruction by even the most competent dietitian cannot do this either. Diet instruction takes time and some follow-through system.

Adherence to dietary modifications is more difficult than adherence to medications, because the change may be unpleasant and often it involves constant use of knowledge and decision making strategies. How does a patient eat at a party, on an airplane, or a cruise ship, at a fast food restaurant, in a school cafeteria, from a refreshment truck at a construction site or at a family reunion? Following dietary advice is the responsibility of the patient and he/she is often ill-equipped in terms of knowledge, motivation and adequate professional support.

The difference in "knowing" and "doing" has been noted by many counselors. In no area does this have a greater impact than in food habit changes. The responsibility for food intake is ultimately and entirely the patient's. The motivation for change in food intake often needs to be stronger than long term health benefits or even the "scare" of getting worse. The lack of success in weight loss programs documents this well. However, some people do change their food habits. These changes can be made compatible with health needs if proper counseling, support, follow-through and information is available. Group dietary counseling is rarely an effective way if used by itself, Zifferblatt and Wilbur have noted:[7]

> Furthermore guard against the suggestion that their time can be used most effectively by counseling patients in groups. Successful change is more likely when nutritional programs can be tailored to individual needs. Although group counseling is often an efficient way to communicate general principles of nutrition and behavioral change, individuals within a group differ considerably in personal characteristics and life style.

COST EFFECTIVENESS

Dietary support of medical practice can no longer be considered a luxury, but must be considered an integral part of treatment even if for no reason other than the prevention of malpractice suits for iatrogenic malnutrition or food drug interactions. In a more positive view, adequate dietary support is necessary for the physician to answer the questions of the consumer conscious patient.

Dietary management is difficult, costly and has not had a high success rate. The benefits of weight control are not questioned in management of many diseases but the cost effectiveness of good dietary counseling for obesity needs to be documented. It has been demonstrated that the public is willing to pay exorbitant prices for food and nutrition information of highly questionable value. Although the actual pamphlets and advice may be "free," people pay inflated prices for ordinary foods in health food stores, pay lecturers and so-called nutrition experts for group and individual advice and buy large quantities of vitamin and mineral supplements with unknown and possibly life threatening consequences. The skill of these faddists and charlatans is enhanced by their lack of need to be scientifically sound and ability to employ scare techniques and the promise of miraculous results. Their ability to draw followers willing to pay large amounts of money for their services may involve an added cost to patient care in at least the short term.

Optimum dietetic support may divert some of the money spent for fads and faddists to improve total health habits and enhance the patient's evaluation of the physician as a focal point of health information. The old "ask your doctor before starting a diet" is often ignored now because of the mass of information available to the lay public.

No real studies of cost benefits of dietary support have been done. Does good dietetic counseling cut down the number of hospitalizations, save physician and nurse time, increase patient comfort and peace of mind and prevent some complications and disease states? If any or all these are so, how much money does this save? The lack of many prepaid programs of medical care, and the lack of third-party payments of dietetic services may make the physician reluctant to demand adequate dietary care for patients.

The cost benefits of treatment of nutrition related conditions such as obesity are obvious if not documented. Similarly, the treatment of constipation whether contributing to debilitation or merely discomfort can be influenced by good dietary care even to being cost effective in terms of fewer enemas and laxatives.

Although cost effectiveness can be demonstrated in some cases, the fact remains that although adequate dietetic support is recognized as being important, it is one service that may be "cut" when crisis situations are considered.

THE CHALLENGE

One of today's major challenges for the physician is providing adequate nutritional care for his/her patients. The determination of food intake, energy use and life patterns of eating is time consuming and requires special skills. Equally difficult is providing the knowledge and climate for change. Diet counseling is hampered by:

1. Lack of precise evaluation methods to determine nutritional adequacy.
2. The scarcity of information regarding the nutrient contributions of foods.
3. The prevalence of "free" information, much of it not true industry inspired or involving "scare" or threat.
4. The social messages regarding food habits which are not compatible with health needs.
5. The limited number of appropriately educated dietary personnel.

The explosion of information in all areas of medicine has left physicians with some impossible choices. If they "keep up" with all areas of medical practice, they have no time to see patients. If all the courses "necessary" were included in medical school, it is conceivable that medical school could be extended interminably.

In order to keep up in nutrition and food science, the physician needs technical and continuing support. The physician then has the right to expect the registered dietitian to furnish adequate dietary support if the following conditions are met:

1. Sufficient dietetic professionals are employed and allowed to function as professionals.
2. Adequate information and time are given to the dietitians to determine the patient's food pattern and preferences, to prepare the instructional materials and to teach and follow through with the patient.
3. Assessment of actual food intake is monitored and the data used in determining the patient's treatment.
4. The dietary restrictions, laboratory tests and drug prescriptions, and other orders such as for physical therapy and psychiatric consultations are all considered as part of the total care and reviewed in terms of the patient as a human being, not a group of medical problems.
5. The physician is available to discuss the effects of the dietary orders and need for change when other factors take precedence.

REFERENCES

1. SCHNEIDER, H.A.; ANDERSON, C.E., and COURSIN, D.B.: Nutritional Support of Medical Practice, Harper and Row, Maryland, 1977.
2. BLACKBURN, G.L., and BISTRIAN, B.R.: Nutritional Support Resources in Hospital Practice, Nutr. Sup. of Med. Pract., 139–159, 1977.
3. FERGUSON, J.: Dietitians as Behavior-Change Agents, J. Am. Diet. Assoc. 73:231–238, 1978.
4. WADE, J.: Role of a Clinical Dietitian Specialist on a Nutrition Support Service, J. Am. Diet. Assoc. 70:185–189, 1977.
5. AMERICAN DIETETIC ASSOCIATION: Position Paper on Recommended Salaries and Employment Practices for Members of The American Dietetic Association, J. Am. Diet. Assoc. 71:641–647, 1977.
6. THE PRESIDENT'S PAGE: J. Am. Diet. Assoc. 68:557, 1976.
7. ZIFFERBLATT, S.M., and WILBUR, C.S.: Dietary Counseling: Some Realistic Expectations and Guidelines, J. Am. Diet. Assoc. 70:591–595, 1977.

16

NUTRITIONAL CARE OF THE PATIENT IN OFFICE PRACTICE

Jeanne R. Rackow, M.S., R.D.

Nutritional care is increasingly an integral part of the total care of patients.[1] Malnutrition—either undernutrition or overnutrition—is one of the most common and vexing problems a physician observes in practice. When a patient is hospitalized, chances are that the nutritional care will be good if the physician has the resources of an effective health team available and utilizes them. But the nutritional needs of a patient do not suddenly appear when he enters the hospital. Nor do they disappear when he is discharged. In many practices 75% to 90% of patient care takes place in the office, away from the hospital resources. Although there is a need for continuing nutritional care in the office, frequently the subject never comes up or efforts to meet this need fail dismally. Hewitt *et al.*[2] maintain that less than one half of the patients continue for more than four weeks with weight reduction programs. Other studies[3–5] indicate that the success rate is even less.

This article discusses the role of nutrition in office practice. It examines the reasons for failure of efforts to provide nutritional care of the patient. Finally, it examines some alternative approaches for incorporating nutritional care into practice effectively, and at a cost the patient can afford.

ROLE OF NUTRITION IN MEDICAL PRACTICE

The role of nutrition in medical practice today is changing because the focus on the relationship of nutrition to health is changing. Nutrition

Ms. Rackow is Professor of Nutrition, University of South Florida, Tampa.

affects health in at least three ways: it is curative of disease, it may prevent disease, and, it is one of the therapeutic measures employed to treat disease.[6]

First, the intake of certain nutrients is curative of a small group of diseases which were prevalent at the turn of the century. Today it is rare to find any of these deficiency diseases except in individuals whose food intake is really bizarre. The almost magic vitamins are available in the corner drug store, in processed foods which have been restored or enriched with them, and even in foods fortified with nutrients not present in the natural state. More sophisticated processing, storage and distribution of foods in this country have made our diets more varied, thus minimizing the possibility that a nutrient will be deficient.

About the only place the symptoms of deficiency diseases appear is in medical textbooks. This can be illustrated by pointing out that pellagra was epidemic in Georgia in the summer of 1922, with 10,000 deaths and another 100,000 reported cases. A few years ago, a medical school in Georgia was unable to find one case in the state to show medical students first-hand the symptoms of pellagra. Thus, it is logical that physicians no longer concern themselves with nutritional care in order to cure disease.

However, nutrition is still important in a second ancillary way; it is one of the therapeutic measures that can be employed to treat illness. Some of the newer modalities of nutritional care have achieved notable results with patients with cancer, hypertension and gastrointestinal disorders. Also, good nutritional status may improve patient response to other therapies that the physician may use by reducing the incidence of infection and complications and by shortening the time of convalescence.[7]

Third, faulty nutrition may be one of the underlying causes of illness. There are still diseases with unexplained, complicated etiologies. Often, there is a close association of the incidence of these diseases with poor dietary intake.

The focus on nutrition has moved from its role as curative of deficiency disease to that of therapeutic intervention in and prevention of disease, and this affects the focus in medical practice. Nutritional care of the patient in the office is still important. However, the role it plays has changed. But all too often, it is ignored because of the press of other therapeutic needs.

NEED FOR NUTRITIONAL CARE IS THERE

The public today is more aware than ever before of the effect of adequate nutrition on health. The newspapers and television talk shows devote considerable space to the claims and counterclaims about nutrition, and even the comic strips have their commentary.

A recent study showed that a majority of the people would prefer getting their information on nutrition from their family physicians.[8] Another study revealed that, in fact, they most often get their information from what can be called paperback nutrition. Current estimates indicate that we waste $½ billion a year on food faddism. Failure to meet the public's need for nutrition information in medical practice has created a vacuum which has allowed the diet hucksters to flourish. Actually, the old-time medicine man has simply taken on a new guise as the natural food store proprietor or the author of the latest paperback.

REASONS FOR INADEQUATE NUTRITION COUNSELING

One reason that physicians do not instruct patients about diet is patient noncompliance. Nutrition counseling is often a frustrating, nonproductive experience for both the physician and the patient. Why is noncompliance such a common failing of nutrition counseling?

Patient Noncompliance Because of Poor Assessment

First, no two people are alike. They do not look alike, but the difference is more than skin deep. Each person has a nutrition individuality. In part, what makes one patient different from the next are the food habits he has acquired. Unless the counselor works within the framework of a person's food habits, his chances of changing nutritional status are minimal. When a patient is given an injection, the physician knows that the medication is where it belongs. All too often, a patient is given a set of dietary suggestions. It is the same set that is given to every other patient, with no attempt to fit it into his usual pattern of living. It is a safe estimate that the recommendations are ignored more often than they are followed.[9] A physician cannot make a patient follow instructions so the challenge is to make him want to follow them. The only way to do this is to make a patient comfortable with those changes that are needed, and this means finding out what determined his food habits in the first place.

Next, people have many beliefs and feelings about food. Identification of those beliefs and feelings may be more important than determining nutrition information that the patient may have. A study by Schwartz[10] showed that attitudes toward nutrition do mediate dietary practice. It is surprising to find out how much the average person knows about nutrition, or thinks he knows. All too often the information he has is wrong. Whether it is right or wrong, the important thing is to find out how he believes it applies to him. Carruth and associates[11] showed that an identification of attitudes and a change of those attitudes resulted in a change of eating habits.

Finally, it is important to determine what a patient is capable of learning. If instruction does not begin at his level, or if the expectations are set too high, the patient may not be able to reach the goals set for him. Often, he may not be willing to admit he cannot follow the instructions for he does not want to disappoint the physician, or he is afraid that he will be considered ignorant.

It takes good assessment to obtain information about present food habits, beliefs and feelings about food, and the ability of a person to learn. Unless these factors are taken into account, in essence the physician is telling the patient to go home and use his willpower which has not been effective to date. It is not surprising to find noncompliance with dietary instructions that are not based on patient assessment.

Failure to Initiate Discussion of Need for Dietary Change

Certainly the use of a diet sheet without assessment is high on the list of office practice which is counterproductive to delivery of good nutritional care. Equally bad is the practice of ignoring a person's need for help altogether.

For example, when a patient comes into the office with a problem of overweight, there are often a myriad of associated, recurring problems. The physician knows that the patient has a weight problem. The patient knows he has a problem. If the physician does not bring the subject up, chances are that the patient will not either. The physician may assume that if the patient really wants to lose weight he will ask for help. Also the physician may hesitate to make the patient feel guilty. Most people already feel guilty about excess weight and they are reticent to admit to anyone, including their family physicians, that they have a problem that they cannot handle. A patient has a role to play in his own care, and a physician needs to promote that ability to care adequately for himself. But the patient needs help in planning this role.

Lack of Up-to-Date Nutrition Information

Many physicians in private practice are ill equipped to work with patients who have nutritional needs. Studies[12,13] have shown that physicians who had received nutrition instruction in medical school or had continuing education training scored significantly higher in knowledge and use of nutrition in practice.

A survey in 1976 conducted by the Department of Foods and Nutrition of the American Medical Association[14] revealed that less than one fifth of the medical schools offered nutrition as a required course of study. Furthermore less than one third of the schools offered postgraduate or continuing education studies in nutrition. The number is growing rapidly, but the fact remains that a majority of physicians in practice today were not given information in medical school on nutrition or how to use it. Opportunities to gain information through continuing education are limited.

Olson[15] believes that clinical nutrition cuts across all branches of medical practice, and nutritional sciences are pertinent to all the basic preclinical sciences. Nutrition should be included in the medical school curriculum so that it correlates with practical application in the clinical setting. Also, continuing education workshops should be available which will provide current information on nutritional care and in addition present ways to utilize that information and develop tools for nutritional assessment of the patient.

Lack of Time and Cost of Effective Counseling

Good nutritional counseling takes time, and time is money. At one time people were not willing to pay what it would cost to work with a counselor but today they are spending hundreds of thousands of dollars to other sources for that same help. Studies have shown that they would prefer being helped by the physician who traditionally is the one to whom they look for health care delivery.

Physician's Role in Nutritional Care of Patients in Office Practice

The constraints of time and the high cost to the patient prevent most physicians from supplying the necessary nutritional support by themselves. There are alternative ways in which nutritional support can become part of office care. Just as the utilization of a team of health professionals has proven to be the most effective way to care for patients when they are hospitalized, team approach to nutritional care for the office patient is also efficient and economical.[16]

However it is the physician who has been charged with the major responsibility for medical care in his community. He must be the initiating force. Without his visible support and encouragement, the effectiveness of any health care team that he may develop will be minimal. The physician should screen his patients to identify those who need counseling. He then should discuss the problem and develop a program for intervention with the patient. Once he has accomplished this, he has a number of alternatives. He may elect to work with the patient if the change in diet is minimal and little follow-up care will be necessary. Many physicians prefer to give initial instruction to the patients. Often however the patient cannot afford the cost of dietary assessment and continuing reinforcement which is necessary for successful therapy when these tasks are performed by the physician.

An excellent resource is the consulting nutritionist who is trained to provide the continuing dietary management the patient needs, thus maximizing the work begun in the physician's office. She may be an employee of a group of private practitioners. She will supply professional therapy at a cost the patient can afford as well as updated nutrition information for the physicians. Some consulting nutritionists have private practices and see patients by referral from physicians in the community.[17]

Often the resources for nutritional support are available already in the office. The expanded role of the professional nurse includes the nutritional care of patients. The development of assessment and counseling skills in the nursing staff already in the practice may provide the continuing care which is needed. Tools for nutritional assessment and strategies used successfully to modify food intake and maintain results are available. They can be incorporated into existing private practices with little effort.[18–20]

CONCLUDING COMMENTS

Patients need help with their nutritional problems not only when they are hospitalized but on a continuing basis as part of the care they receive in office practice. A majority of the public would prefer information on nutrition from their family physicians but most often they get information from other sources. Patient noncompliance is common when dietary counseling without sufficient assessment and follow-up is attempted. This is a frustrating experience for both the physician and the patient. This plus the constraints of time and the high cost to the patient of adequate counseling have deterred many physicians from providing nutritional care. Alternatives are available for delivery of nutritional care. Nevertheless it is the physician who has been charged with the major responsibility for medical care in his community who should initiate therapy. He should discuss the problem with the patient and choose the appropriate approach for incorporating nutritional care into the total care for his patient.

REFERENCES

1. MEDICAL NEWS: Nutrition—No Longer a Stepchild in Medicine, JAMA 238:2245, 1977.
2. HEWITT, M.I.; O'DELL, D.S.; SCHELMAS, K.P., and KOTNOUR, K.D.: Predictability of Patient Compliance With a Weight Reduction Program, Obesity Bariatr. Med. 6:218, 1977.

3. ROSENSTOCK, I.M.: Patients' Compliance With Health Regimens, JAMA 234:402, 1975.
4. CARRUTH, B.R.; MANGEL, M., and ANDERSON, H.L.: Assessing Change-Proneness and Nutrition-Related Behaviors, J. Am. Diet. Asso. 70:47, 1977.
5. GIFFT, H.H.; WASHBON, M.B., and HARRISON, G.G.: Nutrition, Behavior, and Change, Prentice-Hall, Inc., Englewood Cliffs, N.J., 1972.
6. SCHNEIDER, H.A.; ANDERSON, C.E., and COURSIN, D.B.: Nutritional Support of Medical Practice, Harper & Row, Hagerstown, Md.: 1977.
7. COPELAND, E.M.; GASTINEAU, C.F.; SHILS, M.E., and MOERTEL, C.G.: Nutrition in the Cancer Patient, Dialog. Nutrit., Vol. 1, No. 4, 1976.
8. FOX, H.M.; FRYER, B.A.; LAMKIN, G.H.; VIVIAN, V.M., and EPPRIGHT, E.S.: The North Central Regional Study of the Diets of Preschool Children, J. Home Econ. 62:241, 1970.
9. SCHWARTZ, N.E., and BARR, S.I.: Mothers—Their Attitudes and Practices in Perinatal Nutrition, J. Nutr. Ed. 9:169, 1977.
10. SCHWARTZ, N.E.: Nutritional Knowledge, Attitudes, and Practices of High School Graduates, J. Am. Diet Asso. 66:28, 1975.
11. CARRUTH, B.R.; MANGEL, M., and ANDERSON, H.L.: Assessing Change-Proneness and Nutrition-Related Behaviors, J. Am. Diet. Asso. 70:47, 1977.
12. JOHNSON, E.M., and SCHWARTZ, N.E.: Physicians' Opinions and Counseling Practices in Maternal and Infant Nutrition, J. Am. Diet. Asso. 73: 246, 1978.
13. PODELL, R.N.; GARY, I.R., and KELLER, K.: Profile of Clinical Nutrition Knowledge Among Physicians and Medical Students, J. Med. Educ. 50:888, 1975.
14. CYBORSKI, C.K.: Nutrition Content in Medical Curricula, J. Nutr. Ed. 9:17, 1977.
15. OLSON, R.E.: Clinical Nutrition, An Interface Between Human Ecology and Internal Medicine, Nutr. Rev. 36:161, 1978.
16. KINDL, M., and BROWN, P.: Team Approach in Treatment of Obesity, J. Canad. Diet. Asso. 38:278, 1977.
17. TRITHART, E.S., and NOEL, M.B.: New Dimensions: The Dietitian in Private Practice, J. Am. Diet. Asso. 73:60, 1978.
18. JACOBSON, H.N.: Diet in Pregnancy, N. England J. Med. 297:1651, 1977.
19. CRISTAKIS, G., ed.: Nutrition Assessment in Health Programs, Am. J. Pub. Health 63, Pt. 2, 1973.
20. WING, R.R., and JEFFERY, R.W.: Successful Losers: A Descriptive Analysis of the Process of Weight Reduction, Obesity Bariatr. Med. 7:190, 1878.

17

PEDIATRIC NUTRITIONAL DETERMINANTS OF CHRONIC DISEASES

Anthony G. Kafatos, M.D., M.P.H. and George Christakis, M.D., M.P.H.

We owe the present average life span of approximately 72 years to medical and public health advances which have decreased infant and childhood morbidity and mortality. However, longevity has not actually increased in the last century since chronic diseases continue to doggedly plague technologically advanced societies. These diseases include coronary and hypertensive cardiovascular disease, diabetes, obesity and cancer.

Coronary heart disease (CHD) incidence appears to have plateaued and decreased in the last decade. However, CHD remains a current public health problem and hypertension remains the paramount cause of death among blacks. The prevalence of cardiovascular risk factors in western societies also remains impressive. Approximately one third of all adult males have serum cholesterol levels above 260 mg/dl and are exposed to a six-fold increased risk of having a premature myocardial infarction. According to the Ten-State Nutrition Survey, 10–50% of the total population is obese; 10–30% of adolescents are obese; 20% of all Americans are hypertensive.[1] The concept of risk factors as identified by the Framingham investigators may in fact be a major medical and health discovery of the century, as important as the "one germ-one disease" theory of Pasteur.[2] The elucidation of host and environmental factors which interdigitate and interact in a complex "mosaic" manner remains a

Dr. Kafatos is Associate Professor, Department of Epidemiology, University of Miami School of Medicine.
Dr. Christakis is Chief, Nutrition Division, University of Miami School of Medicine.

most fascinating model of coronary and hypertensive heart disease as a "chronic disease."

It may in fact appear strange to consider CHD as a chronic disease since its clinical manifestations may be as acute as sudden death. However, the metabolic and subcellular pathogenic progression of this disease may occur from infancy or even intrauterine life. Atherosclerosis appears to have a long incubation period; hence, our justified concern with lifestyle and infant feeding practices.

We postulate a "tri-composite" concept of atherosclerosis. One part relates to the aging process and is an expression of the mortality of man yielding to the inexorable press of time, the result of a universal genetic endowment which sets intracellular biological "time clocks" to the Biblical average life span of "three score and ten." The second component is also inherited and can be exemplified by the specific genetic penetrance which results in familial types of hyperlipidemia, i.e. hypercholesterolemia and/or hypertriglyceridemia and results in the acceleration of the atherosclerotic process. Approximately 8% of the population exhibits Type IV hyperlipidemia and from 2–4%, Type II hyperlipidemia. Hyperlipoproteinemia can be identified in childhood and has a prevalence rate of about 1 in 200 newborns in U.S.A. populations.[3] The disease in the homozygote state is associated with premature heart disease before the age of 20, while in the heterozygote state is associated with coronary heart disease in the fourth or fifth decade. Diabetes mellitus, another inherited disorder, has a prevalence of from 2–4% in the general population and also constitutes a considerable public health problem.

The third part of our concept of atherosclerosis is potentially more amenable to control and relates to a complex interplay of host and environmental factors. Against a background of the variable genetic penetrance of the familial or acquired hyperlipidemias, the presence of "national dietary hypercholesterolemia" or "universal hyperlipidemia" results when the nutritional environment or national diet pattern is high in calories, saturated fat, dietary cholesterol, oligosaccharides and alcohol. It is this third component which may be primarily responsible for the widespread elevated lipid levels found in middle-aged man.

Most serum lipid disorders which induce atherosclerosis have their roots in childhood. Some are inborn errors of metabolism and others are acquired or associated with various diseases (hypothyroidism, nephrotic syndrome, hepatic disease, etc.). Changes in infant feeding practices such as bottle feeding vs. breast feeding, early introduction of solid foods, infant overfeeding and baby foods high in sodium and oligosaccharides, may be important contributors to cardiovascular risk factors operating silently in infancy and childhood.

In intrauterine life and infancy, cholesterol and lipids are important participants in the cellular structure and function of the central nervous system, and influence the fragility and permeability of membrane integrity. Serum cholesterol increases dramatically the first few days of life from 97.4 mg/dl in cord blood to 146.6 on the 5th day and to 154.8 mg/dl on the 8th day.[4] The optimal level of serum cholesterol for the support of multiple physiological functions during the infant's growth and development is not known. Suggested "normal limits" of serum lipid and lipoprotein cholesterol concentrations in subjects age 0–19 years have been proposed.[5] (Table 17.1).

Serum triglyceride levels also increase rapidly during the first year of life.[6] By the end of the first year, serum lipid values approach those of young adults and appear to be closely related to early dietary practices. Breast-fed babies were found to have significantly higher cholesterol levels (146.8 mg/dl) at the age of two to four months compared to bottle-fed babies (Similac—128.8 mg/dl).[7] However, after the age of four months, there was not significant difference in serum cholesterol levels.

TABLE 17.1. SUGGESTED NORMAL CHOLESTEROL AND SERUM LIPID VALUES FOR CHILDREN

	Total mg/dl Cholesterol	Triglycerides mg/dl	LDL mg/dl	HDL (mg/dl) Males	HDL (mg/dl) Females
Cord Blood	50–95	10–15	20–45	30–55	30–55
1–19 yrs	120–130	10–140	50–170	30–65	30–70

EFFECT OF INFANT FEEDING PRACTICES ON SERUM CHOLESTEROL AND ADIPOSE TISSUE FATTY ACID COMPOSITION

A comparison of a formula which contains 80% corn oil and 20% coconut oil with unmodified cow's milk fed during the first year of life revealed that the unmodified-milk-fed babies had significantly higher serum cholesterol levels during the first year of life.[8] This was probably due to the hypocholesterolemic effect of linoleic acid found in the modified formula. Linoleic acid is a required fatty acid for normal growth; 2–3% of the total calories should be provided by linoleic acid in order to avoid a deficiency of this essential fatty acid. Human milk provides 4% of its total calories from linoleic acid while the modified formula provides 22.3% of the calories from linoleic acid.[9] (Table 17.2).

A relatively high intake of polyunsaturated fatty acids may affect cell membrane fragility, permeability or function. Animal studies suggest that the lipid composition of the central nervous system is not easily altered by dietary fat. Large amounts of alpha-tocopherol may be required to prevent intracellular peroxidation which may be induced by a high intake of polyunsaturated dietary lipids. In adults, Christakis *et al.* found no statistically significant differences in mean levels of alpha-

TABLE 17.2. COMPARISON OF CALORIC, CHOLESTEROL AND LIPID CONTENT OF BREAST MILK, COW'S MILK AND SIMILAC

	Breast Milk	Cow's Milk	Similac
Calories (per 100 ml)	71	69	67
Fat (g %)	3.8	3.7	3.4
Cholesterol (mg %)	20	14	1.5
Linoleic acid (g/100 g fat)	10.6	2.1	35
Percent calories from fat	54	48	46
Percent calories from linoleic acid	4	1.0	22.3

tocopherol in men who had been on a serum cholesterol lowering diet (P/S ratio 1.25) for up to four years.[10]

Dietary fat intake, in addition to inducing changes in serum lipid levels, induces changes in adipose tissue composition. Widdowson *et al.* found that the relative amount of linoleic acid was the same in Dutch and British infants at birth, i.e. 1–3% of total fatty acids.[8] It increased rapidly in the Dutch infants to 25% of adipose tissue composition the first month, and to 32–37% by the fourth month following intake of corn oil rich formulas. Linoleic acid never exceeded 3% in the fat of the British infants. The differences between the adipose tissue fat composition of the infants in the two countries was attributed to the nature of the fat in the milk they received, as British infants received cow's milk with only minor modifications. For the past ten years, many Dutch infants have received milk in which all of the cow's milk fat has been replaced by corn oil. The relationship between type and amount of dietary lipids and adipose tissue composition in infants may have profound metabolic significance with regard to the atherogenic process.

It is unknown whether highly unsaturated adipose tissue in children may be associated with decreased serum cholesterol levels later in life and may, therefore, be a factor in preventing atherosclerosis. No information is available regarding whether degree of saturation of body fat is related to cell multiplication and the likelihood of obesity later in life. Although dietary fat intake induces changes in adipose tissue composition, it is unknown if similar changes occur in the fatty acid composition of arteries, the central nervous system, cell membrane, and other cellular and subcellular components.

The "safety" of a low saturated fat, low cholesterol diet beginning in infancy has been evaluated; however, no definite conclusions have been reached. Dietary intervention, however, may be necessary in special circumstances such as Type II hyperlipidemia during infancy, although it is not generally recommended by the Committee on Nutrition of the American Academy of Pediatrics before the first year of age. This decision was reached because a low dietary cholesterol diet during infancy may be harmful to the growing brain which requires cholesterol for normal development.

Studies in experimental animals have suggested that high cholesterol feeding in early life will reduce serum cholesterol levels later in life; this, however, has not been proven for human infants. Friedman and Goldberg tested this hypothesis by comparing breast-fed and bottle-fed infants. Breast milk contains 26–52 mg cholesterol per 8 ounces (P/S ratio 0.8) whereas a widely used milk formula contains 4 mg of cholesterol per 8 ounces (P/S ratio 1.2). After 4–6 months, both groups switched to skim milk, taking approximately 200 mg cholesterol daily from all sources. The breast-fed infants had significantly higher cholesterol levels at 2–4 months, but after the first year, approximately the same serum cholesterol levels were found in both groups without any significant difference. It is concluded from this study that no protection against high serum cholesterol in later life is likely to be attained as a result of the feeding of a high cholesterol diet early in life.[7]

SERUM CHOLESTEROL IN PRESCHOOL CHILDREN

After the neonatal and infancy periods, serum cholesterol levels continue rising in normal children up to the prepubertal period, i.e. ages nine to 11. The prevalence of high serum cholesterol levels increase from 0.5% in cord blood to 1.3% in the preschool children due to genetic and/or environmental factors.[11]

A child of a father who had a premature myocardial infarction (M.I.) (under age 50) has a threefold greater chance of having an elevated serum cholesterol level compared to a child of a non-M.I. father. This increased chance of developing an elevated serum cholesterol level continues from the preschool age forward to school age and into adolescence.[12] However, children of parents with premature myocardial infarction in a low coronary heart disease country (such as Greece) do not exhibit significant differences in serum cholesterol and lipid levels when compared to children of healthy parents from the same environment.[13] The differences between these two countries of high (U.S.A.) and low (Greece) risk factor prevalence in childhood may be due to genetic hyperlipidemias with early manifestations in the U.S.A. and later (after age 20) in Greece.[13] However, the extent to which ethnic diet patterns may modify, prevent or predispose to hyperlipoproteinemia is also a likely factor.

Other risk factors such as smoking or type A behavior may play a more serious role in the etiology of CHD in the USA than in Greece.

Serum cholesterol levels of children one to 17 years of age have been obtained as part of the Health and Nutrition Examination Survey. The mean serum cholesterol was found to increase rapidly from 165 mg/dl in the first year to 176 mg/dl the second year for boys and girls. The mean serum cholesterol ranged from 168 to 180 mg/dl during the preschool years (two to six years). Girls were found to have higher serum cholesterol levels than boys in every age group. Black boys had higher mean serum cholesterol levels than white boys for every age group. Similar patterns were found for black girls compared to white girls.

SERUM CHOLESTEROL IN THE PRE-ADOLESCENT AND ADOLESCENT PERIODS

Although most studies appear to agree that one in 150 to 200 newborns have hypercholesterolemia, the prevalence increases with age. A study of school children six to 14 years of age in the Southern California Conference of Seventh Day Adventists Church Schools revealed that 7% had serum cholesterol levels above 220 mg/dl.[14] The mean serum cholesterol ranged from 161.2 mg/dl to 184.9 mg/dl for the age groups nine to 14 years. A peak level of serum cholesterol was found at the ages of ten to 12 followed by a subsequent dip. A similar dip in serum cholesterol levels was also reported by Hennekens *et al.*; thereafter, cholesterol levels continue to rise to adulthood.[12] The dip in serum cholesterol at midpuberty may be related to growth spurt and to the rapid increase of serum testosterone and estrogens but those relationships have not been elucidated. Schilling *et al.* studied the serum cholesterol and triglyceride levels of the late teenage period starting at age 18.[15] An accelerated rate of increase in serum cholesterol was noted between ages 19 and 30. They advanced the concept of "cholesterol-years" of exposure to rising levels of serum cholesterol which was hypothesized as linked to the atherogenic process. A study of serum cholesterol levels of adolescents, however, suggests substantial variability among divergent ethnic and racial groups in adolescent boys and girls in New York City.[16] Table 17.3 summarizes recent studies of serum cholesterol levels in childhood.

Serum cholesterol levels appear to be closely related to sociocultural characteristics of the eating patterns of children. As an example, the mean serum cholesterol level of 5–15 year old Mexican children was found to be 99.9 mg/dl in contrast to the mean cholesterol level of comparable Wisconsin pupils which was twice as high (186.5 mg/dl).[17] The conclusions of this study suggest that the cholesterol level characteristics of these two populations have been developed by elementary school age as there were no differences in mean serum cholesterol between the 5–9 year age group and the 10–14 year age group in either study population. There are, however, no longitudinal data in children and adolescents indicating changes of serum lipid levels by age and relationships to their nutrition and sociocultural environment.

TABLE 17.3. MEAN CHOLESTEROL LEVELS IN CHILDREN BY AGE

Investigators	Sex/Age	Cholesterol (mg%)
Harrison & Peat 1975	M/F Cord blood	98.5±22.1
"	M/F 5th day	146.6±24.6
"	M/F 8th day	154.8±24.3
Beal 1970[52]	M/F 1–6 yrs	168 (95–246 range)
"	M/F 6–14 yrs	167 (107–249 range)
"	M 14–18 yrs	156 (155–206 range)
Wiese *et al* 1966[53]	M/F 1–5 yrs	156±38
"	M/F 5–10 yrs	157±27
"	M/F 10–15 yrs	172±22
Owen *et al* 1971[11]	M/F 1–2 yrs	159
"	M/F 2–6 yrs	165
Clarke *et al* 1970[54]	M/F 16–18 yrs	166±30
Baker *et al* 1967[55]	M/F 10–13 yrs	154±32.5
Schilling *et al* 1964[15]	M 16–20 yrs	199±3.6
Friedman & Goldberg 1975[7]	M/F 2–4 mos breast fed	146±4.6
"	M/F 12 mos breast fed	145.8±1.5
"	M/F 18–24 mos breast fed	155.8±6.0
"	M/F 2–4 mos formula fed	123.8±8.3
"	M/F 12 mos formula fed	141.4±1.6
"	M/F 18–24 mos formula fed	154.6±4.5
"	M 15–19 yrs	156.2±7.9
"	F 15–19 yrs	154.9±5.7
Glueck *et al* 1972[56]	M/F 12 mos	129
Rosanen *et al* 1977[57]	M 5–19 yrs	234
Leonard *et al* 1976[58]	M 2–13 yrs	165.3±38.6
Hennekens *et al* 1976[12]	M/F 1–21 yrs (children of healthy men)	176.6+27.9
"	M/F 1–21 yrs (children of men affected by M.I.)	185.1±45
Hodges and Krehl 1965[59]	M 14–19 yrs	160±34
Frerichs *et al* 1977[60]	M/F 5–14 yrs	165.3
"	M/F 5–14 yrs (blacks)	170
"	M/F 5–14 yrs (whites)	162
Friedman & Goldberg 1973[61]	M/F 9–19 yrs	157
Webber *et al* 1978[6]	M/F Cord blood	70
"	M/F 6 mos	135
"	M/F 12 mos	145
Friedman 1975[62]	M/F 0–5 yrs (Arizona)	169
"	M/F 0–5 yrs (Mexico)	148

HIGH DENSITY LIPOPROTEIN (HDL) AND LOW DENSITY LIPOPROTEIN (LDL) CHOLESTEROL AS CHD RISK VARIABLES

Until recently, most lipid studies of childhood and adolescence included total serum cholesterol and/or triglycerides as a risk factor for CHD in later life. It is unknown, however, whether adult serum cholesterol levels can be predicted from serum lipid values in infancy and childhood.[18] It has now been determined that LDL is positively correlated with CHD risk. It thus appears plausible that total cholesterol may have incomplete value for CHD risk prediction and that future studies should differentiate between cholesterol fractions, i.e. HDL and LDL cholesterol. These fractions in childhood and adolescence may enhance or complement the predictive value of adult cholesterol and triglyceride levels as related to later CHD risk. This concept has been supported by recent studies in the U.S.A. and New Zealand.[19,21]

It has also been shown that by measuring the concentration of beta or LDL rather than total cholesterol in cord blood, the diagnosis of hyperbetalipoproteinemia can be made more reliably in the newborn who has an affected parent.[22] Further research is required in order to determine the effect of environmental factors on HDL, LDL and total serum cholesterol early in life.

SERUM CHOLESTEROL BINDING RESERVE (SCBR) CONCEPT AS ANOTHER CHD RISK FACTOR DETERMINANT

It has been proposed that two serum lipoprotein subfractions separated from very low density and HDL have physiological roles in retarding atherogenesis by removing cholesterol from the arterial intima and transporting it back to the circulating serum.[23] Accordingly, individuals having low SCBR, being deficient in those subfractions, may be at higher CHD risk. This hypothesis was tested with patients having premature myocardial infarction.

SCBR was found to be significantly lower in M.I. patients than in controls.[23,24] Further support for this hypothesis was provided by measuring SCBR in diabetic adults in comparison to nondiabetic normal controls of the same age range and sex. These results indicated that the SCBR of diabetic subjects was significantly lower (71.9 mg/dl) than the control subjects (88.9 mg/dl). The SCBR hypothesis as a predictor of future CHD merits testing in children.

HYPERTENSION is a major risk factor associated with coronary heart disease in developed countries of the world. The risk is continuous, i.e. the greater the blood pressure, the greater the risk of the CHD event. Hypertension occurs in family aggregates, suggesting a genetic basis; perhaps up to 60% of the population variance may be attributed to genetic differences.[25] Environmental factors on the other hand may account for 10–15% of the total population variance. Many host and environmental factors are apparently responsible for striking differences in blood pressure prevalence patterns throughout the world. These differences are reflected in the widespread diversity of prevalence rates of hypertension and coronary heart disease among various peoples and in various countries. It is unclear when and how these host and environmental factors are combined to trigger or cause hypertension. It is still unknown what blood pressure level is normal for a given population in a specific geographic area. This is especially true for infants and children where normative blood pressure data has only recently been published for children two to 18 years of age but has not been established for younger children.[26]

BLOOD PRESSURE AND SALT INTAKE

The epidemiology of hypertension and the influence of salt intake, obesity, physiological and social stress has recently been reviewed.[27] It has been proposed that excess salt intake over a number of years may trigger the appearance of hypertension in genetically susceptible individuals. Dahl *et al.* (1968) fed commercially prepared baby food to rats, most of which subsequently died of hypertension.[28] (Commercial baby food preparations were soon modified to limit salt content.) In addition to baby foods, infants ingest four times higher salt intakes when fed cow's milk compared to breast milk. Children in developed countries of the world appear to be nutritionally exposed to a sodium-rich environment.

The average salt intake in the U.S.A. is estimated to be 10–12 g per day which is well above the human requirement of approximately 4 g daily. However, the relationship of salt intake to hypertension is not clear. Dahl's population studies indicate that the higher sodium intakes are associated with a greater prevalence of hypertension.[29,30] On the other hand, experiments in adults with mild, untreated essential hypertension have shown that the administration of 6 g NaCl daily from two to nine weeks did not cause edema or significant changes in body weight or blood pressure.[31] However, only a moderate amount of salt was given for a short period of time during the course of this study. In a similar study of adults, large amounts of sodium were given (37 g NaCl above the usual salt intake) to normotensive adults, resulting in facial puffiness with progressive increase in blood pressure.

Epidemiologic observations suggest a relationship between salt ingestion and hypertension but fail to support the hypothesis that salt consumption is a major factor.[32] Indeed, there is no direct evidence to support the hypothesis that hypertension can be produced in a normotensive man ingesting the usual intake of salt.[31,33] On the other hand, the blood pressure of hypertensive individuals can be reduced by a diet that is low in salt.[34,35] Whether arterial hypertension develops from ingestion of a high-salt diet may depend on genetic predilections, time of exposure and sociologic factors such as crowded living conditions and socioeconomic mobility.

Studies correlating the sodium intake in infancy to blood pressure have been recently initiated (Table 17.4). Such studies are difficult to conduct because many years of follow-up are required. A recent study demonstrated a significant association between the type of infant feeding and diastolic blood pressure.[36] The mean diastolic blood pressure was significantly lower in breast-fed babies compared to bottle-fed babies. The significantly higher blood pressure in the whole-milk-fed babies was attributed to higher sodium content of cow's milk vs human milk. The determination of blood pressure levels in infancy has been the focus of work by Levine *et al.* who by the use of Doppler sphygmomanometry have found that infants who exhibit specific upper percentile of blood pressure levels at birth remain in the same "track" by the end of the first year.[37] It remains to be determined whether infants in the higher percentiles of blood pressure continue to follow the same percentiles in childhood and adolescence.

The studies of Zinner *et al.* suggest that hypertension in adults could be predicted from blood pressure patterns in children and adolescents.[38] Zinner states that it is uncommon to find hypertension after the age of 30 in previously normotensive persons. This strongly suggests the origin

TABLE 17.4. PREVALENCE OF HYPERTENSION IN CHILDREN

Author	Population	Age	Prevalence of Hypertension %
Masland *et al* (1956)[63]	1,795	12–21	1.4
Londe (1966)[64]	1,473	4–15	2.3
Kimura and Ota (1965)[65]	2,728 (Japanese)	0–19	0.6 (hypertensive) 9.2 (borderline)
Heyden *et al* (1969)[66]	435	15–25	11.0
Christakis *et al* (1968)[16]	74 (obese)	10–13	11.0
	556 (non-obese)	10–13	2.5
Johnson *et al* (1975)[67]	168 (white males)	15–29	19.0
	106 (black males)	15–29	34.0
Lauer *et al* (1976)[68]	1,315	14–18	8.9 (systolic) 12.2 (diastolic)
de Castro *et al* (1976)[69]	320	15–19	3.6
Kilkoyne *et al* (1974)[70]	434	12–20	6.9
Cretens (1977)[71]	1,183	college students	5.4 systolic 1.9 diastolic
Cassimos *et al* (1977)[72]	4,428	7–18	3.1
Webber *et al* (1973)[73]	457	15–19	5

of hypertension to be early in life. Although this may be due to genetic influences, early environmental factors may also contribute to hypertension. In a recent longitudinal study, adult blood pressure tracking correlations are reached by age 20, a finding which may have important implications for understanding the natural history of elevated blood pressure and perhaps for decisions concerning intervention.[39]

Briefly summarizing, hypertension is a major risk factor associated with coronary heart disease in Western populations but not in Japan or the Bahamas.[40] Hypertension occurs in family aggregates, thus suggesting a genetic basis. Environmental factors, on the other hand, also play an important role. Sodium intake and obesity are also related to hypertension. Longstanding hypertension appears to alter arterial structure to increase peripheral resistance. Elevation of systolic or diastolic pressure or both promote atherogenesis and myocardial infarction.

NUTRITIONAL DETERMINANTS OF OBESITY

There is a contemporary tendency of all age groups of both sexes to gain excessive weight. The mean birthweight doubling time is 3.8 months today compared to 5–6 months reported several years ago.[41] Bottle-fed infants double their birthweight much earlier compared to breast-fed infants. The reason appears to be that solid foods were introduced earlier to bottle-fed infants than to breast-fed infants. Bottle-fed infants may become overfed because the mother determines feeding termination by encouraging the infant to empty the bottle. On the other hand, breast-fed babies are more active, spend less time in bed, and receive more attention from their mothers. Early introduction of solid food having high caloric density may also contribute to obesity.

The prevalence of obesity, i.e. having a relative weight over 120%, was 16.7% in 300 infants studied in England.[42] In Sweden, obesity prevalence was 15–23%. In the U.S.A. 14% of preschool children had excessive weight, defined as over the 85 percentile for weight on the Iowa Growth Chart. It is estimated that there are 10 million obese adolescents in the U.S.A.[43]

The above-cited prevalence of obesity is based on different methods used by the investigators in defining obesity. There is indeed a problem defining the degree of fatness which can be called obesity. Children exceeding two standard deviations in weight can be considered overweight but may not be obese. However, an infant whose weight is in excess of three standard deviations, and whose length is not proportionately increased, is much more likely to be obese.

Among seven countries studied, the island of Crete in Greece has been found to have the lowest prevalence of CHD.[44,45] Cretan men, aged

40–65 years, were found to weigh 7 kg less than a comparative group of age-matched New York City residents. Although the incidence of CHD continues to be low in the adult cohort, the prevalence of elevated CHD risk factors, such as obesity, appears to be increased in the current generation of Cretan men.[46] In a recent study of 268 children aged 13 to 15 months in Crete (county C), the prevalence of obesity was investigated in relation to two other counties (A and B) having intermediate and high infant mortality compared to Greece's mean infant mortality rate. (Table 17.5). These data indicate that the county with the lowest infant mortality rate (county C) and the highest socioeconomic level, also has the highest prevalence of obesity (31% of the children over 110% relative weight) compared to the lower socioeconomic areas (counties A and B—10% in county A and 25% in county B with relative weight over 110%).[47]

Overweight or obese infants have a greater frequency of illness, specifically respiratory infections. Although these obese children have increased morbidity, there is no evidence that mortality is higher. The long-term problem is that obesity in the first six months of life may have a high predictive rate for childhood obesity.

Dr. Donald B. Cheek's statement merits quoting: "the fetus exists before the infant and the mother before the fetus." How may maternal nutritional status have a direct impact on the nutritional determinants of chronic disease in the fetus?

TABLE 17.5. RELATIONSHIP OF INFANT MORTALITY TO PREVALENCE OF OBESITY

Counties Having Different Infant Mortality Rates	n	Excessive Relative Weight (110–120%) %	Obesity (over 120%) %
A. 63/1000	101	7	3
B. 32/1000	108	19	6
C. 13/1000	268	24	7
Total	477	19	6

1. The weight of the mother, before and during pregnancy, is related to the size of the newborn. The more weight gained, the larger the fetus and the newborn; however, birthweight is not correlated with later overweight or obesity.
2. Mothers of excess-weight infants are older, have greater parity, are taller and heavier.
3. Mothers who give birth to smaller babies have a greater prevalence of smoking and hypertension.
4. The nutritional patterns of the mother provide the substrate from which the fetus cell number and size are partially determined. Some pregnant women, especially teenagers, have low protein and iron

intake before and during their pregnancies. On the other hand, an intake of excessive saturated fats and refined carbohydrates will result in weight gain, contributed by foods of low nutrient density. Such a diet may predispose to fetal hypercholesterolemia and hypertriglyceridemia as well as result in a newborn with more and/or larger fat cells. A related question emerges—what influence does maternal diet pattern have on the infant's? Is the infant "conditioned" to certain nutritional patterns by the diet of the mother?

5. Amino acid imbalance contributes to growth retardation. In postnatal life, growth hormone increases nuclear number in metabolically active protoplasm while insulin is involved in cytoplasmic growth. Thus factors which control synthesis of these hormones control growth. At term, adrenal enlargement occurs resulting in increased glycogen storage. Since the many steroid hormones elaborated by the adrenal may require adequate vitamin C for synthesis and/or release, overall nutritional status is patently important.

CONCLUSION

Chronic diseases such as coronary heart disease, hypertension, obesity, diabetes and cancer appear to exhibit a long latent incubation period and metabolic pathogenesis. Atherosclerosis may have precursors early in life and may progress at a variable rate dependent upon many genetic and environmental factors. Fatty streaks appear in the endothelium of the aorta in infancy; they may remain unchanged, disappear or ultimately develop into fibrous streaks which may progress to atherosclerotic plaque. In populations having a high prevalence of CHD, fibrous plaques appear in the aorta during adolescence.[48,49] These lesions contain more lipid, more inflammatory cells and more extracellular lipid and necrotic debris than did lesions in adolescents from populations with less severe atherosclerosis.[50] Recent studies demonstrate definite regression of the atherosclerotic lesions of the arteries after relatively brief periods of nutritional intervention.[51] Such findings have been confirmed by experiments in primates; they provide unequivocal evidence that plaque regression could occur as a result of a low saturated fat and low cholesterol diet.

Should a "Prudent Diet" be initiated in school-age children in an effort to prevent premature cardiovascular disease? Should a lowered salt intake be recommended? Should not regular physical activity be part of school and home life? Arterial blood pressure measurements should be part of the pediatric clinical examination as hypertension has its roots in childhood and adolescence. The Prudent Diet and antismoking attitudes in childhood may also tend to prevent lung and colon cancer.

Finally, breast feeding and late introduction of solid foods appear to be the most appropriate nutritional pattern in infancy which may prevent the later onset of obesity and hypertension.

REFERENCES

1. TEN-STATE NUTRITION SURVEY: United States Department of Health, Education and Welfare, Anthropometric data, D.H.E.W. Publication No. (HSM) 72-8130, 1972.
2. KANNEL, W.B. and DAWBER, T.R. Hypertensive cardiovascular disease: The Framingham study, in Hypertensive Mechanisms and Management, ed. by Onesti, G., Kim, K.E., Moyer, J.H., New York. Grune and Stratton, pp. 93–110, 1974.
3. GLUECK, C.J., HECKMAN, F., SCHOENFELD, M., STEINER, P., PEARCE, W.: Neonatal familial type II hyperlipoproteinemia: Cord blood cholesterol in 1800 births. Metabolism 20, 597, 1971.
4. HARRISON, W.C. and PEAT, G.: Serum cholesterol and bowel flora in the newborn. Am. J. Clin. Nutrition 28, 135, 1975.
5. LEVY, R.I. and RIFKIND, B.M.: Diagnosis and management of hyperlipoproteinemia in infants and children. Amer. J. Cardiol. 31, 547, 1973.
6. WEBBER, L.S., SRINIVASAN, S.R., FRERISHS, R.R., BERENSON, G.S.: Serum lipids and lipoproteins in the first year of life—The Bogolusa newborn cohort study (Abstract) 18th Annual conference on cardiovascular disease epidemiology, Orlando, Florida, 1978.
7. FRIEDMAN, G. and GOLDBERG, S.J.: Concurrent and subsequent serum cholesterol of breast and formula fed infants. Amer. J. Clin. Nutr. 28, 42, 1975.
8. WIDDOWSON, E.M., DAUNCEY, M.J., GARDNER, D.M.T., JONXIS, J.H.P., PELICAN-FILIPKOVA, M.: Body fat of British and Dutch infants. Brit. Med. J. I, 654, 1975.
9. SCHUBERT, W.K.: Fat, nutrition and diet in childhood. Amer. J. Cardiol. 31, 58, 1973.
10. CHRISTAKIS, G., RINZLER, S.H., ARCHER, M., HASHIM, S.A., and VAN ITALLIE, T.B.: Effects of a serum cholesterol-lowering diet on composition of depot fat in man. Am. J. Clin. Nutr. 16, 243, 1965.
11. OWEN, G.M., LUBIN, A.H., GARRY, P.J.: Nutritional status of preschool children. Midwest Society for Pediatric Research, November 1971.
12. HENNEKENS, C.H., JESSE, M.J., KLEIN, B.E., GOURLEY, J.E., BLUMENTHAL, S.: Cholesterol among children of men with myocardial infarction. Pediatrics 58, 211, 1976.
13. KAFATOS, A.G., NIKOLAIDIS, G., KAFATOS, E., HSIA, S.L., FORDYCE, M.K., CASSADY, J., CHRISTAKIS, G.: Risk factor status of myocardial infarction (MI) and non-MI subjects and their children in Crete (Abstract) Proceedings of the Symposium "The Child in the World of Tomorrow," Athens, July 2–8, 1978.

14. STARR, P.: Hypercholesterolemia in school children. Amer. J. Clin. Path. 56, 515, 1971.
15. SCHILLING, F.J., CHRISTAKIS, G., BENNETT, N.J., COYLE, J.F.: Studies of serum cholesterol in 4,244 men and women: An epidemiological and pathogenetic interpretation. Amer. J. Public Health, 54, 401, 1964.
16. CHRISTAKIS, G., MIRIDJANIAN, A., NATH, L., KHURANA, H.S., COWELL, C., ARCHER, M., FRANK, O., ZIFFER, H., BAKER, H., JAMES, G.: A nutritional epidemiologic investigation of 642 New York City children. Amer. J. Clin. Nutr. 21, 107, 1968.
17. GOLUBJATNIKOV, R., PASKEY, T., INHORN, S.L.: Serum cholesterol levels of Mexican and Wisconsin school children. Amer. J. Epidemiol. 96, 36, 1972.
18. KANNEL, W.B. and DAWBER, T.R.: Atherosclerosis as a pediatric problem. J. Pediatrics 80, 544, 1972.
19. TYROLER, H.A., HAMES, C.G., KRISHAN, I., HEYDEN, S., COOPER, G., CASSEL, J.C.: Black-white differences in serum lipids and lipoproteins in Evans County. Preventive Medicine 43, 541, 1975.
20. STANHOPE, J.M., SAMPSON, V.M., CLARKSON, P.M.: High-density-lipoprotein cholesterol and other serum lipi-s in a New Zealand Biracial adolescent sample. The Warroa College Survey. Lancet 1, 968, 1977.
21. RHOADS, G.G., GULBRANDSEN, C.L., KAGAN, A.: Serum lipoproteins and coronary heart disease in a population study of Hawaii Japanese men. New Engl. J. Med. 294, 293, 1976.
22. KWITEROVICH, P.O., LEVY, R.I., FREDRICKSON, D.S.: Neonatal diagnosis of familial type II hyperlipoproteinemia. Lancet 1, 118, 1973.
23. HSIA, S.L., CHAO, Y.S., HENNEKENS, C.H., READER, W.B.: Decreased serum cholesterol-binding reserve in premature myocardial infarction. Lancet 2, 1000, 1975.
24. HSIA, S.L., BRIESE, F., HOFFMAN, J.: Cholesterol binding reserve and myocardial infarction (Letter to the editor). Lancet 1, 799, 1976.
25. FEINLEIB, M.: Genetic and familial aggregation of blood pressure. Fifth Hahneman International Symposium on Hypertension, January 1977, San Juan, Puerto Rico.
26. PEDIATRICS: Standards for children's blood pressure. Blood Pressure Control, Supplement 59, 802, 1977.
27. CHRISTAKIS, G.: The enigmas of essential hypertension. Monograph, Roche Laboratories, Hoffman-LaRoche Inc., Nutley, New Jersey, 1977.
28. DAHL, L.K. *et al*: Effects of chronic salt ingestion: modification of experimental hypertension in the rat by variations in the diet. Circ. Res. 22, 1, 1968.
29. DAHL, L.K. and LOVE, R.A.: Evidence for relationship between sodium intake and human essential hypertension. Arch. Internat. Med. 94, 525, 1954.
30. DAHL, L.K.: Possible role of chronic excess salt consumption in the pathogenesis of essential hypertension. Amer. J. Cardiol. 8, 571, 1961.
31. GROSS, G., WELLER, J.M., HOOBLER, S.W.: Relationship of sodium and potassium intake to blood pressure. Amer. J. Clin. Nutr. 24, 605, 1971.

32. AMERICAN ACADEMY OF PEDIATRICS, Committee on Nutrition: Salt intake and eating patterns of infants and children in relation to blood pressure. Pediatrics 53, 115, 1974.
33. BROWN, W.J., BROWN, F.K., KIRSHAN, I.: Exchangeable sodium and blood volume in normotensive and hypertensive humans on high and low sodium intake. Circulation 43, 508, 1971.
34. CONCORAN, A.C., TAYLOR, R.D., PAGE, I.H.: Controlled observations on the effect of low sodium diet therapy in essential hypertension. Circulation, 3, 1, 1951.
35. DOLE, V.P., DAHL, L.K., COTZIAS, G.C.: Dietary treatment of hypertension: II sodium depletion as related to the therapeutical effect. J. Clin. Invest. 30, 584, 1951.
36. ELLISON, R.C., GORDON, M.J., SUSENKO, J.M., LERER, T.J.: Breast feeding and later blood pressure in the child (Abstract) 18th annual conference on Cardiovascular Disease Epidemiology. March 13–16, Orlando, Florida, 1978.
37. LEVINE, R.L., HENNEKENS, C.H., KLEIN, B., COURLEY, J., BRIESE, F.W., HOKANSON, J., GELBAND, H., JESSE, M.J.: Tracking correlations of blood pressure levels in infancy. J. Pediatrics. 61, 121, 1978.
38. ZINNER, S.H., LEVY, P.S., KASS, E.H.: Familial aggregation of blood pressure in children. N. Eng. J. Med. 284, 401, 1971.
39. ROSNER, B., HENNEKENS, C.H., KASS, E.H., MIALL, W.E.: Age-specific correlation analysis of longitudinal blood pressure data. Amer. J. Epidemiol. 106, 306, 1977.
40. LUNN, J.A., MIRIDJANIAN, A., FONTANARES, P., JACOBS, E., ROSEN, S., CHRISTAKIS, G.: Epidemiological reconnaissance of hypertension in the Bahamas: with special reference to depot fat composition and its implications in relation to cardiovascular disease prevalence. Mount Sinai J. Medicine 41, 444, 1974.
41. NEWMANN, C.G. and ALPAUGH, M.: Birthweight doubling time: A fresh look. Pediatrics 57, 469, 1976.
42. SHUKLA, A., FORSYTH, H.S., ANDERSON, C.M., MARWAH, S.M.: Infant overnutrition in the first year of life—A field study in Dudley, Worcestershire. Brit. Med. J. IV. 507, 1972.
43. WILSON, N.L.: Obesity. F.A. Davis Company, Philadelphia, 1969.
44. CHRISTAKIS, G., SEVERINGHAUS, E.L., MALDONADO, Z., KAFATOS, F., HASHIM, S.A: Crete: A study in the metabolic epidemiology of coronary heart disease. Amer. J. Cardio. 15, 320, 1965.
45. KEYS, A. (Ed.): Coronary heart disease in seven countries. Circulation, 41, suppl. 1, 1970.
46. ARAVANIS, C. and CORCONDILAS, A.: Atherosclerotic cardiovascular mortality in the island of Crete study, in Atherosclerosis, Metabolic, Morphologic and Clinical Aspects. Advances in Experimental Medicine and Biology, Edited by G.W. Manning and M.D. Haust, Plenum Press, New York and London, Vol. 84, 1977.
47. KAFATOS, A.G., BADA, A., PANTELAKIS, S., DOXIADIS, S.: Infant morbidity and mortality in three counties of Greece. Relationships of infant

morbidity and mortality to medical and sociocultural factors. Iatriki 33, 39, 1978.
48. TEJADA, C., STRONG, J.P., MONTENEGRO, M.R., RESTREPO, C. and SOLBERG, L.A.: Distribution of coronary and aortic atherosclerosis by geographic location, race and sex. Lab. Investig. 18, 509, 1968.
49. STRONG, J.P. and McGILL, H.C.: The pediatric aspects of atherosclerosis. J. Atheroscler. Res. 9, 251, 1969.
50. McGILL, H.C.: The lesion in children. In Atherosclerosis, Metabolic, Morphologic and Clinical Aspects, edited by G.W. Manning and M.D. Haust. Advances in Experimental Medicine and Biology, Plenum Press, New York and London Vol. 84, 1977.
51. BUCHWALD, H., MORE, R.B., VARCO, B.L.: The partial ileal bypass operation in treatment of hyperlipidemias. In Lipids, Lipoproteins and Drugs, edited by D. Kritchevsky, R. Paoletti, W.I. Holmes. Advances in Experimental Medicine and Biology, New York and London. Vol. 63, pp. 221–230, 1975.
52. BEAL, V.: Nutritional intake. Human growth and Development, Cannon, R.W.M. ed. Charles C. Thomas, Springfield, Ill. 63–100, 1970.
53. WIESE, S.H., BENNETT, M.O., BRAUM, I.H., *et al*: Blood serum lipid patterns during infancy and childhood. Amer. J. Clin. Nutr. 18, 155, 1966.
54. CLARKE, R.P., MERROW, S.B., MORSE, E.H. *et al*: Interrelationships between plasma lipids, physical measurements and body fatness of adolescents in Burlington, Vermont. Amer. J. Clin. Nutr. 23, 754, 1970.
55. BAKER, H., FRANK, O., FEINGOLD, S., CHRISTAKIS, G., ZIFFER, H.: Vitamins, total cholesterol and triglycerides in 642 New York City school children. Amer. J. Clin. Nutr. 20, 850, 1967.
56. GLUECK, C.J. and TSANG, R.C.: Pediatric familial type II hyperlipoproteinemia: Effects of diet on plasma cholesterol in the first year of life. Amer. J. Clin. Nutr. 25, 224, 1972.
57. ROSANEN, L. *et al*: Nutrition survey of Finnish rural children. IV. Serum cholesterol values in relation to dietary variables (for publication) 1977.
58. LEONARD, J.V., FORBROOKE, A.S., LLOYD, J.K., WOLFF, O.H.: Screening for familial hyperlipoproteinemia in children in hospitals. Arch. Dis. Child. 51, 842, 1976.
59. HODGES, R.E. and KREHL, W.A.: Nutritional status of teenagers in Iowa. Amer. J. Clin. Nutr. 17, 200, 1965.
60. FRERICHS, R.R., SRINIVASAN, S.R., WEBBER, L.S., BERENSON, G.S.: Serum cholesterol and triglyceride levels in children from a Biracial community. The Bogalusa heart study, In Atherosclerosis, Metabolic, Morphologic and Clinical Aspects, *in* Advances in Experimental Medicine and Biology, edited by G.W. Manning and M.D. Haust, Plenum Press, New York and London, Vol. 84, 1977.
61. FRIEDMAN, G. and GOLDBERG, S.J.: Normal serum cholesterol values percentile ranking in a middle class pediatric population. JAMA 225, 610, 1973.
62. FRIEDMAN, G.M.: Atherosclerosis and the pediatrician in childhood obesity, edited by M. Winick. Vol. 3 in the Wiley Series on Current Concepts in Nutrition, New York, 1975.

63. MASLAND, R.P., HEALD, F.P., GOODALE, W.T., GALLAGHER, J.R.: Hypertensive vascular disease in adolescence. N. Engl. J. Med. 225, 894, 1950.
64. LONDE, S.: Blood pressure in children as determined under office conditions. Clin. Pediatr. 5, 71, 1966.
65. KIMURA, T. and OTA, M.: Epidemiologic study of hypertension, comparative results of hypertensive surveys in two areas in northern Japan. Amer. J. Clin. Nutr. 17, 381, 1965.
66. HEYDEN, S., BARTEL, A.G., HARMERS, C.G., McDONOUGH, J.R.: Elevated blood pressure levels in adolescents. Evans County, Georgia, Seven-year follow-up of 30 patients and 30 controls. JAMA 209, 1683, 1969.
67. JOHNSON, A.L., CORNONI, J.C., CASSELL, J.C., TYROLER, H.A., HEYDEN, S., HAMES, C.: Influence of race, sex and weight on blood pressure behavior in young adults. Amer. J. Cardiol. 35, 523, 1975.
68. LAUER, R.M., FILER, L.J., REITER, M.A., CLARKE, W.R.: Blood pressure, salt preference, salt threshold and relative weight. Amer. J. Dis. Child. 130, 493, 1976.
69. DE CASTRO, F.J., BISBROECK, R., ERIKSON, C. *et al*: Hypertension in adolescents. Clin. Pediatr. 15, 24, 1976.
70. KILKOYNE, M.M., RICHTER, R.W., ALSUF, P.A.: Adolescent hypertension. I. Detection and prevalence. Circulation 50, 758, 1974.
71. CRETENS, M.S.: A hypertension screening program of children in Delta and Menominee Counties (Michigan) J. Am. Med. Wom. Assoc. 32, 216, 1977.
72. CASSIMOS, C., VARLAMIS, G., KARAMPERIS, S. and KATSOUYANNOPOULOS, V.: Blood pressure in children and adolescents. Acta Paediatr. Scand. 66, 439, 1977.
73. WEBBER, M.A., STROKES, G.S., MOSES, M. *et al*: Hypertension survey in a central free chest x-ray clinic: The Sydney hospital hypertension project. Med. J. Austr. 2, 529, 1973.

18

FEEDING CHILDREN

Lewis A. Barness, M.D.

I. INFANT NUTRITION

Nutrition remains a cornerstone in the wellbeing of infants for the first years. Many believe that early nutrition and establishment of good feeding practices may influence the later development of the child, even to the extent of affecting the onset of degenerative diseases in later life. All those providing medical care for children can and should provide information to parents regarding present understanding of infant nutrition in the hope that some illnesses in children may be lessened and the goals of prolonged better health attained.

For the past several decades infant feeding practices have been largely directed by parents who have occasionally based these practices on unsound information. While in most instances such happenstance practices have resulted in infants who thrive, some instances of illness could have been prevented had more careful practices been instituted early in life. The large majority of infants are resilient and can correct minor errors in nutrition. For the 5% or 10% of infants who are more subject to illness, early aids may avoid the illnesses.

BREAST FEEDING?

For eons it was recognized that newborn infants lived only when fed breast milk. With technical advances in artificial formula making and adequate refrigeration, over the last 30 or 40 years it was widely believed that infants thrived equally well when nourished with breast milk or

---

Dr. Barness is Professor and Chairman, Department of Pediatrics, University of South Florida College of Medicine, Tampa.

simulated human milk formulas. Even the most recent studies comparing breast and bottle-fed infants indicate that in a highly developed area, Cooperstown, New York, breast-fed infants have a significantly lower morbidity than those fed simulated human milk formulas.[1]

Among the advantages of breast milk are the following:

Breast milk is less likely to be associated with allergic manifestations in infants. It has been suggested that the lower level of casein and the unique qualities of human lactalbumin are responsible for the lower allergenicity compared with cow's milk or soybean protein.[2]

Iron in breast milk is readily absorbed; that in cow's milk formulas is less easily absorbed.[3] Evidence has been presented to indicate that even though breast milk contains little iron, breast-fed infants not supplemented with iron-containing foods are unlikely to become iron-deficient or anemic. Bottle-fed infants must receive iron supplementation to prevent anemia not only because nonhuman milks contain little iron but also because excessive ingestion of unmodified cow's milk may cause gastrointestinal bleeding.

Zinc and perhaps other trace minerals are also more readily available from breast milk than other milks.[4] Infants with acrodermatitis enteropathica, a severe and often fatal diarrheal disease, frequently survived when fed breast milk but not other milks. Initially this was attributed to the essential fatty acid content of breast milk. Subsequently, it was recognized that this condition was associated with zinc deficiency secondary to poor absorption of zinc in formula-fed infants; zinc absorption was found to be facilitated in breast-fed infants, accounting for their survival.

Breast-fed infants have increased resistance to gastrointestinal and respiratory infections. This is and probably will remain for some time the least likely to be duplicated property of formulas. Specific antibodies which effectively suppress viruses and bacteria in the intestinal tract, e.g. IgA, nonspecific factors such as lysozyme and lactoferrin, as well as human macrophages in human milk which grow in the intestinal tract help improve resistance to infections. Artificial or synthetic sources of these substances do not seem to be on the horizon.[5]

Cretinism may be mitigated by breast feeding, perhaps because of significant thyroid hormones in milk.[6] Low birth weight infants also seem to benefit from fresh breast milk. The better response of low birth weight or prematurely born infants has been attributed to the presence of specific antibodies, the unique characteristics of the protein and fat, or the lower osmolality of human milk.

Less certain advantages of breast feeding have been suggested. Emotional attachment of the infant and parents can be equal whether the infant is bottle of breast fed. Obesity seems less frequent in breast-fed infants but can occur. Calcium absorption, which is poor when cow's milk is fed, is corrected by presently available formulas. The protein content in formulas is lowered to approach that of human milk and the carbohydrate is limited to lactose which produces an acid milieu in the intestine. Scurvy and rickets which are rare in the breast-fed infant[7] are eliminated in the simulation human milk formula-fed infants since these contain added vitamins C and D.

WHAT CAN THE DOCTOR DO?

The most positive influence in the encouragement of breast feeding is in the hands and thoughts initially of the obstetrician. The most negative influences have been found to be discouragement by the obstetrician or the nursery nurses. Many pediatricians also have not encouraged nursing, and this negative or neutral feeling has been transmitted to mothers. Encouragement by the pediatrician, husband, grandmother, and others helps, even though many of these may have been bottle fed.

The recent increase in the number of nursing mothers compared to the last two decades indicates that society is ready to accept nursing after a 20 year decline. First started in the middle and upper classes, nursing has been accepted by the activist groups, and more recently by some of the lower socioeconomic families. Nursing mothers may have problems which differ from those of bottle-feeding mothers. Encouragement and support by the obstetrician, nurses, and physicians caring for the children are necessary. Convincing mothers with fissured nipples and breast abscesses to continue nursing is difficult, but suitable shields or antibiotics can help. Explanation of the benefits of nursing to the baby frequently overcomes the mother's doubts.

Some mothers will not nurse. Social, psychological, economic, and health reasons may prevent nursing. Such mothers should be advised to use a formula which closely simulates human milk, in which the protein and electrolyte contents are lowered, where the saturated fat has been replaced with polyunsaturated fats, and where the formula is supplemented with iron and vitamins.

Breast feeding or formula feeding continues until the baby conveniently drinks from a cup and eats a varied diet, usually at 9–12 months of age.

SOLID FEEDINGS

The time for introducing solid feedings has been clouded by social, sociological, and developmental considerations. Early introduction of solid feedings has no known nutritional basis for infants fed human milk.

Human milk apparently contains sufficient nutrients as a sole food until nine to 12 months of age. Cow's milk or formulas may not be complete foods; for example, zinc, iron and vitamin D supplementation are needed. Other deficiencies may be found but, as stated by the Committee on Nutrition of the American Academy of Pediatrics in 1958, there are no known advantages to introducing solid feedings before 3–4 months of age or even later in the breast-fed.

There are recognized harmful effects of early introduction of solid foods. The more foods introduced in the first six months of life, the more likely the development of food and other allergies either in infancy or later.[8] Many of the home prepared foods and some of the commercial foods may contain excessive quantities of salt. Some evidence in animals indicates that early introduction of high salt foods is related to later hypertension. Feeding an infant who cannot support himself properly in a sitting position is difficult and frequently results in an unnecessary battle. Obesity in infancy can be harmful to the infant himself even if later obesity is avoided. Obese infants, it has long been recognized, combat respiratory infections much less well than lean ones.

Doctors must convince parents that there are no known advantages to early introduction of solid feedings and some undesirable effects. Solid feedings may begin at 4–6 months of age and should be with single foods. Rice cereal can be started at 4–6 months, followed by single fruits such as apple, pears, peaches at 4–7 months, vegetables such as peas, beans, carrots at 5–8 months, meats such as beef, lamb, liver at 6–9 months, egg yolk at 7–10 months, and then finger foods or junior foods. No new food should be introduced more frequently than one each week. Such a regimen should decrease the incidence of infantile diarrhea as well as food allergies.

COLIC

Colic is a poorly defined syndrome in which the baby, two weeks to two months of age, seems to have abdominal pain, draws his legs up, becomes distended, and may pass flatus. Crying decreases usually when the baby is given more attention. The syndrome disappears spontaneously at about three months of age.

Causes of this syndrome are largely unknown. Of the known nutritional causes that produce such irritable infants, the most common is overfeeding and the next most common is underfeeding. Therefore, it behooves the physician first to get an accurate dietary feeding history. Too frequent or too sparse feedings also may contribute. Food intolerance may be a cause of colic but changing the diet should not be tried until other causes are eliminated.

DIARRHEA

Diarrhea is the presence of loose, watery stools. Infants normally may have as few as one stool every three days up to eight stools daily. Frequent stools can be normal and do not indicate diarrhea.

Diarrhea can have multiple causes. In infancy the most common cause is overfeeding, but underfeeding, viral or bacterial gastroenteritis, food intolerance of multiple etiologies, irritable colon, cystic fibrosis of the pancreas, neural tumors and others may cause diarrhea.

In the treatment of diarrhea, the infant's hydration must be maintained. If diarrhea is severe, parenteral fluids are required.

In mild diarrhea or in realimentation after diarrhea has lessened, clear fluids should be given followed by slow reintroduction of the previous diet. After the onset of diarrhea, lactase disappears from the brush border of the intestine making the infant temporarily intolerant to lactose and the intestine wall becomes more permeable to protein. Many with food allergy can date the onset of the allergy to an episode of diarrhea. Therefore, a varied diet should not be reinstituted until several days after the diarrhea has ceased.

JUICES

The purpose of fruit juice in the infant diet is simply to vary the diet. Fruit juices contain vitamin C but this is available from other sources. Fruit juice, even natural fruit juice, has a caloric density almost equal to that of milk or formula, and these calories are mainly composed of carbohydrate. Therefore, early introduction of juice may displace other needed calories.

Bottles containing formula or juices should not be used as pacifiers. The practice of feeding fruit juice through a nipple and bottle is bad, as they may be used as a pacifier which keeps a high carbohydrate mixture nearing the budding teeth and contributes to "milk-bottle caries."

CARIES

Two factors have helped reduce the incidence of caries. In areas where the water supply is fluoridated, caries is decreased. If the water supply is not fluoridated, infants should be given fluoride drops to contain about 0.25 mg daily.

Parents should be warned about milk-bottle caries. When the bottle containing milk or sweetened liquids is kept in the mouth for long periods, development of caries is encouraged. Pacifiers or bottles containing only water should be used for those infants who have extra need for sucking. Weaning from bottle or breast can be accomplished at 9–12 months. Unsweetened water should be given to satisfy thirst.

SKIM MILK

Concerns about obesity and saturated fatty acids have led some to recommend skim milk in the diets of infants. This can be dangerous, especially in infants less than a year of age.

Obese infants should not be made to reduce, but to limit the rate of gain. This is a more satisfactory and less potentially harmful method of producing a more desirable physiognomy. This can be accomplished by decreasing the caloric density of nutritionally good foods. If one ounce of water is added to 4 ounces of complete formula, the caloric density is equal to that of 2% skim milk, and generally satisfies the hunger of an infant at this lower caloric intake. Water can be given between feedings or mixed with solid feedings.

In contrast, skim milk has produced a high osmolar load for the infant and satisfies neither thirst nor appetite. Therefore, infants can drink large quantities of this fluid consuming a high electrolyte high protein unbalanced diet. The danger of developing hyperelectrolytemia with subsequent ill effects such as diarrhea or brain damage is real. Dangers are lessened with 2% milk, but use of this is also unnecessary. After the age of a year or two, if the diet is sufficiently varied and the child does consume large quantities, skim milk may be safe. Skim milk should not be used for realimentation following diarrhea.

One proposed purpose for the early introduction of skim milk in the infant diet is to lower the saturated fat in the diet. Both human milk and simulated human milk formulas contain considerable polyunsaturated fat. Furthermore, in reviewing the use of fats in those with hyperlipoproteinemia, the Committee on Nutrition of the Academy of Pediatrics found no good reason to limit type or quantity of fat at such an early age even in high-risk infants. As information accumulates, it may be found that low saturated fat intakes are desirable for the older child, but as yet no good information warrants such a recommendation.

MILK INTAKE

During the first year of life, infants require 100–120 kcal/kg/day. Milk supplies about 67 kcal/dl or 670 kcal/liter or quart, sufficient for about a 7 kg or 15 pound infant. This is usually the maximum recommended intake of breast milk or formula, and additional calories are supplied by other foods. Thus at one year a 10 kg (21 pound) infant gets about two thirds of his calories from breast milk or formula. When the infant is weaned to whole milk, a more varied diet is desirable. This can be accomplished by limiting cow's milk to 500 ml (1 pint) a day. Such infants and children will then seek more varied sources of calories, some of which will contain iron.

CONCLUSION

All who care for infants can help prevent diseases of infancy by recommending good nutritional practices. Most important is the recommendation by obstetricians, nurses, pediatricians and other primary care physicians that breast feeding be utilized for 9–12 months. If the mother will not or cannot nurse, those formulas which most nearly simulate human milk with added vitamins and iron should be utilized.

Solid feedings should not be offered until 4–6 months of age, and should be introduced singly. Overfeeding and underfeeding should be avoided. If diarrhea develops, solid feedings should be reintroduced singly.

Juices are largely carbohydrate, should not be given early, and preferably should not be given by a bottle. No carbohydrate-containing solution, including juices or formula, should be used as a pacifier. The infant should be given his feeding and the bottle removed from the mouth to prevent bottle caries.

In areas where the water supply is not fluoridated, the infant should be given fluoride drops.

Skim milk is dangerous if used as a major nutrient in the first year of life because it provides an unbalanced diet with a high protein and high electrolyte load. Other nutrients can accomplish better the desired effects of skim milk.

After weaning, which should occur at 9–12 months, whole cow's milk intake limited to one pint daily (500 ml) encourages the infant to consume a varied and balanced diet.

II. AFTER THE FIRST YEAR

INTAKE

During the first year infants usually consume most foods offered them and appear to have an unlimited appetite. Beginning with the second year, appetite decreases and may remain low until about four to seven years. Decreased appetite parallels the physiological decrease in growth rate. Parents should be reassured that the child will not suffer ill effects from the markedly lower intake. They should continue to offer varied foods but not force the child to eat. Forced feeding at this age can lead to psychological problems as well as to obesity and other errors of overfeeding. Growth charts can be utilized to show the parents the benignity of the decreased intake.

VARIETY OF FOODS

During the first year of life, when the diet consists largely of human milk or simulated human milk with added vitamins, all known nutrients are consumed in reasonable amounts. After weaning, varying the sources of foods also provides all known nutrients. Selections of foods should be made from different foodgroups. The "basic four" is an easy-to-remember and simplified grouping of foods. The "four" consist of (1) meat, fish, poultry, eggs, (2) dairy products: milk, cheese and similar products, (3) fruits and vegetables, (4) cereal grains, potatoes, rice. In the past, selection from these groups provided a generally satisfactory diet. In recent years the widespread use of fast foods or artificially reconstituted foods has suggested to many that more complex divisions of food groups is necessary, at least to separating fruits from vegetables, and making a separate category for fats and oils. Any grouping which is satisfactory to the physician and family should lead to a varied diet for the growing child.

Limiting caloric intake of each of these groups to no more than ⅓ the total daily caloric intake generally provides the balance needed to supply all nutrients. This requires limiting whole milk ingestion to about one pint a day (or three glasses of skim milk) from one to six years, about three glasses from six to ten years, and a maximum of about one quart thereafter. Adequate fluid intake should be maintained by more liberal use of water. Other beverages which contain sugar are best relegated to occasional use.

Some children after weaning are unable to digest lactose. If gastrointestinal symptoms develop after drinking milk, they should not be urged to drink any milk. High quality protein can be obtained from multiple vegetable and animal sources and vitamins, calcium and other minerals from other sources. Fish, nuts, and legumes are good sources of calcium and the colored vegetables offer ready sources of most vitamins.

Concern about high fat intake has suggested to some that no good has been shown to accrue from the high fat intake of the present American diet. If concerned, utilizing skim milk instead of whole milk and limiting egg ingestion to four per week has been suggested as a reasonable step to the "prudent diet" after the first year. Limiting salt intake may similarly be beneficial and is discussed elsewhere in this issue.[9]

A suitable variety can be obtained by selecting from:

Breakfast—cereal, milk, bread, cheese or other protein source
Mid-morning—fruit or fruit juice
Lunch—meat, colored vegetables, fruit, peanut butter
Mid-afternoon—fruit or juice
Dinner—meat, fish, egg, vegetable, fruit or milk
Bedtime—milk or "snack"

SUPPLEMENTAL VITAMINS

Those children who are eating a varied diet need no supplemental vitamins. In various surveys in this country little evidence was found for any vitamin deficiency and where found the incidence did not differ in those populations given or not given vitamin supplements. The use of supplemental vitamins "as a tonic" or for children with no appetite is likely to foster bad habits including the habit of taking pills to solve problems.

SUPPLEMENTAL FLUORIDE

If the drinking water is fluoridated, no fluoride supplements should be used. In nonfluoridated areas, supplemental fluoride has been found to lower the incidence of caries. Recommended dosage is presented in the articles on dental nutrition.[10,11]

VEGETARIANISM

A vegan is one who eats no animal products. A vegetarian is one who eats eggs or dairy products but does not eat animal flesh. All necessary nutrients are obtainable in a vegetarian diet, but must be varied. For example, proteins of individual vegetables may have low biological value but when mixed with different vegetable proteins the combination has a higher biological value than either of the proteins alone. This may be due, in part, to the combination having a complementary effect on the essential amino acid mix. For example, a grain-legume combination provides much better nutrition than either grains or legumes alone.

Vitamin B_{12} is present almost entirely in foods of animal origin. Therefore, the diet of the vegan is Vitamin B_{12} deficient. The other B vitamins are present in whole grain cereals and in leafy vegetables. Calcium obtained largely from dairy products is also obtainable from fish, nuts, and legumes. The high fiber of vegetables usually causes bulkier bowel movements. Absorption of zinc, chromium, and other trace minerals may be decreased in those eating high fiber diets. Consumption of foods with indigestible fibers may lower cholesterol absorption and may have an effect in preventing later gastrointestinal diseases.

If the diet is selected as a fad, short periods are probably harmless. However, prolonged restricted diets whether of animal or vegetable origin are likely to be associated with the development of deficiencies.

ADOLESCENT NUTRITION

Adolescence is marked by accelerated growth. Undernutrition slows growth and overnutrition can speed it up. Caloric intake must be increased to provide normal growth. Ranges of increased requirements of calories, composition of calories, and minerals and vitamins are outlined in Recommended Daily Allowances.

With a varied diet, the requirements of macro and micronutrients are usually met when the caloric requirements are met. If, however, a large proportion of the calories are obtained from a single food or single group of foods, deficiencies may develop. Refined sugar has received attention as supplying carbohydrate calories without any other nutrients, so-called "empty calories." The dietary need of 40–60% of the calories as carbohydrate can be partially met by sugar as well as by more complex carbohydrates. Sticky sugars or frequent ingestion of sugar especially in confections are factors in the development of caries. Complex carbohydrates may be less atherogenic than simple carbohydrates, but data are not conclusive. The active person, including the athlete, requires calories to maintain energy, and for these supplemental carbohydrates as simple or complex sugars may be convenient, rapidly utilizable sources. However, simple sugars should be limited in total amount so that calories are obtained from multiple sources.

The diet of the pregnant adolescent girl is of special concern. During the active growth period, caloric intake adequate for growth is necessary. The adolescent who becomes pregnant has usually passed her maximum growth period, since menses and ovulation follow this period. If prepregnancy nutrition has been good, recommendations for good nutrition are similar to those for any other pregnant woman.[12] The development of good eating habits is essential before the child becomes pregnant to insure a good outcome of the pregnancy.

ATHLETE NUTRITION

Like all others, child or adolescent, the athlete benefits from a varied diet. Vitamins, minerals, proteins and other supplements are unnecessary and may be harmful. Adequate caloric intake is necessary both for growth and for the increased demands of activity. Children who do not perform well may have limited diets because of expense, lack of sufficient time to eat or because of poor habits.

Short energy spurts utilize stored ATP and phosphocreatine. Prolonged energy expenditure utilizes muscle glycogen anaerobically. Glycogen loading is possible by limiting carbohydrates during training, followed by high carbohydrate intake several days before the competitive event.

Food intake should be regular in pleasant surroundings. Water should be scheduled before and during athletic events. With regular meals and adequate water intake, no electrolyte solution is necessary.

For regular meals, the menu should include familiar foods and should be sufficient to prevent hunger and feelings of weakness. The timing should be such that the stomach is empty at game time. A good pregame meal is high in carbohydrate, low in fat, with abundant liquid and restricted in bulk and salty foods.

Athletes should be informed that exercise tolerance is diminished by smoking or drugs.

Prolonged exercise has been found to be associated with decreasing hemoglobin levels. The precise mechanism is unknown but appears related to an increased blood volume and change in body composition. Hemoglobin levels should be determined periodically and if low, ferrous sulfate should be given.

OBESITY

Multiple factors have been implicated in causing later obesity. Overfeeding, early introduction of solid foods to the infant, infantile obesity, increased fat cell numbers, heredity, psychosocial factors and others have been suggested for causing obesity but it is difficult to document any one cause of late and persistent obesity. Increasing activity, consistent periods of exercise, decreased television watching and active lifestyles seem to be associated with less obesity and better self image than any dietary or other forms of behavior modification, but no extensive series on any regimen is available. Preservation of mental well-being and avoidance of creating a sense of guilt is essential in any dietary manipulation, especially for treatment of obesity.

CONCLUSIONS

For the child after one year of age, decreased intake may cause concern. If the selection of foods is broad and if caloric consumption maintains weight so that normal growth patterns are attained, fears are groundless. Forced feeding at this age helps develop poor eating habits and may be a factor in later obesity. Fluoride supplements are necessary for the first ten or 12 years of life, but vitamin supplements are unnecessary and may be undesirable.

Vegetarian diets can supply all nutrients provided that foods are selected from all food groups. Vegetarian diets have higher fiber content which may be advantageous. Fad diets are not harmful if consumed for short periods, or if selection is not restricted.

Athletes should be reminded that they need sufficient calories and adequate water. Sufficient exercise is prophylaxis against obesity.

REFERENCES

1. CUNNINGHAM, A.S.: Morbidity in Breast-Fed and Artificially Fed Infants, J. Ped. 90:726, 1977.
2. BAHNA, S.L., and HEINER, D.C.: Cows Milk Allergy, Advances in Ped. 25, 1–37, 1978.
3. McMILLAN, J.A.; LANDAW, S.A., and OSKI, F.A.: Iron Sufficiency in Breast Fed Infants and the Availability of Iron from Human Milk, Ped. 58:686, 1976.
4. HAMBIDGE, K.M.: Role of Zinc and Other Trace Metals in Pediatric Nutrition and Health, Ped. Clin. N. Am. 24:95, 1977.
5. HAMBREUS, L.: Proprietary Milk versus Human Breast Milk in Infant Feeding: Critical Appraisal from the Nutritional Point of View, Ped. Clin. N. Am. 24:17, 1977.
6. BODE, H.H.; VANJONACK, W.J.; and CRAWFORD, J.D.: Mitigation of Cretinism by Breast Feeding, Ped. Res. 11:423, 1977.
7. LAKDAWALA, D.R., and WIDDOWSON, E.M.: Vitamin D in Human Milk, Lancet 1:67, 1977.
8. GLASER, J., and JOHNSTONE, D.E.: Prophylaxis of Allergic Disease in Newborn, JAMA 153:620, 1953.
9. KAFATOS, A.G., and CHRISTAKIS, G.: Pediatric Nutritional Determinants of Chronic Diseases, J. Fla. Med. Assn., (April) 1979.
10. GROW, T.E.: Nutritional and Oral Health, J. Fla. Med. Assn., (April) 1979.
11. AMERICAN ACADEMY OF PEDIATRICS, COMMITTEE ON NUTRITION: Fluoride Supplementation: Revised Dosage Schedule, Pediat. 63: 150–152, 1979.
12. MAHAN, C.: Nutritional Concerns in Pregnancy, J. Fla. Med. Assn., (April) 1979.

19

THE SCHOOL LUNCH PROGRAM: ITS PAST, ITS PROBLEMS, ITS PROMISE

Donald Ian Macdonald, M.D.

Almost 1 million Florida students (K-12) participated in the school lunch program on the average day of the 1977–1978 school year. How well did these children fare nutritionally and how much did they learn about food and nutrition? This paper will examine these questions while looking into the history of the program, its problems and changing purposes, and its future.

HISTORY

The National School Lunch Act became law in 1946 having evolved from efforts which began almost 100 years earlier. Three main forces were involved in development of the program which led to the law.

One of these was the concern that many children were too hungry and nutritionally deficient to perform at their optimal levels. The first school lunch program in this country dates back to 1853 when the Children's Aid Society of New York City opened the first of its vocational schools to the poor and served free meals to all who attended. Forty one years later The Starr Center Association provided penny lunches at several Philadelphia schools.

Shortly after the turn of the century Robert Hunter in his book "Poverty" and John Spago in "The Bitter Cry of the Children" focused the spotlight of public attention on widespread poverty in children and its effect on their ability to succeed. It was pointed out that in Europe the problem had been attacked through school feeding programs. By 1913

Dr. Macdonald is a pediatrician in practice in Clearwater. He is a member of the Ad Hoc Committee on Nutrition and Committee on School Health.

there were school lunch programs in 30 cities in 14 states. Soon afterward the National Congress of Parents and Teachers began to push for and assist in school lunch programs.

A second factor leading to the passage of the National School Lunch Act was a surplus of commodities. In the years following the stock market crash of 1929, a huge agricultural surplus developed in a country with millions of hungry children. In 1935 Congress passed Public Law 320 which initiated purchase and distribution of excess commodity foods to school lunch programs. With this law the Department of Agriculture became the overseer of the program, a position it still occupies. A third major push was massive unemployment also related to the Depression. In 1935 the Works Progress Administration (WPA) was formed and among other things provided labor and trained supervisory personnel for school lunch programs.

From these beginnings the program has continued to grow. During World War II high unemployment rates dropped and commodity excess all but disappeared but federal support for school lunch continued. Lewis B. Hershey, Director of Selective Service, estimated that 155,000 war casualties were related to malnutrition. Surgeon General Thomas Parran pointed to the National School Lunch Act as one of the most important health laws of our time. With testimony of this sort the Congress was spurred to act, and in 1944 $50 million was provided for milk and lunch reimbursement. By 1947 all states had programs under the national act. State financial support has followed.

School lunch is big business. It's the second largest away-from-home food market: $7.8 billion is spent annually of which 30% is federal funding; 25 million children are served daily and over 4 billion meals are consumed annually; 30–40% of these meals are free or at a reduced price.

PROBLEMS AND CHANGING PURPOSES

Like many programs which have evolved to solve a variety of problems, there is still a question as to primary purpose. Is it to feed hungry children? The nutritive impact of school lunches unfortunately has never been systematically measured but studies in developing countries have shown benefit in terms of school performance. The Iowa Breakfast Studies showed similar results. Or is the program purpose to teach nutrition, to help consume excess commodities, or provide a place for employment of the unemployed? Should the program still be under the direction of the Department of Agriculuture or should direction come from an agency whose emphasis is more directly on health and education? Other concerns are plate waste, low attendance, lunchroom atmosphere and logistics, the commodity food program and the provision of adequate nutrients.

Plate Waste

A major concern of food service professionals is getting students to use school cafeterias and to eat the food they are served. The latter problem, commonly referred to as plate waste, has become a political, parent and taxpayer issue. It has been estimated that $400 million of food is dumped into school garbage cans each year. CBS's popular "Sixty Minutes" devoted an hour to the issue and school food service journals are filled with related articles.

There are many ways of looking at plate waste. Maybe it is partly a reflection of an affluent society which also has high rates of restaurant and home plate waste. Some of it is related to the fact that with standard portion sizes aimed at the average child's appetite too much food is given to some and too little to others. If food preparation is such that food looks or tastes unappetizing wastage will increase. Quality ingredients prepared and served with an eye to color, texture, taste and avoidance of monotony will lead to conservation of nutrients.

Tastes Change

When burritos were first tried in Tampa four years ago they were largely thrown away. Since then a taco quick service restaurant moved into town and began advertising and now tacos are among the most popular menu items in nearby schools and burritos are back on the menu. Ethnic background and family social habits and customs are also related to food acceptance. Introducing new foods to students has long been an aim of many, but experienced school lunch managers know to reduce portion size for unfamiliar foods. Genetic differences are also important when such things as lactose intolerance of many children, especially blacks, is considered.

More and more schools now have student advisors involved in meal planning. In Florida, school Youth Advisory Councils (YAC) are organized and meet on a statewide basis as well as in their own schools. Some schools have had children rate student acceptance of foods on the basis of matching their feeling about what they have just eaten or drunk with a variety of faces (Fig. 19.1).

Children's tastes and choices of food are often different from adults. Some foods present unusual problems. Most adults like apples and consider them healthful enough to keep the doctor away if taken daily. Younger children who are missing front teeth and adolescents in braces may shun them. When sliced to reduce portion size they turn brown and unappealing. Cafeteria managers don't like them because they are so often used as missiles and at least one school banned them because they plug up commodes.

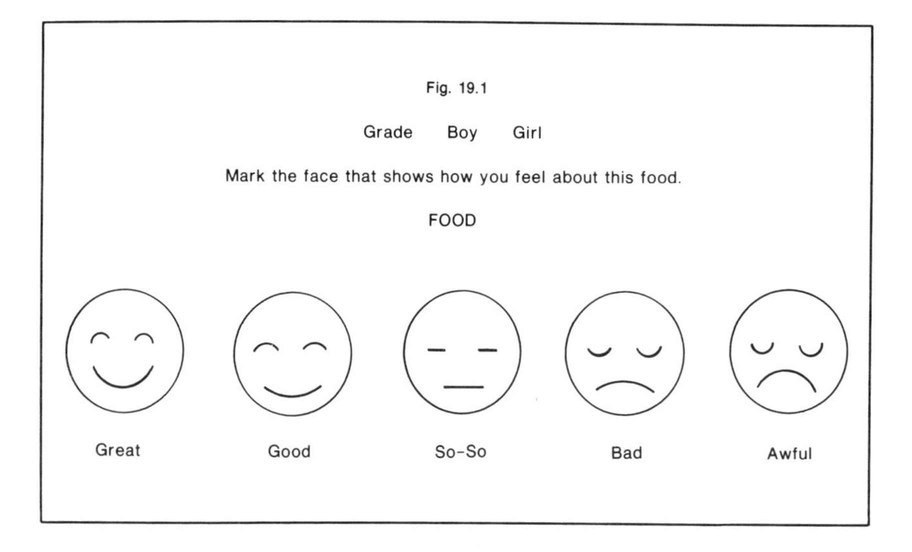

Studies on plate waste are occurring in many places in efforts to reduce the problem. It is agreed that wastage should be measured at each school as a guide to changing preferences, appropriate portion size and reaction to monotony. A study in Leon County, Florida, has shown that plate waste decreases each year from kindergarten through grade 5. It has confirmed studies done elsewhere that plate waste is not the same for all menu items. Most wasted are vegetables followed by fruits and then in descending order dessert, entree, bread and milk. Girls tend to throw more food in the garbage than boys. A study of high school seniors in Hawaii showed that 42% of girls ate no vegetables, 45% no fruit, 10% no meat and 10% no milk. The corresponding percentages for boys were 22, 24, 27 and 3. The Leon County study also showed that allowing choice of salad dressing in older children tended to increase acceptance. The issue of plate waste will continue to be with us and demands further study and evaluation as increasing emphasis is placed on acceptance, nutrition and cost.

Lunchroom Atmosphere and Logistics

The logistics of serving lots of meals to lots of kids in a short period of time can be mind boggling. A well run cafeteria can serve 10–12 students per minute when all students are served the same items. If students are allowed choices the rate may slow to 6–7 students per line per minute. State guidelines for newer construction call for lunchroom capacity to seat approximately one third the student population at a time. Older schools and overpopulated schools may fall well short of this goal.

An example might help illustrate some of the logistical problems. A senior high school meeting state guidelines would be expected to have 700 cafeteria seats if the student body totaled 2,100. Most schools this size would have four serving lines. If each of these lines averaged 11 students served per minute it would take almost 16 minutes to serve 700 students. If food choices were offered it might take 27 minutes. Thirty minutes of release time for lunch are allowed in most Florida counties. According to my calculations 30 minutes would allow the last students through the line between 3 and 14 minutes to eat depending on whether or not a choice is offered. This is well short of the state guidelines suggesting a minimum of 20 minutes eating time for each child. If the child is asked to put away his tray, makes a bathroom stop, or has his next class far from the cafeteria, he is in trouble. There is considerable variation in lunchroom scheduling related to such factors as double sessions and bus schedules which in Pinellas County bring some students to school as early as 7:15 and others as late as 10:00 a.m.

Many students choose not to use the cafeteria. For some, open campuses where they can leave to eat provides an answer. For others, snack bars and vending machines, often placed for fund raising projects, provide an out. Others gobble their food or go hungry. Answers are not easily found. Increasing cafeteria seating is expensive as is increasing labor and the number of serving lines. Extending the lunch break or serving smaller groups over a longer period does not enthuse most principals. Convincing more principals of the importance of the program could lead to major improvements in scheduling, atmosphere, nutrient consumption, and nutrition education.

Vending machines have been blamed by some as a major cause of low attendance in cafeterias and seen by others as a way to lure the students in. A bill to ban vending machines in the schools was introduced in the last Florida legislature. Using the machines to dispense fruit juice or so-called "nutritious snacks" is advocated by others. There are proponents who would put machines in cafeterias to lure students in and others who would use them to dispense meals which could be heated. This emotionally charged issue is far from resolved.

Commodity Foods

Commodity foods, one of the early factors leading to establishment of the school lunch program, have become a problem. Variation in what is available month to month and year to year has led to problems in long range menu planning. A trip to a school food service warehouse may reveal large quantities of such things as cranberries and soy beans. To consume these will require quite a bit of ingenuity on the part of the meal planners. Smaller schools especially have trouble incorporating into their plans commodities which are not shelf stable. Recently contracts for processing commodities into shelf-stable ready to eat foods have been hailed as a major innovation. Despite this there are many who feel it is time to sever the close relationship with the commodities program and instead effect cash savings through combined regional or large area bidding and purchase of foods.

In Florida, Food and Nutrition and Management is in the Department of Education and the Commodity Food Program in the Department of Agriculture. This makes for less than optimal coordination of effort. Nationally there is consideration to remove the School Lunch Program from auspices of the Department of Agriculture and place it under the direction of the Department of Education or Health and Human Services. This makes sense.

Type A Lunch Pattern

In an effort to meet nutritional needs of children it was decided from the program's beginning to try to provide students with one third their daily nutritional requirements at the luncheon meal. To standardize planning and serving, the needs of a child age 10–12, based on the 1968 Daily Dietary Allowances, were chosen as the basis for estimation of portion size. This created problems for the younger child who ended with more on his plate than he needed, for the girls who had lower requirements than boys, and for the older children who needed more. This problem was partially rectified with changes in figuring the 1974 RDA to incude nine age-sex groupings. These have been reduced in school lunch figuring to five groups. Not addressed was the fact that for many low income families the school meal might be the main meal of the day. It also did not consider the problem of the overweight child who would be better with a smaller than average serving.

The Type A Lunch (Table 19.1) until recently included five food groups which must be served with each lunch. There is also funding for Type B and C lunches but these lunches are seldom used. The early menu requirements were later modified to include iron and vitamin A and more recently the butter/margarine requirement has been dropped. Milk was originally acceptable only in its whole form until pressure was applied to allow flavored milk and later skim milk. Fat which earlier was to account for 40% of the calories is now set to provide 35%.

Until 1975 teenagers were being given all five food groups to meet the requirement for federal reimbursement. Many of them had no intention of eating all the things put on their plate. To combat the subsequent plate waste Congress passed what has been called the "offer versus

TABLE 19.1

Type A Lunch: 5 groups

1. Milk - at least ½ pint
2. Meat or fish or eggs or cheese or dry beans or dry peas or soybeans or peanut butter
3. Vegetable and/or fruit
4. Whole grain or enriched bread or cereal
5. Butter or fortified margarine - no longer mandatory

Type B Lunch

1. Milk as above
2. Half portions of other groups

Type C Lunch

1. ½ pint of milk

serve" amendment which allows full Type A funds to senior high schools if students take from at least three of the five designated food groups.

Other lunch patterns than the Type A lunch have been suggested. One of these, referred to as nutrient standard menus, is a computer based approach which works to provide adequate amounts of those nutrients for which requirements have been established. It should allow more meal flexibility and more reliable provision of nutrients than the Type A lunch. Unfortunately the nutrient composition of many foods used is not known and computers are not always easily available. The method does hold promise for the future.

Realizing that students may discard or not select vital nutrients, some advocate fortification of foods which are popular with children. They point out that an added benefit of this method is that a more limited selection of foods would be made available which should reduce cost. Food and labor costs are rising rapidly and it is increasingly difficult to meet the budget with available subsidies without increasing price to students (Table 19.2).

THE FUTURE

Breakfast Programs

The Child Nutrition Act passed in 1966 established a pilot program for schools to serve breakfast to needy children and those with long bus rides. The program was expanded after the 1968 White House Conference on Food, Nutrition and Health. In 1972 there was additional expansion to allow all schools to participate and in 1975 Public Law 94-105 was passed giving permanent authorization to the program. In fiscal year 1978, 115,285 Florida children were served over 21 million

TABLE 19.2

COST PRICE STRUCTURE:	TYPE A LUNCH
Cost per lunch 1978	$ .90
Estimated 1979	1.00
Charge to student	
Full pay elementary	$ .50
Full pay middle/high	.60
Reduced price lunch	.20
Federal support	
All lunches	$ .1525
Free lunches (.1525+)	.6825
Reduced price lunch (.1525+)	.5825
Commodity food support	.15
Florida state funding	
For free and reduced	
price lunch only	$ .019

breakfasts in 915 participating schools. Critics of the program feel that it is the responsibility of parents to provide children with breakfast. Advocates point to the fact that families which eat breakfast together are becoming rarer and estimate that over 30% of all children prepare their own breakfast. It has also been established that 37–50% of all children receive an inadequate morning meal.

Food and Nutrition Education

Emphasis seems to be shifting more and more to using the school lunch program as a teaching tool. The hope is that students will not only learn how to make sensible food and nutrient selection but will develop lifelong eating habits related to this information. It is further hoped that the atmosphere of the lunchroom will be such that students will learn to relax while eating and use the meal table as a place to exchange ideas and thoughts while slowing the pace. There are those who would serve at least some of the meals in the classroom.

There are problems. One is the fact that in recent years teachers have negotiated their contracts so they no longer spend time in the cafeteria with their students. The logistics of scheduling and seating have already been discussed. Another problem is that the cafeteria supervisors are not considered members of the faculty and have little input to curriculum planning or knowledge of what's happening in the classroom. Referred to earlier is the fact that many teachers and principals are lacking enough nutritional education to appreciate adequately the long and short range benefits of the lunch program or the teaching of nutrition.

But nutrition education is an idea whose time has come and there seems to be no doubt that it will be increasingly emphasized. Students are interested in such things as obesity, vitamin supplements, "organic" foods, vegetarian diets and many other food related topics.

The Florida legislature is interested. In its 1978 session it added the requirement that nutrition education be specifically included in the Comprehensive Health Education Bill which it funded categorically in the same session. Congress is also working on a comprehensive health education package. In 1977, President Ford signed into law a bill which gives 50 cents per school child to each state for the purpose of teaching nutrition. Neither of these bills deals specifically with school lunch programs but there is an obvious relationship. Some consider them piecemeal approaches and feel there must be better coordination between food preparation, nutrient delivery and health education.

SUMMARY

The National School Lunch Act became law in 1946. This act which followed approximately 100 years of interest in feeding school age children has acted as the framework for a program which has been growing and changing ever since.

School food service professionals have been looking seriously at such problems as plate waste, nonattendance at school cafeterias, provision of adequate nutrients, coupling of feeding with learning and establishment of sound eating habits. Their job has been made difficult by problems of money, school scheduling and dining area space, and lack of administrative support. Despite these handicaps the program is generally running fairly well and providing real service to many children. The hope for the future is that through research and through education of legislators, parents and school administrators, the problems will lessen. Then eating at school will become a more effective area not just for provision of nutrients but also as a center for comprehensive health education.

BIBLIOGRAPHY

FLANAGAN, T.G.: School Food Services, Education in the States—Nationwide Development Since 1900. National Education Association of US, 1968.

JANSEN, G.R. and HARPER, J.M.: Consumption and Plate Waste of Menu Items Served in National School Lunch Program, J. Am. Diet Assoc. 73:205 (Oct.) 1978.

JANSEN, G.R. and HARPER, J.M.: Nutritional Aspects of Nutrient Standard Menus, Food Tech. (Jan.) 1974: 62.

LACHANCE, P.A.: U.S. School Food Service: Problems and Prospects, School Food Service Research Review, 2:73, 1978.

LaCHANCE, P.A.: Simple Research Techniques for School Food Service; 2. Measuring Plate Waste, School Food Service Journal 30:68, (Sept.) 1976.

PILOT STUDY TO COMPARE TYPE A LUNCHES WITH ALTERNATIVE SUBSIDIZED LUNCHES AMONG HIGH SCHOOL STUDENTS: Departments of Agricultural and Chemical Engineering and Food Science and Nutrition, Colorado State University, Sept. 5, 1978.

PLATE WASTE STUDY: School Food Service, Leon County, Florida, 1978.

PERSONAL COMMUNICATION

GEORGE HOCKENBERY: Administrator, Food and Nutrition Management, Department of Education, Tallahassee, Florida.

RUTH R. KELLY: Assistant Director, School Food Service, Pinellas County, Florida.

BARBARA K. WARCH: Supervisor, School Food Service, Hillsborough County, Florida.

20

THE *WIC* PROGRAM: TYING SUPPLEMENTAL FOODS TO NUTRITIONAL NEEDS

Alvin M. Mauer, M.D.

On November 10, 1978, President Carter signed into law S-3085, the Child Nutrition Amendments of 1978. In this legislation was included provision for continuation of funding for the Special Supplemental Food Program for Women, Infants and Children (WIC). It was characteristic of the history of WIC that this decision by the President was a cliff-hanger, with a real possibility of a veto as urged by the Office of Management and Budget. It appears that only last minute intervention by a coalition of groups interested in child nutrition urging the President to sign the bill saved the day for WIC.

In his statement, the President acknowledged that WIC has had success in improving the health of low income, pregnant and nursing women and young children. He acknowledged that the program is fully consistent with his commitment to preventive health measures and could even result in a reduction of hospital expenditures and Medicaid costs. This program has had enormous support throughout the country and it is difficult to argue against the need for proper nutrition in pregnant and lactating women and growing infants and children. Why, therefore, has the WIC program been such a controversial issue from its very inception and what are its real strengths and weaknesses in providing benefits for those designed to be helped by the legislation?

Dr. Mauer is Director, St. Jude Children's Research Hospital, Memphis.

HISTORY OF WIC LEGISLATION

The history of this legislation began during the late 1960s when three surveys concerning the nutrition and health of the poor in this country were made. Between 1968 and 1970, the Ten-State Survey,[1] A Study of Nutritional Status in Pre-School Children in the United States,[2] and A Nutritional Survey of Pre-School Children From Impoverished Black Families in Memphis[3] were accomplished. Findings were identical. A significant proportion of infants and children were smaller than expected and a dietary deficiency of iron was evident in up to one half of these children between ages one and two years. There was a clear correlation of the findings of undernutrition with income, with an increasingly greater frequency of small stature and evidences of iron deficiency. A review of dietary patterns supported the judgment that the undernutrition was caused by decreased food intake, not inappropriate diet. In none of these surveys were gross evidences of vitamin deficiencies found, nor severe protein-calorie deprivation characteristic of developing countries.

The implication of these findings of undernutrition among the poor of this country for subsequent development and performance of the children is not clear. There is good documentation that severe undernutrition during infancy affects subsequent physical growth and intellectual functioning.[4] The direct relationship between moderate undernutrition and subsequent growth and intellectual development, however, is still unknown.[5,6] It may be that the developing child has great reserves with respect to its developmental capacity and moderate undernutrition will not pose a significant hazard. However, our inability to define the hazards of moderate undernutrition during infancy may also reflect the lack of sensitivity of our current testing instruments to pick up these differences in intellectual capacity. Furthermore, many factors influence a child's development and it is difficult to selectively evaluate nutrition as one among many of these environmental influences.

Even though the findings of moderate undernutrition among the poor of this country could not be assigned a definitive role with respect to health and development, a clear concern was registered in Congress. In 1972, primarily due to the efforts of the late Senator Hubert Humphrey, Congress authorized the development of a pilot program to test the efficacy of special supplemental foods for pregnant and lactating women and infants. The initial program was authorized for two years and was to be supported by funding levels of $20 million annually. The population eligible to receive these benefits were "pregnant or lactating women and infants determined by competent professionals to be nutritional risks because of inadequate nutrition and inadequate income." The Congress also authorized an evaluation of this program so that its results could be reviewed by Congress at the end of the initial two-year period. The legislation was designed to study the efficacy of nutritionally defined food supplements in a special population at high risk for malnutrition.

At this point the perilous journey of the WIC Program began. The United States Department of Agriculture expressed reluctance about being able to administer the program because of the medical evaluation component and for five months tried to convince the Department of Health, Education and Welfare that the administration responsibilities should rest there. After five months of negotiation HEW finally declined and at this point the USDA indicated it would be improbable that the funds could be allocated for programs during the first fiscal year. However, Congress and also interested community people applied pressure and in March 1973 the USDA did convene a Task Force for program development. Subsequently, a suit was filed resulting in a consent order signed by the USDA indicating that the unspent $20 million from the first year would be carried over into the second year, making a total amount of $40 million for fiscal year 1974.

Delays in processing grant applications further slowed implementation of the program. Only a few grants had been made by fall 1973 and in November a second court action was required to order the USDA to announce all of the year's grants by December. Start-up time delays for the designated sites meant that only 110 of the 255 programs were actually in business by March 1974, three months before the end of the second fiscal year. A number of short-term grants were made to commit all the allocated money, but that meant the annualized funding level far exceeded the $40 million. Congress, in June, authorized $100 million for an additional year of funding.

In spite of the difficulties in getting this program underway, by 1974 there were an estimated 204,000 participants in the program. Unfortunately, the contract for evaluation of the WIC Program was not signed until November 1973 and, thus, the results were not available to Congress at a time that action on new legislation was needed. Public Law 94-105 extended this program in 1974 through fiscal year 1978 and increased the authorization of appropriations to a funding level of $250 million for fiscal year 1976 and each succeeding fiscal year through fiscal year 1978.

Presently, there are about 70 agencies in 48 states, Puerto Rico and the Virgin Islands administering the WIC Program. Only six states operate the program on a statewide basis. There are 1,300 operating WIC clinics. There are over 1,600 counties in the United States that have not implemented the WIC Program. At this time it is estimated that 1.124 million women, infants, and children are participating in the WIC Program out of an estimated 8.3 million low income individuals who are potentially eligible but who are not now being reached by the program.

Certainly, the WIC Program has proved to be one of the most popular of governmental programs in recent years. At all levels from national organization through state agencies to the community level and to the participant there has been a consensus concerning the program's value. The programs have been changed to include a provision that there must be association with a health care facility. The new bill stresses once again the need for an ongoing evaluation of the results of the program. There has been an effort to assure the program will be delivered to those most in need by adding the income stipulation. The eligibility criteria have been further refined to define nutritional risk as (a) detrimental or abnormal nutritional conditions detectable by clinical or anthropometric measurements; (b) other documented nutritionally related medical conditions; (c) dietary deficiencies that impair or endanger health; or, (d) conditions that predispose persons to inadequate nutritional patterns or nutritionally related medical conditions including, but not limited to, alcoholism and drug addiction.

Why then was there such a risk of veto for this popular bit of legislation which has been recognized as contributing to the health of pregnant and lactating women and infants and children? The decision to veto this legislation came from the Office of Management and Budget. With increasing concern for governmental expenditures, all programs have come under close scrutiny. Congress had increased the funding level from an apparent $250 million in fiscal 1978 to $550 million in fiscal 1979 and a guaranteed $800 million in fiscal 1980. This seemed to be an enormous jump to OMB. However, the actual level of funding for fiscal 1978 approached $440 million because of court orders requiring a carry over of unspent funds from previous fiscal years. Therefore, the real increase in activity was not as large as it seemed and to the supporters of this bill the added monies were necessary because of the great number of counties still unserved by WIC and the relatively small proportion of potentially eligible people who were receiving its benefits. The guaranteed funding for 1980 was felt necessary because of the difficulties this program had had in the past. It seemed a clear time for providing a period of stability for program development. Perhaps now this program, with its stormy period of gestation and hazardous childhood, can enjoy a period of growth and development with this financial nourishment from Congress.

EVALUATION OF THE WIC PROGRAM

For all the legislative and administrative fireworks what, in fact, has the WIC Program accomplished with respect to improving the health of the women and children involved? The original intent was to mount a pilot project which would provide information about the value of such special supplemental food programs. As indicated, it was unfortunate that the contract for evaluation was not signed until November 1973. At that time, the programs were already getting underway and it was impossible to coordinate data collection prospectively. It was found that even such apparently simple measurements as height and weight were difficult to determine accurately with inexperienced personnel. There was no time for training programs or assessment of quality control for the various measurements. Other problems that arose in this difficult study were the lack of a true control group, the inability to link patients so that initial and follow-up visit data could be analyzed, a large drop-out rate and the inability to always assess reasons for inclusion of an individual in the WIC Program. Under the circumstances, therefore, the inability of this medical evaluation to provide definitive information is understandable.

Conclusions that were reached by the principal investigator of this study were that an acceleration of growth in weight and height was associated with the WIC Program and that there was a consistent increase in the mean blood hemoglobin concentration and a reduction in the prevalence of anemia. Pregnant women participating in the program gained more weight than women in the initial population and there was an increase in the mean weight of babies born to women in the program. A reduction in anemia rate among these women was found. Because of the constraints of the study, these data cannot be accepted as conclusive with respect to the benefits of the program.

There have been individual reports from single programs or state programs indicating that the beneficial effect has been noted in infant weight gain, reduction in anemia rate, increased birth weight of infants born to mothers on the program, and an increase in clinic participation for general health care for participating infants, children, and women. Unfortunately, all this information has been gathered without standardization of procedures and presented in forms which make it impossible to critically evaluate.

Perhaps one of the greatest needs for this program at this time is a careful analysis of benefits. Individual programs have indeed demonstrated that nutritional benefits from Federal Food Assistance Programs occur.[7] A review of the problems of evaluating the nutrition and health benefits of a special supplemental food program has been prepared.[8] In that review, a series of recommendations are made for future evaluations of the WIC Program. There has been no systematic evaluation undertaken by the USDA since the completion of the report of the initial study. The current legislation calls for such an evaluation, which hopefully will be done in such a manner that the data collected can be critically analyzed. This evaluation is going to be absolutely essential if any attempt to assess the cost benefit ratio of the program is undertaken. The current legislation has extended the program for four years. Hopefully, at the end of that time these answers will be available.

For all the difficulties in analyzing medical benefits there is no question about the acceptance of this program. Even if the information available is anecdotal, there are sufficient numbers of testimonies to lend weight to the program's value. According to field experience participants in the program attend clinic more regularly and women enter the program earlier in pregnancy. In some settings the WIC Program has introduced people to a system of health care for their children. Thus, not only has the supplemental food apparently improved the nutritional status but it has served as an inducement for participation in a health care program. The impact of nutrition education as a part of this program is difficult to assess but there is a general feeling that the participants are more knowledgeable about food and its importance. Thus, while the evidence remains soft, it is all supportive of the program's value.

CONCLUSIONS AND FUTURE DIRECTIONS

With support for the program guaranteed for the next two years, there should be time to consolidate the gains made in developing and administering it. Currently the USDA appears to be an enthusiastic defender. Much has been learned in some states about such administrative matters as data collection and processing. Distribution of food has been developed for individual communities according to their needs. Experienced people are now available for the conduct of this program in local communities.

There still remain some basic issues needing resolution. One of the most important, in my opinion, is the problem of eligibility criteria. From the very beginning this program was designed to be preventive rather than remedial in nature. The current eligibility criteria stresses evidences of nutritional deficiences for eligibility rather than the risk of developing these deficiencies. As physicians, we are primarily concerned with preventing growth failure and iron deficiency rather than correcting it when present. Sufficient studies are now available to properly identify the population at high risk for nutritional deficiency.

One of the real advances of this program has been to recognize the relationship of nutrition and health care for pregnant and lactating women, infants, and children. In this country, at this time, we are much aware of the needs for preventive measures with respect to health in order to reduce the increasing health care costs. In many respects the WIC Program is a model for this kind of approach.

Clearly, one of the most important needs of the WIC Program at this time is a solid evaluation of results. It can be hoped that the USDA will mount such an effective evaluation program as soon as possible and avoid the difficulties of the first study.

This program has been a unique effort on the part of Congress to provide a defined food package to a group of people found to be at high nutritional risk. Perhaps one measure of its success has been the ability of the program to weather the storms of the years since its inception. It will be interesting to see its further progress as it enters the relatively tranquil seas of guaranteed support during the next few years.

REFERENCES

1. GARN, S.M., and CLARK, D.C.: Nutrition, Growth, Development, and Maturation: Findings from the Ten-State Nutrition Survey of 1968–1970, Pediatrics 56:306–319, 1975.
2. OWEN, G.M.; KRAM, K.M., *et al.*: A Study of Nutritional Status of Preschool Children in the United States, 1968–1970, Pediatrics 53:597–646, 1974.
3. ZEE, P.; WALTERS, T., and MITCHELL, C.: Nutrition and Poverty in Preschool Children. JAMA 213:739–742, 1970.
4. STOCH, M.B., and SMYTHE, P.M.: 15-Year Developmental Study on Effects of Severe Undernutrition during Infancy on Subsequent Physical Growth and Intellectual Functioning. Arch. Dis. Child 51:327–336, 1976.
5. KALLEN, D.J.: Nutrition and Society. JAMA 215:94–100, 1971.
6. READ, M.S.: Malnutrition, Hunger, and Behavior. J. Am. Diet. Assoc. 63:379–391, 1973.
7. KAFATOS, A.G., and ZEE, P.: Nutritional Benefits from Federal Food Assistance. Am. J. Dis. Child 131:265–269, 1977.
8. USDA ADVISORY COMMITTEE ON NUTRITION EVALUATION: Evaluating the Nutrition and Health Benefits of the Special Supplemental Food Program for Women, Infants, and Children. United States Department of Agriculture Food and Nutrition Service, FNS 165, November, 1977.

21

PUBLIC HEALTH AND THE PRACTICING PHYSICIAN—PARTNERS IN COMMUNITY NUTRITION

Ruth Baker, R.D., M.P.H.
C.L. Brumback, M.D., M.P.H.

A recent cartoon shows a bewildered consumer pushing her cart down the aisle of a supermarket. She passes four signs—"Health Food," "Soul Food," "Junk Food," and "Food Food."

Where do your patients get their information about food—from TV, newspapers, magazines, health food stores, books, family, friends, neighbors, fellow workers or fellow students, teachers, health professionals, weight control groups, health organizations?

This nation is experiencing an explosion of nutrition information and misinformation. Your patients are being bombarded by hundreds of nutrition messages from many sources. Some are valid and scientifically-based; some costly, but neither helpful nor harmful; others actually damaging, and some perhaps even fatal such as the extreme stages of the Zen Macrobiotic diet or some of the liquid protein diets used for weight control. How does the individual select the messages which will determine his food patterns and eating behavior?

Food patterns are the result of numerous forces which operate within the life of each individual. Persons eat as they do because of cultural influences, religion, family background, tradition, socioeconomic factors, education, advertising, and lifestyle. Health and medical advice may determine eating patterns if the individual is convinced of the relevance

Ms. Baker and Dr. Brumback are affiliated with the Palm Beach County Health Department, West Palm Beach, Florida.

of his diet to his health status but, in many instances, considerations other than health and well-being are more cogent influences.

"Nutrition is an emerging art and science which integrates a broad spectrum of disciplines, ranging from biochemistry and medicine to statistics, anthropology, and public health."* Nutrition science has moved rapidly from the dramatic discovery of the vitamins and amino acids and their roles in human health and disease to a better understanding of fats and micronutrients and the interrelationships of all nutrients. Scientists are becoming increasingly aware of the interactions of nutrients and drugs. For example, alcoholism, in addition to its effect upon the liver, may increase primary nutritional deficiencies, and the use of oral contraceptive agents increases the body's need for vitamin B_6 and folic acid. A marked decrease in the prevalence of the deficiency diseases—goiter, pellagra, scurvy, and rickets—has been noted since the food enrichment program has enhanced the value of some of the most basic foods. Nutrition surveys, however, indicate that there is no room for complacency about the nutritional status of the population, for specific cases of clinical and subclinical malnutrition have been identified. Ironically, many of the nutrition problems currently observed are the result of excesses or overconsumption. Among the ten leading causes of death, at least six can be considered to have diet as a major risk factor: heart disease, cancer, stroke, cirrhosis, diabetes, and arteriosclerosis.

With increasing emphasis, practicing physicians and public health leaders are urging individuals to assume greater responsibility for their own health care. In practical terms, this means adopting a lifestyle which will minimize their risk factors—those variables which have been found to be statistically associated with a high incidence of disease. Individuals are being taught to choose an appropriate diet to maintain optimum nutrition and desirable weight, to avoid hyperlipidemia and hypertriglyceridemia, to avoid cigarette smoking, to find healthful ways of handling stress, and to follow a program of physical activity appropriate to their health status.

In early 1977, the Senate Select Committee on Human Needs issued a report, "Dietary Goals for the United States," and revised the goals somewhat in the second edition later that year. Although the goals (Table 21.1) have been disputed by some clinicians and nutritionists, they have received broad acceptance in principle. They are considered a first step toward recommending the kind of food pattern which would aid in reducing the risk of developing certain diseases. The Dietary Goals point to a way of eating similar to the "Prudent Diet" which was developed by the late Dr. Norman Joliffe and his staff of the Bureau of Nu-

* Nutritional Assessment in Health Programs, Proceedings of a conference held October 18–20, 1972, G. Christakis, editor, American Public Health Association, Washington, D.C. 20036, 1973, $4.00.

trition, New York City Health Department. Its effectiveness in lowering elevated blood cholesterol in men and reducing heart attack rates was demonstrated in the experience of the Anti-Coronary Club. The American Heart Association has recently issued an updated statement, "Diet and Coronary Heart Disease" for physicians and other health professionals, and it, too, advocates similar modifications.

TABLE 21.1. DIETARY GOALS FOR THE UNITED STATES[1]

(a) To avoid overweight, consume only as much energy (calories) as is expended; if overweight, decrease energy intake and increase energy expenditures.
(b) Increase the consumption of complex carbohydrates and "naturally occurring" sugars from about 28% of energy intake to about 48% of energy intake.
(c) Reduce the consumption of refined and processed sugars by about 45% to account for about 10% of total energy intake.
(d) Reduce overall fat consumption from approximately 40% to about 30% of energy intake.
(e) Reduce saturated fat consumption to account for about 10% of total energy intake; and balance that with polyunsaturated and mono-unsaturated fats which should account for about 10% of energy intake each.
(f) Reduce cholesterol consumption to about 300 mg a day.
(g) Limit the intake of sodium by reducing the intake of salt to about 5 g a day.

To achieve these goals, the following changes in food selection and preparation are recommended:
(a) Increase consumption of fruits and vegetables and whole grain.
(b) Decrease consumption of refined and other processed sugars and foods high in such sugars.
(c) Decrease consumption of foods high in total fat and partially replace saturated fats, whether obtained from animal or vegetable sources, with polyunsaturated fats.
(d) Decrease consumption of animal fat, and choose meats, poultry and fish which will reduce saturated fat intake.
(e) Except for young children, substitute low fat and nonfat milk for whole milk and low fat dairy products for high fat dairy products
(f) Decrease consumption of butterfat, eggs and other high cholesterol sources; some consideration should be given to easing the cholesterol goal for premenopausal women, young children and the elderly in order to obtain the nutritional benefits of eggs in the diet.
(g) Decrease consumption of salt and foods high in salt content.

[1] Dietary Goals for the United States, Second Edition, Government Printing Office, Washington, D.C. 20402

IS THERE SUCH THING AS A TYPICAL AMERICAN DIET?

One can identify a number of trends or movements, but it is impossible to generalize about or describe a typical diet. Some of the popular trends are described below:

The "Fast Food" Craze.—About 40% of all meals are eaten outside the home. A high percentage of those meals are eaten in fast food restaurants which have proliferated throughout the country. Those meals tend to be high in saturated fat and lacking in fruits and vegetables. An encouraging development has been the addition of the salad bar by some of the fast food chains. Some experts believe that the industry would respond to a demand for leaner beef if the public became more assertive.

Gourmet Cookery.—Devotees of this school seek the exotic, the unusual, the elegant. Most gourmet cooks shun prepared and packaged items, preferring to create every recipe from scratch. Cooking is perceived as a creative, artistic endeavor, and its results challenge and appeal to all the senses. Gourmet cooking has shifted from the very rich, high-calorie menu with many courses to a simpler, more temperate menu.

The "Health Food"Culture.—Many adolescents, young adults and elderly have been attracted to unprocessed, natural, organic foods. While those terms are hard to define and mean different things to different people, the members of this group have come to it from a concern for ecology, a dread of "chemicals," and a sincere belief that foods which they categorize as "health foods" have superior value.

While health food stores provide a wide range of nutritious foods, similar foods can often be found in conventional markets at lower costs. The danger of shopping in health food stores is that the customer is often pressured into purchasing foods or supplements which he does not really need. The validity of health information given the customer is highly variable and in some instances dangerous. Often, people have unrealistic expectations of what health foods can do for their particular problem, and they postpone seeking medical care or discontinue medical treatment.

Vegetarianism.—Advocates of vegetarianism can be divided into at least three categories. First are the ovolactovegetarians who refrain from eating meat of any kind but use milk, milk products, and eggs. Second are the lactovegetarians who avoid meat and eggs but consume milk and milk products. Third are the pure or strict vegetarians who eat only foods from plant sources. Some variations exist among these categories. Vegetarians choose their way of eating for moral, religious, or health reasons. A well-selected vegetarian diet, with suitable combinations of vegetable proteins to complement one another, can be nutritionally adequate. Some vegetarian groups have a very favorable health experience in contrast to the population at large. Strict vegetarians, who eat no food from animal sources at all, should use products fortified with vitamin B_{12}, or a supplement of that vitamin.

Food Fads or Fad Diets.—There are changing fashions in popular diet schemes and it is almost impossible to keep up with them. Most fad diets are promoted glowingly as marvelous, sure-fire, new discovery, "get-thin-quick-without-feeling-deprived" schemes, and the obese are particularly vulnerable. Often the "Guru" is a self-styled "nutrition expert" who knows enough jargon and is sufficiently skilled at merchandising to be very persuasive. Because most fad diets do not lead to the development of new eating habits, weight loss is temporary and the individual waits for the next week's diet to come along.

Moderate Ways of Eating.—Among persons of all ages are those who eat a variety of nutritious foods in moderate amounts, recognizing the importance of eating wisely to maintain health and prevent illness. Some have been convinced by education; some have had the good fortune to be members of a culture that has a tradition of moderation; and others have been persuaded by their health advisors to modify their diets as an important part of a treatment plan.

These groups are not mutually exclusive and there is considerable overlap among them. Many individuals deviate from their usual pattern on special occasions. For example, the normally cautious eater goes on a cruise!

There are psychological, social, and economic reasons for our choosing one style or another, and the health professional can guide the individual to select from the infinite variety of available foods to meet his nutritional needs without abandoning his usual preferences entirely or sacrificing the pleasures of good food.

The health professional should avoid the mistake of assuming that the patient eats as he/she does or of attempting to counsel the patient regarding diet without knowing his present food habits.

PUBLIC HEALTH AND COMMUNITY NUTRITION

Public health or community nutrition is an integral part of a modern public health department. Charged with responsibility for the health of population groups through safeguarding the environment, performing regulatory functions, and controlling communicable diseases, public health also directs its efforts toward prevention of illness and, in some areas, provides primary health care to the medically indigent.

Whether seen in private practice or public health services, some groups are nutritionally vulnerable and require diet counseling. Among those who receive guidance from physicians, nurses, or nutritionists are women during pregnancy, mothers of infants and children, and patients who have diabetes. Patients with heart disease, hypertension, anemia, cancer, obesity, and other diet-related conditions are also high-priority groups. It is important that physicians, nurses, and health educators be equipped with nutrition knowledge so that they may counsel patients when indicated.

Health education and nutrition guidance are important components and, as knowledge and experience increase, concepts of behavior modification and risk factor reduction, applied in group settings, are utilized more frequently and more effectively.

The Palm Beach County Health Department conducted an innovative and effective program in Cardiovascular Risk Factor Detection and

Reversal from 1974–1976 with funding from the Florida Regional Medical Program. Clinic patients 18 to 59 were offered a series of tests to determine their cardiovascular risk factor status. Age, sex, height, weight, blood pressure, and smoking history were recorded. The study included: serum cholesterol, triglyceride, glucose, and uric acid determinations. Patients whose risk factors were extremely elevated were referred to the medical clinic. Those whose risk factors were moderately elevated were enrolled in an intervention program. Through a series of group discussions and demonstrations, participants learned how to make behavioral and dietary changes and thereby lower cholesterol and triglyceride levels, control weight, manage hypertension, and cope with stress.

The project was accomplished with the cooperation and support of the Palm Beach County Medical Society, Palm Beach County Chapter of the American Heart Association, and Florida Atlantic University. It demonstrated that a county health department could successfully mobilize its resources to launch a risk factor detection and reversal program and that individuals of low and middle socioeconomic status would respond favorably with encouraging outcomes.

Such an approach might serve as a model to be used in group practice.

In 1970 the Palm Beach and Lee County Health Departments participated in conducting a Migrant Nutrition Study. That study, described in the monograph, "Families of the Field," revealed that the most common health problems associated with nutrition were iron deficiency anemia and growth deviations, reflected in both underdevelopment and obesity. A unique feature of the study was that it included a nutrition education component. Classes were conducted in specially equipped vans at those migrant camps where the highest incidence of nutritional deficiencies had been identified. Classes for adults and children taught families what foods were best sources of needed nutrients and demonstrated ways of preparing those foods. Resurvey revealed evidence of dietary changes, particularly in increased iron intake in young children and decreased caloric intake by the obese. A short-term educational program helped participants to increase knowledge of food buying practices and community resources.

ARE YOU USING COMMUNITY RESOURCES?

Health Departments and practicing physicians should recognize, utilize, and develop community resources which may actually provide resources for food or may assist in educating patients. For assistance in utilizing these resources, the public health nutritionist or other health department professionals may guide the patient in learning about them.

RESOURCES FOR FOOD ASSISTANCE

Food Stamps.—A national program which provides food stamps to persons below a specified income level, enabling them to purchase a more adequate diet than would be possible otherwise. Patients in need of food stamps should be referred to the local Department of Health and Rehabilitative Services Food Stamp Office where their eligibility will be determined.

WIC.—A special Supplemental Food Program for Women, Infants, and Children. WIC serves pregnant, postpartum, and lactating women, infants up to one year and children up to five years. Patients must be medically indigent and must be certified to be at nutritional risk according to specified criteria. WIC coupons provide designated foods of high nutritional value. WIC is considered "food by prescription." About 70,000 participants in Florida receive the benefits of the WIC program and it is being expanded substantially. This program is generally operated through the county health department.

School Lunch and Breakfast.—The school lunch is almost universally available but school breakfast is less common. Teachers and school nurses have frequently observed that youngsters are more alert and perform better in school if they have had some nutritious food in the morning. The provision of school breakfast should be encouraged in those areas where children come to school without breakfast either because the parent does not prepare it or the busing schedule requires such an early departure that the youngster cannot eat breakfast. Children from low income families may be eligible for free or reduced price meals. With the passage of the Comprehensive School Health Education Act, health education and nutrition education should be strengthened at all grade levels and in all school systems.

Congregate Meals for the Elderly.—This program serves persons over 60. Many elderly persons lack the incentive or sense of self-worth to prepare meals for themselves. Some live on very limited incomes. Preference is given to those who are socially or graphically isolated and may not have the knowledge or resources to eat a nutritious diet. Congregate meals provide good nutrition plus socialization.

In some areas, a pilot program called "Super Suppers" was instituted in 1978 as a supplement to the Congregate Meals Program which operates five days a week. "Super Suppers" are packages of prepared foods in easy-to-manage containers. Each package constitutes a meal which meets the guidelines of the Title VII program by providing one third to one half of the Recommended Dietary Allowances. Eight different menus are available and they are rotated. Prior to weekends and holidays, participants receive "Super Suppers" for those days.

The local Health and Rehabilitative Services District Program Office of Aging and Adult Services will direct persons to the program.

Home Delivered Meals for the Handicapped and Disabled.—The Home Delivered Meals Programs, popularly known as "Meals on Wheels," are limited. This may be a valuable resource for a patient who is convalescing from illness or surgery. Some services are operated by public agencies, others by voluntary groups such as church groups, hospital or medical society auxiliaries, and still others by commercial firms.

Resources for Counseling and Education

In addition to those programs which provide food, or the wherewithal for obtaining it, there are usually other agencies or services which can assist you, the physician, in guiding your patients toward reliable nutrition information. Not all of these services are available in every area, but checking with the local Information and Referral Service or the county health department will help to identify resources.

Outpatient Counseling Services

In some communities, hospitals offer diet counseling, for a fee, on an outpatient basis. The physician whose practice does not permit him to spend sufficient time for effective diet counseling may refer patients to these services.

Dietitians as Members of Group Practice

Some physicians have added a dietitian to the group, on a full-time or part-time basis, and members of the group refer patients for counseling.

Dietitians in Private Practice

Dietitians, working alone or with other dietitians, have set up private practice and accept referrals from all physicians in the community. Area physicians should make contact with dietitians and nutritionists through their District Dietetic Associations or through the staff of the hospital with which they are affiliated.

The terms "dietitian" and "nutritionist" refer to the same discipline and describe persons who are trained in the science of nutrition and have as their goal the optimal nourishment of people. The term "dietitian" is often considered the generic term. Usually, the dietitian is involved in food service as well as therapeutics, while the nutritionist, who has had additional educational preparation, is involved in community programs for the promotion of health and control of disease.

Visiting Nurse Association, Visiting Homemaker Service, and Other Home Health Care Agencies

These agencies provide bedside care in the home under the orders of the patient's physician. The nurses have had preparation in nutrition and can help the patient and/or his family interpret and apply dietary instruction. Home health care may be available under various auspices. Staff have had some training and should be skilled in preparing recommended foods for the patient.

American Heart Association (Local Chapter)

This national organization has shown outstanding leadership in developing materials for professional and lay use. Leaflets and booklets are available on diet and coronary heart disease, diet modification to control hyperlipidemia in childhood and adolescents, sodium restriction, the fat controlled diet, risk factor reduction, exercise, smoking cessation, hypertension, and other related subjects. In many counties they conduct community screening programs, always referring those individuals with elevated risk factors to their own physicians for care. In some areas, the Heart Association provides diet counseling by a registered dietitian, upon referral by a physician. Community education programs and seminars for professional and lay persons are offered.

American Diabetes Association (Local and State Affiliates)

In cooperation with the American Dietetic Association, the national organization has revised the Exchange Lists for Meal Planning, a useful plan for counseling patients in diabetes or weight control. The bimonthly magazine, "Forecast," has an upbeat, positive tone which provides information and encouragement to readers. Regular meetings of the local group offer individuals who have diabetes, and their family members, the opportunity to hear speakers on a variety of subjects which concern them and to participate in group discussion. At least one meeting each year is devoted to diet.

Cooperative Extension Service (Affiliated with University of Florida)

Each county has agents trained in home economics. Some have Expanded Nutrition Projects through which trained aides and materials are available for information on normal nutrition, food budgeting, marketing, and preparation. Since many families lack basic skills, they may obtain practical help from this resource.

Adult Education—Community Schools

Schools may offer courses in normal nutrition in their evening programs. If combined with courses in other health-related topics, this may be valuable. Local medical societies and health departments should check content of such courses and qualifications of the instructors before endorsing or recommending such courses.

Weight Control Groups

The overweight patient presents a great challenge to physician and nutritionist. Many individuals respond better to group efforts at weight control based on behavior modification than to individual counseling and/or instruction. Referral to a recognized, soundly-based group may be an effective procedure. Special food promotions are not essential.

CLINICAL PRACTICE AND NUTRITION

Public health and clinical medicine face the nutritional problems of "too much" and "too little," of malabsorption or impaired utilization of nutrients, of imbalance, of interfering interactions with alcohol or drugs.

Steps in approaching and dealing with nutritional problems are comparable to procedures in dealing with any health problem. They include awareness of the nutritional determinants of disease; nutritional assessment; diagnosis based on physical examination, laboratory data, and diet history; treatment, and follow-up. These nutrition items should be an integral part of a comprehensive medical assessment.

Diet History.—When diet counseling is indicated, the first step is to learn the patient's present food pattern. Many diet history forms are available and the form may be self-administered or filled out by the health staff. It may be simple or complex. The physician or other health professional needs to know the patient's home situation, who prepares the food, what resources are available (cooking equipment, refrigeration, storage facilities), access to markets, approximate amount of money available for food. A diet record of several days gives a more complete picture than a 24-hour recall, but is harder to obtain. The combination of the 24-hour recall plus frequency information (how often do you eat green leafy vegetables? for example) is useful in making the patient more aware of his eating behavior and enabling the therapist to evaluate strengths, weaknesses, deficiencies, and excesses in his food pattern. A food diary of seven to 14 days is valuable for weight control, diabetes, and other situations where food consciousness is critical. Its value is enhanced if the patient records time of day at which food or beverage is taken, the environment (work, home, restaurant), other person or persons present, the kind and amount of food, how it was prepared, and the individual's mood or emotional state as he consumed the food or beverage. If a diet modification plan is to be effective, it must include setting of goals, learning new food behaviors, and some follow-up for reinforcement and/or evaluation.

CONTINUITY OF CARE

The diet counselor should interpret the diet in terms of the patient's home and work situation and lifestyle. If necessary, there should be referral to another agency or a suggestion that the patient call for further explanation. Recommendations may seem clear in the office, clinic or hospital, but very fuzzy when the patient is on his own.

It is desirable that the spouse or another family member participate in the instruction, especially if the patient is not the one who purchases and prepares the food. If the patient's diet can be adapted to the family's meals, the entire family may benefit and the patient may find it easier to follow dietary recommendations.

When a patient is hospitalized, the hospital experience should be educational as well as a treatment opportunity. The hospital food should exemplify the type of diet which the patient should have—for all his health needs. The patient should learn kinds of foods to eat and size of servings. Recently, a 70-year-old man who had been on a fat-controlled, cholesterol-restricted diet since his coronary eight years ago was terribly upset because he was served eggs and butter for breakfast when he was hospitalized for surgery of the prostate!

The hospitalized patient should receive diet instruction early in his hospitalization, not when he is about to be discharged. Too often the dietary department receives the request for diet instruction just prior to discharge. "Suitcase counseling," when the patient is packing to go home, is apprehensive about paying the bill, about leaving a protected environment or about a dozen other things, can hardly be effective. In the coronary care unit of a well-known teaching hospital, the policy states that the physician must order diet instruction at least three days before the patient's discharge or the dietary department does not provide it. The majority of patients do receive diet instruction.

In conditions which require modification of diet, the following principles are important:

1. The diet should be as nearly adequate as possible. If it is deficient, appropriate supplements should be prescribed.
2. Only those components of the diet which affect the patient's condition should be modified.
3. The diet should be individualized according to his likes and dislikes, present food habits, resources, and lifestyle.
4. The patient needs to know what to eat—kinds of food and amounts—and what not to eat. Such admonitions as "don't eat salt," or "watch carbohydrates," "try a 1000 calorie diet" or "eat a lot of fiber" mean little to the worried patient who has no knowledge of food composition and caloric values.
5. The patient needs to know whether a diet modification is short-term or long-term. If it is the latter, he needs help in developing a new eating pattern—one with which he can live for the rest of his life.
6. The counselor must strike a balance between an attitude that is too casual and an attitude that is so rigid and punitive that the patient feels frightened and terribly guilty if he deviates from the food plan at all.

SUMMARY

Some current nutrition issues and concerns have been discussed from the perspective of a county health department. The practicing physician and the health department should try to help individuals assume responsibility for their own health care and develop a lifestyle which includes, among other things, a prudent diet, based on moderate amounts of a variety of nutritious foods. Resources exist in every county to aid the individual who needs reliable information in understanding and following sound dietary recommendations. Making wise food choices is more than having information—although that is fundamental—because the behavior of people is altered through knowledge, understanding, and motivation.

There are opportunities for close working relationships among all health professionals, and private practitioners and public health practitioners will profit from a sharing of knowledge and experience. Continuing education in nutrition for prevention as well as for treatment should be encouraged.

The challenge of improving nutrition is an enormous one, but the promise of reducing illness and increasing wellness makes it an exciting one.

22

ALCOHOL, MALNUTRITION AND LIVER DISEASE

Charles S. Lieber, M.D.

Interrelationships between alcoholism, malnutrition and liver disease are complex; alcoholism commonly causes both malnutrition and liver disease, and hepatic dysfunction may be engendered by malnutrition per se. Traditionally, the disorders affecting the liver have been attributed exclusively to nutritional deficiencies accompanying alcoholism, but recent studies, summarized here, indicate that in addition to dietary deficiencies, alcohol itself can be incriminated as a direct etiologic factor in the pathogenesis of alcoholic liver disease.

MALNUTRITION IN ALCOHOLISM

The alcoholic derives a major portion of his caloric intake from alcohol and consequently has a much reduced demand for other foods to fulfill caloric needs. For example, alcohol (ethanol) provides 7.1 kilocalories/g; thus, 600 ml (20 oz) of 86-proof liquor represents about 1,500 calories or approximately one half to two thirds of the daily caloric requirement. Alcoholic beverages differ little in nutritional value except for carbohydrate content, trace amounts of B vitamins (especially thiamin and niacin) and iron. Harmful amounts of lead, cobalt and iron may rarely be present. The significance of other congeners in beverages remains largely unexplored. Though calorimetrically the combustion of ethanol liberates 7.1 cal/gram, ethanol does not provide equivalent caloric food value when compared with carbohydrate[1]; this discrepancy is most likely the

Dr. Lieber is Chief, Section of Liver Disease and Nutrition and the Alcoholism Research and Treatment Center, Veterans Administration Medical Center and the Mt. Sinai School of Medicine of the City University of New York, Bronx, N.Y.

result of a metabolic effect of alcohol. Since alcoholic beverages do not contain significant amounts of protein, vitamins and minerals, the intake of these nutrients may readily become borderline or insufficient. Alcohol also has direct effects on the gut[2] and pancreas, part of which are concentration-dependent. Furthermore, alcoholics have been shown to display malabsorption for a number of essential nutrients, including vitamins such as thiamin and B_{12}.[2] One of the most common vitamin deficiencies in the alcoholic is the lack of folate; it is a cause for macrocytic anemia and intestinal malabsorption.

ROLE OF DIETARY FACTORS IN THE PATHOGENESIS OF LIVER DISEASE IN THE ALCOHOLIC

Prevailing concepts concerning the pathogenesis of alcoholic liver injury have undergone a striking evolution. In the forties and fifties, it was generally accepted that "there is no more evidence of a specific toxic effect of pure ethyl alcohol upon liver cells than there is for one due to sugar."[3] This view was virtually universally espoused and until recently most textbooks of medicine reiterated that there was no evidence supporting the toxicity of ethanol itself. As stated in the 1958 edition of Harrison, it was "generally agreed that alcohol is not a hepatotoxin and that its effects on the liver probably are secondary to an associated nutritional disturbance."

This concept of the exclusively nutritional origin of alcoholic liver injury was based on both experimental and clinical studies. In rats, it has been shown that alcohol given in the drinking water was not capable of producing liver damage unless associated with a deficient diet.[3] However, rats display a natural aversion for ethanol and under the experimental conditions used, intake is relatively small and blood ethanol level negligible. When the alcohol aversion was counteracted by incorporation of ethanol in a totally liquid diet, and the ethanol consumption was thereby increased to 36% of total calories (an intake still less than that of many alcoholics) fatty liver resulted despite otherwise nutritious diets.[4] The clinical data supporting the lack of hepatotoxicity of alcohol consisted of several studies according to which alcohol could be administered without apparent untoward effects in a hospital setting.[4]

These studies however had several shortcomings. In some, alcohol was administered to heavy drinkers in amounts clearly below those consumed spontaneously. In other studies, larger amounts were given but in doses carefully calculated not to exceed the alcohol oxidizing capacity of the individual, thereby preventing a significant increase in the blood level of alcohol; furthermore no control studies were carried out simultaneously. Moreover, virtually all of these patients had underlying cirrhosis. Therefore, in these studies it must have been difficult to assess further changes, especially since no chemical measurements were carried out in these biopsies.

Role of Protein and Lipotropes

That dietary factors can modify the effect of alcohol on the liver has been clearly shown in rodents. Alcohol increases choline requirements, possibly by enhancing choline oxidation; choline supplementation reduces (but does not fully prevent) steatosis after chronic and acute alcohol administration.

Though in growing rats, deficiencies in dietary protein and lipotropic factors (choline and methionine) can produce fatty liver, primates are far less susceptible to protein and lipotrope deficiency and clinically, administration of choline to patients with alcoholic liver injury is ineffective in the face of continued alcohol intake. Furthermore in subhuman primates some fibrosis but, in virtually all studies, no cirrhosis was produced with protein deficiency alone. To cause cirrhosis, one has to create dietary conditions not normally achievable with natural foods (such as an association of a low protein and a high cholesterol content). Actually, to what extent nutritional deficiencies may potentiate the alcohol induced liver damage in the primate has not been as yet determined. In some patients subjected to intestinal bypass for obesity, lesions similar to those present in some alcoholics, namely hepatitis and fibrosis, have occurred, and it has been concluded therefore that in both situations, a similar pathogenesis, namely malnutrition, may pertain. Such reasoning "by analogy" is hazardous, however, since pathogenesis of the liver lesion after bypass is still unsettled. Even if malnutrition were shown to be the culprit in the latter situation, extrapolation to the alcoholic is not necessarily warranted. It could be argued, for instance, that similar liver lesions have also been engendered by chemical agents in man, not to mention the experimental evidence referred to subsequently of the production of liver damage after alcohol and an adequate diet. Under those conditions, plasma branched chain amino acids are increased,[5] whereas after bypass, these are depressed. This illustrates one of the many differences between these two conditions.

In children, protein deficiency causes hepatic steatosis, one of the manifestations of kwashiorkor, but this disease does not lead to cirrhosis. Acute and prolonged starvation (as treatment for obesity or as a consequence of anorexia nervosa) even to the point of cachexia (as seen during times of war) do not necessarily lead to fatty liver. In adolescent baboons, a low-protein, low-fat diet (7% and 14% of total calories) did not result in liver injury on either biochemical analysis or light and electron microscopic examination, even after 19 months.[6] Severe protein restriction (4% of total calories) did, however, produce steatosis in the baboon.[6] Protein deficiency could potentiate the effect of ethanol. Administration of ethanol with a diet deficient in protein and lipotropic factors had more pronounced effects than that of either factor alone,[7] at least in rodents.

Role of Dietary Fat

Chronic alcohol ingestion leads to deposition of dietary fat in the liver.[8] Furthermore, for a given alcohol intake, much more steatosis developed with diets of normal fat content than with a low-fat diet.[8] The chain length of dietary fatty acids also affects the degree of fat deposition in the liver after alcohol feeding. Replacement of long-chain triglycerides with medium-chain triglycerides markedly reduced the capacity of alcohol to produce fatty liver in rats,[9] probably because of the propensity of medium-chain fatty acids to undergo oxidation instead of esterification. The applicability of these findings to clinical practice has not as yet been assessed.

ALCOHOL AS A DIRECT CAUSE OF LIVER CHANGES

Under metabolic ward conditions, it was shown that administration of ethanol caused not only a fatty liver as assessed morphologically, but also a striking increase in liver triglycerides measured chemically.[8] This was associated with marked ultrastructural changes of the mitochondria and endoplasmic reticulum, although the alcohol was administered with an adequate regimen supplemented with minerals and vitamins,[10] or even with a high protein diet. It was also shown that alcohol administration prevents the disappearance of the fatty liver. The question was then raised whether lesions more severe than steatosis, particularly cirrhosis, can be produced by alcohol in the absence of dietary deficiencies. Studies in rodents had been unsatisfactory because even when given with a liquid diet, the intake of alcohol in rodents does not reach the level of average consumption in the alcoholic, namely 50% of total calories. Such a consumption was achieved in the baboon, again through incorporation of ethanol in totally liquid diets.[11] The nonalcohol calories of the diet were provided by protein (36% of total nonalcohol calories), fat (42%) and carbohydrate (22%). All of the other nutrients were calculated to exceed the normal requirements of the baboon (National Academy of Science, 1978). Choline was given at twice the level recommended for the baboons. This diet was also liberally supplemented with minerals and vitamins. The fat and carbohydrate composition of the baboon diet was calculated to mimic an optimal clinical situation in which the alcoholic may be trying to achieve a high protein diet (36% of calories) with available natural foods while drinking. In fact, even if the alcoholic tried hard it would be difficult for him to consume a diet richer in protein than the one administered to the baboons (36% of calories). Nevertheless, the baboons developed not only fatty liver, but after 2–5 years, one-third also had progression of liver damage to cirrhosis.[12] Therefore it was concluded that in addition to dietary factors, alcohol itself plays a key etiological role in the development of liver injury. If one can extrapolate from these baboon data to the human situation, it would seem that heavy drinkers, even if they make an extra effort to maintain a high protein diet, will not necessarily succeed in preventing the development of cirrhosis unless they also control their alcohol intake.

The demonstration of the hepatotoxicity of ethanol also raises the question of a possible "threshold" of this action. As in the case of many other toxins, the effects of alcohol are subject to great individual variability. The response to ethanol varies as a function of hereditary factors, associated diseases, and particularly dose and duration of alcohol intake. Various epidemiological studies clearly showed a relationship between the incidence of cirrhosis in an alcoholic population and amount of alcohol intake, whereas no role for dietary deficiency was revealed. Such a statistical relationship of the incidence of cirrhosis to the amount of alcohol consumed (but not to protein malnutrition) was shown for instance by Pequignot *et al.*[13] In fact, the individuals surveyed had developed cirrhosis despite an average daily dietary protein intake of 100 grams or more. In other epidemiological studies, hospitalized alcoholics reported a history of a poorer protein intake. However one cannot conclude from such observations to what extent, if any, the low protein intake contributed to the liver complications. In addition to showing that even diets relatively rich in protein do not preclude the development of alcoholic cirrhosis, earlier studies of Pequignot also revealed that the incidence of cirrhosis increased markedly when the daily intake of alcohol reached 160 grams. This was interpreted by some to indicate a "threshold" of toxicity of alcohol at that level. However, more recent studies of Pequignot *et al.*[13] have also shown that daily intake of alcohol as low as 40 grams in men and 20 grams in women resulted in a statistically significant increase of the incidence of cirrhosis in a well nourished population. Obviously, because of individual variations, the exact toxic level for a given subject is usually unknown. However, the public should be made aware of the fact that even with adequate diets, amounts of alcohol considered before as innocuous may indeed harm the liver. This is particularly pertinent in the case of women, whose increased susceptibility was also indicated by a higher incidence of cirrhosis for a given alcohol intake: Wilkinson *et al.*[14] indeed found women to be more susceptible than men to the development of alcoholic cirrhosis. Nutrition again did not play an appreciable part in the causation of liver disease and cirrhosis was not found to be more common among the lowest socio-economic groups.[14]

SUMMARY AND RECOMMENDATION

Experimental, clinical and epidemiological evidence indicates that even when adequate diets are consumed, ethanol exerts liver toxicity, whereas the role of malnutrition in the development of human cirrhosis remains elusive. At present, the optimal diet for the alcoholic is not established. Obviously, specific nutritional deficiencies such as lack of thiamin and folate should be avoided and when present corrected. Concerning protein, however, the situation is less clear. In rats, carbon tetrachloride-induced cirrhosis can be prevented by a low protein diet. Early studies relating beneficial effects of high protein diets were uncontrolled. Subsequently the risk in cirrhotic patients of dietary-induced encephalopathy has become more apparent. Therefore, in the absence of experimental data to the contrary, high protein diets do not seem indicated at the present time, and until this issue is resolved it may be prudent to settle for an intake of proteins which does not exceed the individual protein tolerance of the cirrhotic or the RDA recommended amount (0.8−1 g/kg), whichever is lower. Similarly, there is no indication for choline supplementation, especially in the absence of information regarding choline requirements in the primates and in view of the disappointing results with choline supplementation in the alcoholic. In addition to correction of the diet one must also focus on the control of the alcohol intake. Recent studies have shown that even in well-nourished populations, amounts of alcohol much lower than hitherto suspected must be considered as potentially cirrhogenic, particularly in women.

REFERENCES

1. PIROLA, R.C. and LIEBER, C.S.: The energy cost of the metabolism of drugs, including ethanol. Pharmacology 7:185, 1972.
2. LINDENBAUM, J. and LIEBER, C.S.: Effects of chronic ethanol administration on intestinal absorption in man in the absence of nutritional deficiency. Ann. N.Y. Acad. Sci. 252:228, 1975.
3. BEST, C.H., HARTROFT, W. S., LUCAS, C.C. and RIDOUT, J.H.: Liver damage produced by feeding alcohol or sugar and its prevention by choline. Brit. Med. J. 2:1101, 1949.
4. LIEBER, C.S., JONES, D.P. and DECARLI, L.M.: Effects of prolonged ethanol intake: Production of fatty liver despite adequate diets. J. Clin. Invest. 44: 1009. 1965.

5. SHAW, S. and LIEBER, C.S.: Plasma amino acid abnormalities in the alcoholic: Respective role of alcohol, nutrition and liver injury. Gastroenterology 74:677, 1978.
6. LIEBER, C.S., DECARLI, L.M., GANG, H., WALKER, G. and RUBIN, E.: Hepatic effects of long term ethanol consumption in primates. *In* Medical Primatology 1972, (E.I. Goldsmith and J. Moor-Jankowski, Eds.) S. Karger, Basel, Part 3, pp. 270.
7. LIEBER, C.S., SPRITZ, N. and DECARLI, L.M.; Fatty liver produced by dietary deficiencies: Its pathogenesis and potentiation by ethanol. J. Lipid. Res. 10:283, 1969.
8. LIEBER, C.S. and SPRITZ, N.: Effects of prolonged ethanol intake in man: Role of dietary, adipose, and endogenously synthesized fatty acids in the pathogenesis of the alcoholic fatty liver. J. Clin. Invest. 45:1400, 1966.
9. LIEBER, C.S., LEFEVRE, A., SPRITZ, N., FEINMAN, L. and DECARLI, L.M.: Difference in hepatic metabolism of long- and medium-chain fatty acids: The role of fatty acid chain length in the production of the alcoholic fatty liver. J. Clin. Invest. 46:1451, 1967.
10. LANE, B.P. and LIEBER, C.S.: Ultrastructural alterations in human hepatocytes following ingestion of ethanol with adequate diets. Amer. J. Path. 49:593, 1966.
11. LIEBER, C.S. and DECARLI, L.M.: An experimental model of alcohol feeding and liver injury in the baboon. J. Med. Primatology 3:153, 1974.
12. LIEBER, C.S., DECARLI, L.M. and RUBIN, E.: Sequential production of fatty liver, hepatitis and cirrhosis in sub-human primates fed ethanol with adequate diets. Proc. Nat. Acad. Sci. 72:437, 1975.
13. PEQUIGNOT, G., TUYNS, A.J. and BERTA, J.L.: Ascitic cirrhosis in relation to alcohol consumption. International J. Epidemiology 7:113, 1978.
14. WILKINSON, P., SANTAMARIA, J.N. and RANKIN, J.G.: Epidemiology of alcoholic cirrhosis. Aust. Ann. Med. 18:222, 1969.

23

HYPERACTIVITY AND THE FOOD-ADDITIVE-FREE DIET

Esther H. Wender, M.D.

Hyperactivity, and frequently associated learning disabilities, is the most common behavorial-developmental problem in childhood, affecting, by the most conservative estimates, at least 5% of the childhood population. This psychiatric syndrome, most frequently referred to as hyperkinesis or minimal brain dysfunction, has been the subject of much controversy in both the medical and lay literature. Some of the more important issues concern the true incidence of the disorder, diagnostic criteria, and appropriate treatment, particularly treatment with stimulant medication. Negative feelings about the use of medication has stimulated interest in other forms of treatment, some of them nutritional. Probably the most widely publicized nutritional treatment for hyperkinesis involves the elimination of certain food additives from the diet. In this article the food-additive-free diet is described and the rationale for its use explained. Possible mechanisms of action for this and other nutritional therapies are discussed. Finally, the article reviews recent research on the food-additive-free diet and its effect on hyperkinesis. Conclusions are discussed regarding the efficacy and potential hazards of this nutritional treatment and, lastly, recommendations are presented for discussing these issues with patients and their families.

Rationale for the Diet

The term "food additive" is a general one, referring to any non-nutrient added to food for a variety of reasons including food preservation, or

Dr. Wender is Assistant Professor of Pediatrics, University of Utah College of Medicine, Salt Lake City.

enhancing the food's palatability or appeal. The diet in question, however, is designed to remove only some food additives, specifically, all artificial food coloring and flavorings. Salicylates that occur naturally in some foods are also eliminated. The diet was originally developed to treat patients who are sensitive to salicylates. Salicylate-sensitive persons react not only to the salicylates found in medicines but also to those occurring naturally in foods. Some of these patients also react to chemicals in certain artificial food dyes, particularly tartrazine which is the chemical constituent of the most commonly used yellow dye. Artificial flavorings that contain salicylate products (oil of wintergreen) as their base must also be eliminated. The food-additive-free diet, therefore, comes from, and is essentially the same as, the diet used in the treatment of salicylate-sensitive patients. Why is this particular diet thought to help children with hyperkinesis? The diet was first recommended by Ben Feingold, M.D., an allergist.[1] He states that he observed several adult salicylate-sensitive patients whose psychiatric or behavioral problems improved while on this diet. On the basis of these observations he wondered if the diet might help children with common behavioral problems. He began employing the diet in the treatment of children with hyperactivity and/or learning disabilities. According to his reports several children improved dramatically on this special diet, which led him to speculate that hyperactivity and learning disabilities were caused, in a substantial percentage of children, by food additives. He claims that the incidence of hyperactivity and learning disability is increasing in recent years (an undocumented assumption) as the result of the greater use of food additives in the American food industry.

Proposed Mechanisms of Action

Dr. Feingold does not feel that food additives produce behavioral change on the basis of allergic mechanisms. Instead he thinks that hyperactive children are sensitive to the chemicals in food additives. Others disagree, however, and argue that some children are allergic to food additives as well as to specific foods, for example, corn, chocolate, wheat and milk. Some of these arguments can be clarified by understanding the differences between food allergy and food sensitivity. These differences are outlined in Table 23.1. In the case of definite food allergy, the reaction is immediate and the signs and symptoms are atopic regardless of the type of allergen. The reaction is IgE mediated, antibodies to the offending food can be clearly demonstrated, and the patient is skin test positive. A different type of food allergy results in a delayed reaction that may involve gastrointestinal as well as atopic symptoms. Such symptoms commonly include diarrhea, vomiting and/or abdominal pain

TABLE 23.1. FOOD ALLERGY

Immediate	Delayed
1. IgE mediated	1. Perhaps IgE or lymphocyte mediated
2. Definite atopic symptoms	2. Skin test ± positive
3. Skin test positive	3. Allergic and/or GI symptoms
	4. ± demonstration of antibodies
	5. Diagnosis by elimination diet and rechallenge

1. No increase in IgE, antibodies, or positive skin tests
2. Multiple symptoms—may be only behavioral
3. Diagnosis—must use placebo controls

or else allergic skin reactions or wheezing. Milk allergy in the infant and toddler is the most common example of delayed-reaction food allergy. This phenomenon is thought to be mediated by lymphocytes. Elevated IgE levels and antibodies to the offending food are inconsistent manifestations and positive skin tests may or may not be seen. A specific mechanism for this type of allergic reaction has never been demonstrated, so most experts agree that accurate diagnosis requires amelioration of symptoms following an elimination diet and a return of those symptoms following challenge and rechallenge with the offending food. An elimination diet may produce changes in vague complaints on the basis of suggestion or positive expectation. Therefore, signs and symptoms must be fairly specific or objective for this diagnostic technique to be trusted. This point will be mentioned again in the discussion of food sensitivity.

In contrast to either the immediate or delayed type of food allergy, the symptoms of "food sensitivity" are said to be quite variable and may include only behavior or such vague complaints as fatigue and chronic aches and pains. Food sensitivity is not thought to be mediated by allergic mechanisms. Instead the symptoms are thought to be produced by specific reactions to chemicals contained in food. Such reactions are said to occur only in patients who are susceptible, probably on the basis of inherited biochemical traits.

Since these specific chemical reactions cannot be demonstrated by objective tests, the existence of food sensitivity is very controversial. As in the case of delayed-type food allergy, clinicians attempt to diagnose food sensitivity by demonstrating change in symptoms following an elimination diet plus a return of these same symptoms when the patient is challenged with the suspected food. The problem is that changes in vague complaints and/or purely behavioral symptoms may occur following dietary change due to the nonspecific effects of expectation and suggestion. These nonspecific effects are collectively known as "placebo effects."[2] In order to know whether changes in symptoms are due to nonspecific, placebo effects or to the elimination of a specific chemical, diagnostic procedures must include a placebo control. This means that the patient is given two different diagnostic tests. In one instance the specific food is eliminated. In the second instance a similar dietary change is made, but the specific food is not eliminated (the placebo control). Neither the patient nor the diagnostician should know which diagnostic test is being given. This way neither the patient nor the diagnostician can be influenced by the expectation of change or else the expectation is spread evenly between the two diagnostic tests. In my opinion food sensitivity cannot be accurately diagnosed without employing such placebo controls.

THE FOOD-ADDITIVE-FREE DIET

The specific requirements of the food-additive-free diet are outlined in Table 23.2. Group 1 specifies the fruits and vegetables that must be eliminated on this diet because they supposedly contain salicylates. Recently, three items on this list—oranges, almonds, and strawberries—have been found to contain no appreciable amounts of salicylates.[3] This highlights one of the problems in specifying the food-additive-free diet. Information about the salicylate content of food is based upon old literature and needs to be reviewed using modern day techniques of food analysis. Until that is done these dietary restrictions must be considered tentative. The food items in group 2 are eliminated because, in general, they contain either artificial food colorings or flavorings. This list can only be specified in a general way since the same food item prepared by different manufacturers sometimes contains artificial colorings and flavorings and sometimes does not. All food labels must be carefully checked and, even then, manufacturers must be consulted to determine the exact techniques of preparation for many food items. A review of Table 23.2 will indicate why the diet is very difficult for most families to follow. Most preprocessed foods must be eliminated and many commonly consumed foods must be prepared "from scratch." Drinks are a particular problem because of the popularity of manufactured beverages, and because fruit juice substitutes often come from fruits eliminated in group 1. It should be noted that for a family to adhere to this diet requires major changes in shopping habits and in food preparation.

RESEARCH DESIGN

In order to study the theory that hyperactivity and/or learning disabilities are caused by the ingestion of specific food additives, the general effect of dietary change on behavior must be separated from the specific effects of food additives by the use of placebo controls as previously

TABLE 23.2. FEINGOLD'S ADDITIVE-FREE DIETS—FOODS TO BE ELIMINATED

Group 1—Natural salicylates		
Fruits—	*Almonds Apples Apricots **Berries Cherries Currants Grapes & Raisins Nectarines	*Orange (Grapefruit, Lime and Lemon Permitted) Peaches Plums and Prunes
Vegetables—	Tomatoes Cucumbers	
Group 2—Artificial colorings and flavorings		
Cereals—	All with artificial colors and flavors All instant breakfast food	
Bakery Goods—	Manufactured baked goods Frozen baked goods Most packaged mixes Commercial breads permitted except eggbread and whole wheat	
Luncheon Meats—	Bologna Salami **Sausage **Ham, bacon and pork	Frankfurters Meat loaf
Other Meats and Fish—	All barbecued meats Prestuffed poultry Frozen precooked fish	
Desserts—	Manufactured ice creams, sherbets, etc. Powdered puddings Flavored yogurt Dessert mixes	
Candies—	All manufactured types	
Beverages—	All soft drinks except 7-Up Instant breakfast drinks Quick-mix powdered drinks Canned drinks except pure grapefruit or pineapple juice Prepared chocolate milk	
Miscellaneous foods—	**Margarine **Butter Mustard Soy sauce Commercial chocolate syrup Barbecue chips Cheeses (except natural, white) Cloves Catsup Chili sauce	
Sundries—	Toothpastes and powders Mouthwashes Cough drops Many medicines and vitamins Aspirin products Perfumes	

*Note that oranges, almonds and strawberries are free of salicylates according to recent food analysis. See text.
**Check labels.

mentioned. One way to provide such placebo controls would be to treat comparable groups of hyperactive or learning disabled children with either the specific food-additive-free diet described in Table 23.2 or else a constrasting diet (control diet) requiring similar changes in shopping patterns and food preparation but indistinguishable from the food-additive-free diet. It is very difficult to devise this type of contrasting diet. It is reasonably easy to construct a diet requiring similar shopping and food preparation but it is very difficult to disguise the differences between the contrasting diet and the real food-additive-free diet, particularly since this diet has received so much publicity. Still, in a couple of studies an attempt was made to provide a control and an experimental diet. A different approach to the research problem is illustrated in Figure 23.1. In this type of study the hyperactive or learning disabled children are first treated with the food-additive-free diet, making no attempt to disguise the treatment. The assumption is made that a certain percentage of these children will respond favorably to this dietary change but the experimenter, at this stage of the study, cannot tell whether the effect is due to the removal of specific food additives or whether it is due to nonspecific psychological factors. The group that responds favorably is then studied further. While remaining on the food-additive-free diet this group of children is then challenged with a specific food that may contain food additives or else is completely free of such substances. The food item that contains the additives must be indistinguishable from the one that does not. If Dr. Feingold's claims are correct, when challenged with the food containing additives, these diet responsive children should show a deterioration in behavior while those who ate the food free of additives should remain improved. A special food has been manufactured for the purpose of scientifically testing the food-additive-free diet theory. This challenge food contains a mixture of the nine most commonly used food dyes in the American food industry at a dose which is equal to half the average daily consumption of artificial food colorings in the American diet. This challenge food is in the form of a cookie or candy bar disguised with chocolate color and flavor to make the bar that contains food coloring indistinguishable from the one that does not. This challenge material contains artificial food colorings but does not contain either salicylates or artificial flavorings, which means that any conclusions drawn from studies using this challenge material are valid only for the colorings. Most of the adequately designed research studies have employed this type of research design.

SUMMARY OF RESEARCH FINDINGS

Of the studies that have been completed so far, two employed a control diet.[4,5] Combining information from the two studies, a total of 51 school

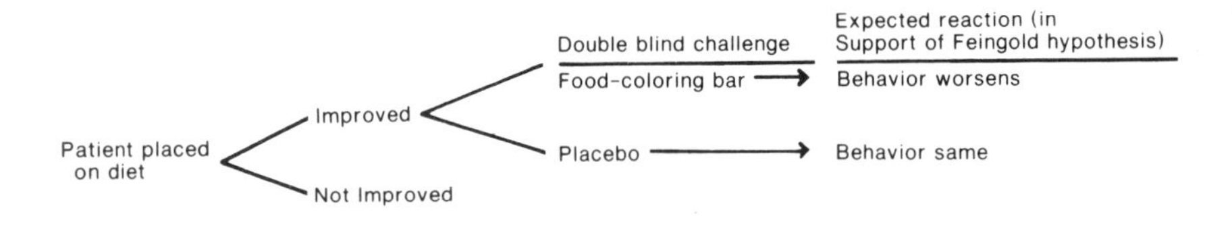

FIG. 23.1. RESEARCH DESIGN OF CHALLENGE STUDIES

age children and ten preschool children were tested. In both studies some improvement was seen on the food-additive-free diet as compared to the control diet, but only when the additive-free diet followed the control diet, and not when the order of these two treatments was reversed. This is known as an order effect and has been noted previously in behavioral research. The explanation for this finding is the subject of controversy but may be due in part to the family's expectations. If only mild changes are seen throughout the experiment, families are likely to interpret the second treatment as the "real treatment" when the first one had relatively little effect. In only one of these two studies was the improvement statistically significant.[4] In this study the control diet was not very adequately disguised. In the other study, where the control diet was fairly cleverly disguised, the only improvement was seen in the preschool children and there only in the parents' responses and not on more objective, but perhaps less sensitive, laboratory tests.

Several well designed challenge studies have been completed, testing a total of about 80 children.[6–11] These studies have yielded the following results: First, several studies have demonstrated that the food-additive-free diet under uncontrolled (open trial) conditions does produce behavioral improvement that can be documented by behavioral questionnaires.[6,7] As mentioned previously, however, at this stage of the study one cannot tell whether the improvement is due to the elimination of food additives or to psychological factors. When these patients have been challenged with artificial food colorings under controlled (double-blind) conditions no deterioration of behavior has been noted. This strongly suggests that the initial behavioral improvement was due to psychological factors (placebo effects) since behavior does not worsen when artificial colorings are added back into the diet. It is not known whether the behavior would deteriorate if salicylates or artificial flavorings were added back also. A third finding was not expected and its significance is still being studied. When the food bar containing artificial food colorings is ingested, some of the studies have demonstrated a very short-lived (lasting one hour) effect that seems to bear no relationship to overall behavior or learning.[6-10] The nature of this effect has not been well described but seems to consist of a transient period of irritability and inattentiveness. This transient response may be the pharmacological effect of a single, large dose of food colorings and, if so, would probably also be detected in normal children. Further work needs to be done to specify the characteristics of this effect, to find out if it is related to the dose of food colorings, and to see if all children, not just hyperactive and learning disabled children, would show this type of response. It is clear, however, that this brief response does not affect the hyperactive or learning disabled child's overall behavior as measured by teachers, parents, or objective evaluations done in the laboratory or classroom.

REMAINING PROBLEMS

Some problems remain that have not been answered by the studies completed so far. First, the challenge studies have employed only artificial food colorings as the challenge material. Perhaps the expected deterioration in behavior would be seen if the challenge materials also contained salicylates or artificial flavorings. Second, there is still considerable controversy over the issue of the appropriate dose of food colorings and their frequency of administration. Some argue that the dose used in studies so far has been too low based upon an underestimation of the average daily intake of these additives, and that the food containing coloring should be given more frequently to more closely simulate the usual eating pattern of children. Though both arguments have some merit, there are reasonable replies to both criticisms. First, though both salicylates and artificial flavorings should be tested, the artificial food colorings are probably the most important additive excluded in this diet—important because the exclusion of colorings eliminates some of the most popular and most frequently purchased food items. Researchers are justified, therefore, in testing this category of additives first. The controversy concerning dose of food coloring is based upon different ways of estimating the average intake of colorings in children's diets. One author argues that children ingest more colorings, on the average, than do others in the general population. However, the ingestion of food colorings does not ordinarily occur in one or two large bolus amounts but instead is taken in small amounts spread over time. A dose larger than that contained in the specially manufactured food bar probably represents a very high single dose of food coloring and does not, therefore, mimic the usual pattern of dietary intake. Also, Dr. Feingold frequently says that even one minor dietary infraction usually results in a significant deterioration in behavior. If this is so, the challenge food bar which contains approximately half the total daily intake of food coloring should certainly produce a noticeable effect, but, under controlled conditions, it does not.

Finally, many questions have been raised over the issue of dietary compliance. This is an important issue in the studies that employed a control diet since these studies were aimed at finding out whether any children might respond to the food-additive-free diet. If children do not comply with the diet, any favorable dietary effect would be obscured. However, compliance is not an important issue in the challenge studies since children selected for these studies were already ostensibly diet responsive, which makes compliance irrelevant unless one argues that even greater improvement would be seen with stricter adherence to the diet. Also, in most studies careful diet diaries were kept in an attempt to correlate dietary infractions with behavioral changes but no such correlations could be found, suggesting that compliance with diet is not an important issue.

CONCLUSIONS

It is my conclusion on the basis of the studies done so far that there is no good evidence linking artificial food colorings to the occurrence of the hyperactivity syndrome or minimal brain dysfunction. There does seem to be a pharmacological effect—which is brief and probably of no significance to overall behavior—of food colorings when given in single, large doses. This effect needs to be more clearly described and studied more carefully to see if it is dose related and if it occurs in normal children.

RECOMMENDATIONS

Given these negative conclusions, what do I tell parents? First, the answer to this question depends on whether the parent is asking me for advice or telling me that they have tried, or want to try, their child on this diet. If they are asking me for advice I give them information much like that contained in this article. If the family is motivated to try this treatment and seems anxious to have my permission, I see no reason to discourage their efforts since the diet is basically nutritious and since favorable, nonspecific psychological effects may be genuinely helpful to some families. The only nutritional concern relates to the intake of vitamin C since most popular vitamin C containing fruits are eliminated from the originally published form of the diet. It is also important to observe if the family continues to pursue other aspects of treatment that may have already been prescribed. For example, if the family tries the diet but also discontinues the child's medication and his or her behavior deteriorates, enthusiasm for the diet may keep the family from noticing the effect of discontinued medication. A third potential problem is that of arguments between parents who are pushing the diet and the child who is resisting. In this situation the child may develop a hostile, rebellious attitude that may have a harmful effect on his overall problem. It should be mentioned that this same type of hostile reaction can develop towards medication or psychotherapy as well as dietary treatment.

REFERENCES

1. FEINGOLD, B.F.: Why Your Child is Hyperactive, Random House, New York, 1975.
2. SHAPIRO, A.K.: Placebo Effects in Psychotherapy and Psychoanalysis, J. Clin. Pharmacol. 10:73–78, 1970.
3. HARLEY, J.R., *et al.*: An Experimental Evaluation of Hyperactivity and Food Additives. Phase I, Private Publication, University of Wisconsin, Madison, Wisconsin, 1977, pg. 15.
4. CONNORS, C.K.; GOYETTE, C.H., and SOUTHWICK, D.A., *et al.*: Food Additives and Hyperkinesis, A Controlled Double-Blind Experiment, Pediatrics 58:154–156, 1976.
5. HARLEY, J.P.; RAY, R.S.; TOMASI, L., *et al.*: Hyperkinesis and Food Additives: Testing the Feingold Hypothesis. Pediatrics 61:818, 1978.
6. GOYETTE, C.H.; CONNORS, C.K.; PETTI, T.A., *et al.*: Effects of Artificial Colors on Hyperkinetic Children: A Double-Blind Challenge Study. Psychopharmacology, Bulletin 14:39, 1978.
7. LEVY, F.; DUMBRELL, S., *et al.*: Hyperkinesis and Diet: A Double-Blind Crossover Trial With a Tartrazine Challenge, Med. J. Australia 1:61, 1978.
8. MATTES, J., and GITTELMAN-KLEIN, R.: A Crossover Study of Artificial Food Colorings in a Hyperkinetic Child. Am. J. Psychiatry 135:987, 1978.
9. SHAYWITZ, B.A., and GOLDENRING, J.R., *et al.*: The Effects of Chronic Administration Food Colorings on Activity Levels and Cognitive Performance in Normal and Hyperactive Developing Rat Pups. Ann. Neurology 4:196, 1978.
10. SWANSON, J.M., and KINSBOURNE, M.: Artificial Color and Hyperactive Behavior. To appear in Knights, R. M. and Bakker, D. (Eds). Rehabilitation, Treatment and Management of Learning Disorders, University Park Press (in press).
11. WILLIAMS, J.I., and CRAM, D.M., *et al.*: Relative Effects of Drugs and Diet on Hyperactive Behaviors: An Experimental Study. Pediatrics 61: 811, 1978.

24

FOOD ADDITIVES

William J. Darby, M.D., Ph.D.

Widespread public concern regarding food additives stems, in large measure, from the fear resulting from lack of understanding or knowledge. Such lack pertains to information in the following areas:

the chemical nature of all food;

the identity of "food additives";

the historical roles of food additives as ingredients of traditional foods;

failure to differentiate between "adulteration," "contamination," and food additives as desirable, beneficial components of traditional foods; and

the regulatory controls and safeguards that assure the safety and nutritive value of our food supply through federal, state and local regulatory agencies.

Finally, there abound unrealistic concepts and proposals for the prevention or cure of disease states through simplistic, impractical alterations of food patterns or of food production techniques. Not only are these without scientific validity but they are naively unattainable in today's industrialized, urbanized society.

CHEMICAL NATURE OF FOOD

It is trite to remind us that all components of foods are chemicals: carbohydrates, including a variety of simple sugars; lipids, including fats,

Dr. Darby is President, The Nutrition Foundation, New York and Washington, D.C.

fatty acids, sterols, waxes; proteins, amino acids, peptides, and derivatives of amino acids; minerals, ranging from essential ones required in gram quantities to trace substances needed in microgram amounts and others for which a nutrient role is not identified; vitamins and precursors of vitamins; and water. Foods naturally contain substances other than nutrients including naturally occurring emulsifiers, thickeners, buffers, chelating agents, pigments or colors, organic acids, flavors, antioxidants, antimycotic materials.

Complex chemical interactions occur during home processes, as well as industrial ones, of drying of foods, cooking or, indeed, even storage of foodstuffs. During the latter, naturally occurring enzymes frequently alter the chemical composition of the food. For example, the increased ripening of fruits during storage usually generates additional quantities of sugars.

Upon storage and/or heating, the widest variety of chemical changes occur. Examples of these are: the interaction of protein derivatives with simple sugars or the so-called "browning (or Maillard) reaction" responsible in part for the desirable flavor of many cooked meats; alcohol and carbon dioxide may be expelled as in the process of baking of leavened bread; oxidative changes may destroy labile substances including nutrient essentials such as vitamin C or alter colors of ingredients or products such as Tabasco sauce; oxidative and hydrolytic changes in lipids result in rancidity accelerated by heat and other conditions; some types of bacterial actions, such as lactic acid fermentation of milk, inhibit or prevent undesirable bacterial alterations by putrefactive organisms. Such microbial processes include compositional changes, the chemical nature of which changes, and the metabolic import of the resultant compounds remain to be fully elaborated.

The unstandardized, uncontrolled variable conditions of home or domestic storage, preservation and preparation result in a less uniform, less identifiable series of changes in the food product than does the defined, controlled conditions of industrial processing.

Modern, sophisticated analytical techniques enable food scientists increasingly to identify and ofttimes quantitate the miniscule trace compounds, organic and inorganic, present in foods and the complex assortment of these responsible for certain desirable properties such as flavor. Mussinan notes that prior to 1939 ten volatile compounds had been identified as constituents of raspberry juice, but that since that time more than 100 additional compounds have been identified and reported.[1] In other studies of blackberry essence, earlier investigators had identified 23 compounds. Modern studies separating the concentrate by column chromatography resulted in 33 fractions, each analyzed separately by GC-Mass spectroscopy. One of these fractions was found to contain 66 compounds not previously identified as a constituent of blackberries. The total number from all 33 fractions far exceeds this.

The numerous important volatile flavor components of foods constitute a wide range of complex alcohols, aldehydes, ketones, acids, esters, amines and other nitrogen-containing compounds, sulfur-containing compounds, oxygen, nitrogen or sulfur heterocyclics, halogenated compounds, cyanides, phenols and so on.[2] Similarly diverse constituents are responsible for numerous other properties of foods such as colors.

It is of much interest that the so-called artificial flavors frequently are comprised of but 4–10 or so of the dominant naturally occurring flavor-contributing compounds. Such artificial flavors then become "food additives." Indeed, many substances, in addition to flavoring agents that have given rise to major controversies when added to foods, occur widely in various traditional foods in nature, for example, benzoic acid, coumarin, saffrole, salicylates, caffeine, oxalates, acetic acid, salt, phosphates, various alkaloids, nitrates and, most recently, nitrosamines. Natural foodstuffs contain a wide variety of substances that are not now known to have nutritive value and which, if taken in amounts substantially larger than those encountered in normal usage, may be toxic.[7] Concerning these, Dr. J.M. Coon, Professor of Pharmacology, Thomas Jefferson University, has written: "Viewing all chemicals that are present in our food supply—the natural components, agricultural chemicals, food additives and natural and man-made contaminants in perspective—it is clear that the greatest area of unknown involves the natural and normal components of our foods."

WHAT ARE FOOD ADDITIVES?

The Committee on Food Protection of the National Academy of Sciences has identified food additives as follows:[4]

> In addition to those chemicals that constitute foodstuffs per se, chemicals may be incorporated—either directly or indirectly—during the growing, storage, or processing of foods. These chemicals may be described for convenience as 'food additives.' When they are purposely introduced to aid in processing or to preserve or improve the quality of the product, they are called intentional additives. Such materials as vitamins and minerals for enrichment, mold inhibitors, bactericides, antioxidants, colors, flavors, sweeteners, and emulsifiers are intentional additives. They are added to the food product in carefully controlled amounts during processing, and the amounts necessary to achieve the desired effect are usually very small.

Common types of intentional food additives include acid ingredients, such as potassium acid tartrate, tartaric acid, monocalcium phosphate, sodium bicarbonate, citric acid, lactic acid, malic acid. These are used as acidifying, buffering or neutralizing agents.

Upon storage, wheat flour loses its pale yellow tint, becomes white and undergoes "aging" in a manner to improve its baking qualities. Small amounts of oxidizing agents accelerate this process and reduce storage costs and hazards of spoilage and insect and rodent infestation. These agents include oxides of nitrogen, chlorine dioxide and similar compounds.

Traditionally, sources of lecithin and other naturally occurring emulsifying agents such as egg yolk are used to improve the volume, uniformity and fineness of grain and bakery products, some breads and frozen desserts. Commercially, lecithin and mono- and diglycerides and related compounds similarly are utilized as "additives." Both of the latter occur in large quantities in the gut during digestion of a fat-containing meal.

Traditional as well as so-called artificial flavoring agents have been employed throughout recorded history, and the conquests arising from efforts to obtain desired spices and flavoring agents have influenced the course of history. Many of the traditionally utilized spices and condiments are often termed additives.

The limited number of preservatives permitted in foods are added to prevent or inhibit microbial growth. These include sodium diacetate, the propionates of sodium and calcium and acidic substances such as acetic acid, lactic acid and monocalcium phosphate, which are added to baked products to retard the growth of fungi and bacteria which in bread produce "rope," rendering the bread inedible. Similarly, benzoic acid and sodium benzoate inhibit bacterial or fungal growth in oleomargarine, certain fruit juices, pickles and confections. Sugar, salt and vinegar are time-honored preservatives when used in sufficient quantities.

In addition to the intentional additives, certain other chemicals may find their way into foods as a result of their use in some phase of the production, handling, or processing of food products. They are known as "incidental additives." Under provisions of the federal food and drug laws, such additives are permitted in foods only if they cannot be avoided by invoking good production and processing practices and, then, only if the amounts that occur under these conditions are known to be safe.[4]

Circumstances Governing Use of Food Additives

National regulatory agencies long have codified the regulation of use of food additives. The first international codification of circumstances governing their use appears to be those elaborated in the first report of the joint FAO/WHO Expert Committee on Food Additives.[8] This Committee was convened in 1956; I was privileged to chair it. This international group formulated general principles concerning the use of food additives and these principles serve, with little modification, as guidelines for national regulatory and advisory groups. For example, the National Academy of Sciences has summarized as follows situations in which food additives are acceptable and those in which they should not be used:[4]

Several circumstances justify the use of food additives to the advantage of the consumer. Every chemical used in food processing should serve one or more of these purposes:
—improve or maintain nutritional value
—enhance quality
—reduce wastage
—enhance consumer acceptability
—improve keeping quality
—make the food more readily available
—facilitate preparation of the food.
Apart from the question of safety, the use of food additives in some situations is not in the best interests of the consumer and should not be employed when:
—used to disguise faulty or inferior processes
—used to conceal damage, spoilage or other inferiority
—used to deceive the consumer
—otherwise desirable results entail substantial reduction in important nutrients
—the desired effects can be obtained by economical, good manufacturing practices
—used in amounts greater than the minimum necessary to achieve the desired effect.

DISTINCTION BETWEEN "ADULTERATION," "CONTAMINATION" AND "FOOD ADDITIVES"

It is evident from the stated situations in which additives should not be used that consumer deception or debasement of product constitutes situations where food additives "should not be employed." The purposes served by acceptable food additives are beneficial and contrast strikingly with the self-serving debasement of products perpetrated by dishonest members of society in all ages prior to the establishment of effective regulatory codes. As these codes have evolved, they have included not only prohibition of adulteration but also have effected the reduction of undesirable or aesthetically objectionable contamination.

British regulations against deception and adulteration originated in the 12th century as controls of weights and measures to prevent deceptive practices and weights involving imported spices. Indeed, this is the origin of the avoirdupois system of weights commonly used for many centuries in English-speaking countries. In early industrialization, adulteration of food and use of even poisonous substances in coloring or disguising inferior foods occurred. These practices were exposed in a classical series of articles that appeared in the medical journal "Lancet" and in the mid-1850s members of the medical profession in Britain gave leadership to subsequent enactment of food regulations.

PURE FOOD AND DRUG LEGISLATION IN U.S.

The English experience served to stimulate and accelerate similar interest in the United States, culminating in the passage of the Pure Food and Drug Law of 1906 signed by President Theodore Roosevelt. The campaign for this was led by Dr. Harvey W. Wiley, chemist in the U.S. Department of Agriculture. This law made illegal the transport across state borders of adulterated foods and drugs, the inclusion of poisonous substances in foods or concealing of inferiority. Food and drugs locally produced and consumed were left under local jurisdiction. The Food and Drug Administration ultimately came into being to enforce provisions of the Act of 1906 and subsequent regulatory legislation. This act was drastically revised by the Congress in 1938 in what is known as the Federal Food, Drug and Cosmetic Act which still serves as the basis of food legislation in the U.S. It prohibits adulteration and misleading labeling. Major amendments to the 1938 law include the 1954 Miller Pesticide Act which established procedures for setting safe amounts of residues of pesticides that unavoidably may remain on raw fruits, vegetables and other agricultural products. In 1960 the Color Additive Amendments were enacted covering both synthetic and natural colors. Synthetic colors must be certified, batch by batch, by analyses in the FDA laboratories. Any color additives carcinogenic for man or animals are prohibited by this legislation through what has come to be widely known as the "Delaney Clause." This Clause applies also to other intentional additives.

A Food Additives Amendment to the Food, Drug and Cosmetic Act adopted in 1958 requires proof of safety to be furnished by the manufacturer based upon extensive animal tests before a substance may be added to a food. When this Act was passed many substances then used in food processing were widely regarded by scientists as safe, although they may not have been subjected to as rigorous experimental animal testing as has increasingly been required since the passage of the 1958 amendment. Numerous of these substances were items traditionally considered ingredients of food and long used without recognized evidence of injury. The Food and Drug Administration surveyed an appreciable body of scientific opinion and developed positions concerning these previously used substances that became classified as "Generally Recognized As Safe" or GRAS. Substances not recognized as GRAS and substances newly introduced since the 1958 Food Additives Amendment cannot be used without safety testing and approval by the Food and Drug Administration.

The scientific community, academic institutions, industry and regulatory agencies repeatedly review and re-examine substances considered GRAS as well as substances that have been approved under existing regulatory requirements. As methods have evolved for detecting new biological phenomena or toxic effects, long used materials are restudied. Where new findings give rise to cautions, further scrutiny of compounds and, in some instances, removal of these from approved lists have occurred. Examples of these include the cyclamates; a number of food colors including, most recently, FD & C Red 2; and the currently contested action relating to saccharin. The 1977 revision of the Code of Federal Regulations lists more than 600 substances considered to be GRAS. The Food Additives Amendment specified that judgments concerning GRAS status would be made by those "qualified by scientific training and experience to evaluate the safety of substances based on scientific data derived from published literature." Promptly the Flavor Extract Manufacturers' Association formed a panel of experts to evaluate the natural and synthetic substances and compounds used as flavoring materials. As of 1978, some 1400 substances were identified, about 800 being included in the Code of Federal Regulations under the title "Synthetic Flavoring Materials and Adjuvants." The use of these substances, not GRAS substances in the strict sense, is administered by FDA as though they are GRAS.

Action by FDA in further evaluation of GRAS substances has not been static. In 1970 they contracted with the Franklin Institute of Philadelphia to search the scientific literature from 1920 and to prepare for FDA bibliographies and abstracts which were in turn sent to several institutions for examination and evaluation, including preparation of literature reviews. The FDA contracted with the National Academy of Sciences to survey the food industry in order to determine levels of use in foods of each of the substances and thereby estimate human daily intakes. Studies were initiated under contract with nongovernment laboratories to assess by special tests such properties as mutagenicity and teratogenicity of many GRAS substances and also contracted with the Federation of American Societies for Experimental Biology (FASEB) to evaluate the information so obtained and to provide FDA with reports on the health aspects of each of the nearly 400 such food ingredients. These evaluations are being conducted by a group of qualified scientists designated as the FASEB Select Committee on GRAS Substances (SCOGS).

Reports prepared by SCOGS subsequently serve to guide the Food and Drug Administration in decisions or revisions of positions concerning GRAS substances. By mid-1978 final evaluatory reports on 262 GRAS substances had been submitted to FDA and tentative evaluation reports on 89 others were awaiting completion of hearings or were in the hands of FDA. Tentative reports on 48 remaining GRAS substances were near completion.

It is of considerable interest to note the results of this intensive effort, as summarized by Dr. George W. Irving, Jr., Chairman of the Select Committee on GRAS Substances.[6]

> Of the 351 GRAS substances covered in final or tentative evaluation reports:
>
> Seventy-one percent were found to be without hazard when used in food at current levels or at levels that might reasonably be expected in the future (Conclusion 1).
>
> Fifteen percent were found to be without hazard if use is limited to levels of addition now current (Conclusion 2).
>
> Six percent were found to be without hazard when used in food at current levels, but due to uncertainties in the existing data, specific studies need to be conducted promptly (Conclusion 3).
>
> Four percent were found to exhibit adverse effects when used in food at current levels requiring that safe usage conditions be established (Conclusion 4).
>
> Four percent were found to be unevaluatable due to the inadequacy of available data (Conclusion 5).
>
> FDA has proposed regulatory action on 60 GRAS substances and has taken final regulatory action on 28 others, based in part on the Committee's reports. FDA actions have consistently reflected the conclusions reached in SCOGS reports.

OTHER SAFEGUARDS

This brief outline of existing regulatory organization and activities is focused on the structure of the Food and Drug Administration. The U.S. Department of Agriculture has similar major regulatory responsibilities for meat and meat products and raw agricultural commodities; the U.S. Treasury Department's Bureau of Firearms and Alcohol has the major responsibility for alcoholic beverages; the newer agency, the Environmental Protection Agency (EPA), has wide-ranging regulatory and tolerance setting activities that pertain to numerous aspects of the environment and include the review and setting of tolerance levels for residues of environmental chemicals, particularly pesticides, in foodstuffs. The enforcement of these tolerances set by EPA becomes the responsibilities of the Food and Drug Administration and/or the U.S. Department of Agriculture.

While these governmental protective controls pertain, the first line of assured compliance lies within the food and agriculture industry itself.

Food and animal production is subject to wide monitoring by processors in order to minimize problems of compliance. Control laboratories routinely monitor products to assure compliance.

Where legitimate questions are raised concerning the need for new scientific evaluation of safety of additives, ingredients or residues, industry, government and the academic community share in the support and responsibility for seeking answers to these questions. Major programs of research are currently in progress to obtain new information on a wide variety of long-used additives. These include *inter alia* food colors, a number of flavoring materials, caffeine and related compounds, non-nutritive sweeteners and representatives of all classes of nutrients.

As new scientific evidence accrues, interpretation and extrapolation of its significance for man involve objective assessment of the scientific evidence concerning the nature of any detectable toxicologic effect in properly designed laboratory investigations, the level of intake or the concentration at which such effects become manifest, the relationship of those levels to realistic use levels within the population, and other aspects of the so-called risk:benefit ratio. Ultimate decisions involve not only scientific judgment but the societal judgment or expression of acceptable risk, societal wants and political expediency. Conflicts that arise, such as the current confrontation regarding saccharin, reflect in varying degrees these several forces involved in decision-making. That this is so is evident from the fact that saccharin, the ban of which is proposed by the Commissioner of the Food and Drug Administration in the United States, is not banned in Canada (although restricted in its distribution) nor in European countries; cyclamates, banned in the U.S. some years ago by the Secretary of HEW, are readily available throughout Europe; FD & C Red 2, used in the United States for some 80 years with no evidence of human injury, was banned by action of the Food and Drug Administration two years ago, and the newly approved FD & C Red 40 has been substituted in large measure for it in the U.S. Based upon the same scientific evidence, the judgment of regulatory agencies in Canada and abroad has been not to approve FD & C Red 40 and to retain use of FD & C Red 2. Such divergent regulatory actions from nation to nation reflect less the scientific evidence and its interpretation than the political and populace pressures brought to bear upon decision makers. Where such pertains, it is highly probable that the scientific evidence of safety is reassuring.

REFERENCES

1. APT, C.M.(ed.): Flavor: Its Chemical, Behavioral and Commercial Aspects. Proceedings of the Arthur D. Little, Inc., Flavor Symposium, 1977. Westview Special Studies in Science and Technology, Westview Press, Boulder, Colo., 1978.

2. BIRCH, G.G.; BRENNAN, J.G., and PARKER, K.J.: Sensory Properties of Foods, Applied Science Publishers Ltd., London, 1977.
3. NATIONAL ACADEMY OF SCIENCES—NATIONAL RESEARCH COUNCIL: Chemicals Used in Food Processing, Publication No. 1274, Washington, D.C., 1965.
4. NATIONAL ACADEMY OF SCIENCES—NATIONAL RESEARCH COUNCIL: Use of Chemicals in Food Production, Processing, Storage, and Distribution. Committee on Food Protection, Food and Nutrition Board, Division of Biology and Agriculture, National Research Council, Washington, D.C., 1973.
5. DARBY, W.J.: History of Food Protection Committee, Activities Report—1976, Food and Nutrition Board, National Research Council, National Academy of Sciences, 1976.
6. IRVING, G.W: Safety Evaluation of The Food Ingredients Called GRAS, Nutrition Reviews 36:351–356 (Dec.) 1978.
7. NATIONAL ACADEMY OF SCIENCES—NATIONAL RESEARCH COUNCIL: Toxicants Occurring Naturally in Foods, Publication No. 1354, 1966; Second Edition, 1973.
8. WORLD HEALTH ORGANIZATION: General Principles Governing the Use of Food Additives, WHO Technical Report Series No. 129, WHO, Geneva, 1957.

25

MIAMI MULTIPLE RISK FACTOR INTERVENTION TRIAL (MRFIT)

AN EXPERIMENT IN CORONARY HEART DISEASE PREVENTION IN HIGH RISK MEN AGE 35–57

PRELIMINARY REPORT

Janice M. Burr, M.D., Terence A. Gerace, Ph.D.,
Mary Ellen Wilcox, R.D., M.Ed., and George Christakis, M.D., M.P.H.

In 1971 a Task Force on Atherosclerosis appointed by the National Heart and Lung Institute recommended the development and support of a preventive trial in men with multiple coronary heart disease risk factors.[1] Previous studies in the United States and abroad have shown that elevated serum cholesterol, hypertension and cigarette smoking are clearly associated with a high incidence of coronary disease.[2] The Multiple Risk Factor Intervention Trial (MRFIT) was therefore initiated to test the hypothesis that significant reduction of these three key variables through an intervention program would be associated with decreased morbidity and mortality from coronary heart disease. From 1972 to

From the Nutrition Division, Department of Epidemiology and Public Health, University of Miami School of Medicine, and the Dade County Department of Public Health, Miami. Dr. Burr is Co-Principal Investigator; Dr. Gerace is Director of Intervention and Co-Investigator; Ms. Wilcox is Project Chief Nutritionist, and Dr. Christakis is Principal Investigator.

1974, 20 clinical centers were selected to participate.[3] The Dade County Department of Public Health in Miami was one of these centers and the only county health department to be included in the national program. In 1976 the Miami MRFIT also became associated with the Nutrition Division of the Department of Epidemiology and Public Health at the University of Miami School of Medicine.

The program office for MRFIT is at the National Heart, Lung and Blood Institute (NHLBI) in Bethesda, Maryland. The Coordinating Center is located at the University of Minnesota. This Center collects data and periodically distributes reports concerning changes in risk factor status of the participants of all clinics. Clinical end points of myocardial infarction, angina, intermittent claudication and disability or death from any cause are not published. The Central Laboratory, monitored by the Center for Disease Control in Atlanta, is at the Institute for Medical Sciences in San Francisco. Cassette tapes of electrocardiograms of all MRFIT participants are read by computer at Dalhousie University in Nova Scotia. The electrocardiograms are also received by physicians at the University of Minnesota.

The administration of national MRFIT includes a Steering Committee composed of one or more investigators from each center and representatives from NHLBI. There are a number of special committees which report to the Steering Committee. They are Design and Analysis, Quality Control, Publication and Presentation, Intervention, and the Executive Committees. A Policy Advisory Board of prominent biomedical scientists monitors the scientific and operational aspects of study. The MRFIT includes a truly multidisciplinary staff of physicians, psychologists, epidemiologists, biochemists, nutritionists, nurses, health counselors, technicians, and administrative and clerical personnel. All are working together closely to meet the research objectives of the six year intervention effort. Periodic regional and national meetings are held for all staff involved in the intervention program to enhance these efforts.

MRFIT SCREENING AND ADMISSION CRITERIA

By November 1, 1975, 370,599 men aged 35 to 57 across the country had participated in the first screening visit and from these 12,866 were ultimately selected.

Eligibility for second screen was based on a combination of risk factors placing the candidate in the upper 10–15% of coronary heart disease risk according to criteria established from experience in the Framingham Study.[4] Individuals with a diastolic blood pressure level in excess of 114 mm Hg, serum cholesterol over 349 mg/dl, history of heart disease or treatment for diabetes mellitus were excluded from the study. Of all men initially screened, 29% had diastolic pressures of 90 mm Hg or greater, 15% had a serum cholesterol level of 260 mg/dl or greater, and 37% smoked cigarettes. The "average" MRFIT man, based on data for all 20 centers, was age 46.7, weighed 189 pounds, had a first screen serum cholesterol level of 257 mg/dl and a diastolic pressure of 99 mm Hg. His forced vital capacity was 3,699 cc with a one-second forced volume of 2,966 cc. Sixty four percent smoked an average of 36.7 cigarettes a day.[5]

Extensive histories of socioeconomic background, dietary habits, physical activity and personality traits were obtained. Eight centers administered the Roseman-Friedman Interview for Type A Coronary Prone Behavior.

At the second and third screening visits, each participant received a physical examination, pulmonary function test, electrocardiogram and blood studies. A treadmill exercise stress ECG test was performed at the third screen; however, no one was excluded on the basis of the results. A candidate free of clinical coronary heart disease or other major illness who expressed willingness to cooperate in the six-year MRFIT study was invited to participate. At the second and third screening visits every individual was informed that if he joined MRFIT, he would be randomly assigned to either the "usual care" (UC) group or the special intervention (SI) group. The UC participant is examined by MRFIT annually but referred to his usual source of health care for control of risk factors. The SI participant visits a MRFIT center at least every four months for risk factor reversal. The coordinating center sends a schedule of code number names and dates for the annual physical examinations of each participant with a "window" of two months on either side of the randomization anniversary. Copies of all electrocardiograms and laboratory results from annual examinations are sent to each private physician, if the participant grants permission to send these records.

At the Miami Center 11,613 men of varied demographic background were screened; 414 were randomized, half to the UC and half to the SI group. The number of men at the Miami Center has continued to increase as participants from northern cities move to Florida and are transferred here for follow-up.

PSYCHOSOCIAL CHARACTERISTICS OF SPECIAL INTERVENTION: MEN

The Miami MRFIT Center has a heterogenous study population derived from a screening program which included such diverse sites as public utilities, electronic corporations and unemployment lines. Seventy-four percent of the participants are white, 5% are black, and 21%

are white with Spanish surnames. Less than half of those with Spanish surnames are facile in English. The economic and educational status of the SI men at the Miami Center is summarized in Table 25.1.

At the second annual examination 41% of the SI men reported having a physician to whom their results would be forwarded. Forty-three percent reported having a physician at entry into the study. Forty-five percent scored low on the Knutsen's scale for assessing self-esteem; 33% had high coronary prone behavior (Type A) scores as measured by the Jenkins Activity Survey.[6] Forty-three percent reported having five or more significant life events (divorce, serious job or family incidents, etc.) during the 12 months prior to entry into the program.

INTENSIVE INTERVENTION PROGRAM

The initial Intervention Program formally began at the third screening visit immediately following the randomization process. At that time all SI men received a MRFIT Participant Guide, a "Weight Control Message" and an opportunity to briefly discuss their risk factors with a physician. Smokers heard a special "Smoking Message" from one of our physicians immediately following the treadmill test. Each SI participant was assigned to either a nutritionist or smoking specialist, depending on his risk factor status. The participant and his specialist set goals related to serum cholesterol reduction or smoking cessation such as "cold turkey" cessation of smoking and limiting eggs to two weekly. Participants who had a diastolic blood pressure of 90 mm Hg and above or who were taking antihypertensive medication were scheduled to return to the Miami MRFIT Center within four weeks for a hypertension confirmation visit.

Initially, ten consecutive weekly group meetings comprised the Intensive Intervention Program. Groups of five to nine men and their wives convened at the Miami MRFIT Center. Seventy-three percent of the SI men attended group sessions. The sessions included (1) educational films, slides and talks which described the relationship between risk factors and coronary heart disease, and (2) discussions and practical experience related to the methods of lowering risk factors. The small group format allowed for some of the characteristics found in self-help groups such as testimonials, role models, peer pressure, competition, group support and practical lay suggestions. The group meetings were conducted by a three member intervention team composed of a health counselor, smoking specialist and nutritionist. The ten sessions began with orientation in which the group leader described the risk factor profiles of the men in attendance. The participants were shown the theoretical reduction in risk of having a myocardial infarction if a fictitious man having the mean

TABLE 25.1. INCOME AND EDUCATIONAL LEVEL OF MIAMI MRFIT SPECIAL INTERVENTION: MEN

Income from Job	Percent SI Men	Education Level	Percent SI Men
< $10,000	24	Less than high school graduate	24
$10,000–$14,999	33	High school graduate or high school plus trade or business school	31
$15,000–$22,999	28	Some college or bachelor degree	34
> $22,999	14	Graduate or professional education, or graduate or professional degree	11

values of the group's risk factors were to stop smoking, lower his cholesterol 10% and reduce his diastolic blood pressure to 80 mm Hg.

During the first five sessions participants had the opportunity to describe their reasons for coming to MRFIT, changes they had made during the week and problems they were having making the desired changes. Group leaders acted as facilitators for these discussions with specific responsibility for maximizing the chances that changes in health related behaviors would follow each meeting.

Role playing in a cafeteria or restaurant scene also provided opportunity for participants to practice assertive behavior such as inquiring about the type of margarine the restaurant offered. A mock-up grocery store allowed the participants to practice choosing foods and reading nutrition information on labels in a situation where they could receive immediate feedback from the staff. Food models were used to help participants learn to estimate the amounts of food they eat. Participants also learned to use a special Brand Name Grocery Guide which provided the information required to shop according to MRFIT guidelines.

Each group had one session devoted to hypertension in which the film "What Goes Up" (American Heart Association) was shown. The meeting was conducted by the group's Health Counselor and a MRFIT physician. An important part of the hypertension session was the question and answer period that followed the movie. Hypertension visits were held prior to group meetings between 5:00 and 7:00 p.m. The group's health counselor and a physician conducted these visits.

Although certain information was communicated to all groups, the specific programs and emphases were tailored to the risk factor profile, particular needs and the week-to-week progress of each group. Prior to the group meetings held from 7:00 to 9:00 p.m., private counseling evening sessions were conducted by the nutritionist and smoking specialist.

Four month follow-up visits are generally conducted in the evening for each intervention group. At follow-up visits, new risk factor reduction goals and strategies are proposed to the participant and an assessment is made of the participant's motivation in the relevant risk factor areas. About four weeks later when the results of tests are available, the group reconvenes for discussion of its progress and future intervention plans.

At the end of each annual examination, the primary counselor reviews the life events check list which was filled out by the participant. This gives the counselor an opportunity to probe into the events and their possible influence on the risk factor status of the participant. In addition, the counselor sets up the appointment for the annual medical conference held four weeks after the annual physical examination. This is a special meeting in which the MRFIT physician reviews the progress of the participant from his visit to the present. The half hour conference includes a review of the participant's current risk factor status, an assessment of his motivation, opportunity for the participant and spouse to ask questions relative to his intervention progress, and a modification of the participant's current risk reversal program or initiation of a new program. Nearly 90% of the SI men who attend the annual physical examination return for an annual medical conference.

RECENT INTERVENTION EFFORTS

Following the tenth intervention session, each participant was paired with a primary counselor, health counselor, nutritionist, or smoking specialist, depending on his particular risk factor status. Further intervention was then carried out through individual counseling, either at the clinical center, via mail or telephone, or through special groups which met at the Center. The number of intervention contacts following the intensive intervention phase was determined by the participant's risk factor status and motivation level.

Among the intervention methods for smokers, we have used One-Step-at-a-Time Smoking withdrawal system filters by Water Pik, stress management and relaxation groups. A campaign was also initiated to encourage "hard core" smokers to avoid cigarettes for as many hours as possible during the American Cancer Society's "Great American Smoke Out."

Nutrition intervention modalities have included (1) application of behavior modification techniques, (2) continued cholesterol and weight reduction efforts for both individuals and groups, (3) "shape-up" exercise and weight reduction groups, (4) food give-a-ways to men who increase their intake of fish, (5) ladies' groups which maintain interest of the wives of the program, and (6) a 26 consecutive weekly phone call program to discuss weight and cigarette status. Other specific clinic events such as group reunions, holiday open houses and food demonstrations are used as educational experiences. These also serve to motivate and sustain a sense of comradeship among participants. A participant oriented newsletter called "The Beat Goes On" is published for the SI group to convey news about Miami SI participants and the Miami Center.

RISK FACTOR INTERVENTION MODALITIES AND PRELIMINARY RESULTS

1. Nutritional Program

The MRFIT Basic Eating Pattern embodies the most recent and applicable information from previous studies directed toward lowering serum cholesterol through dietary measures alone. It is an eating style based upon rational food choices in keeping with the free-living status of the participants. The primary goals are to lower intake of dietary saturated fat and cholesterol while increasing the intake of polyunsaturated fats. Moderation in total calories and a varied intake of whole grain cereals, low-fat dairy products, vegetables, legumes, and fruits are also included in the nutritional program.

Approximately 35% of calories are derived from fat, 8% from saturated fat, 10% from polyunsaturated fat and not more than 250 mg of dietary cholesterol is permitted. The portion size of meat is limited to 6 ounces. Leaner cuts of beef, pork, and lamb are recommended as well as more frequent use of fish, seafood and poultry. Egg yolks are restricted to two per week; substitution of vegetable oils is urged.

The Nutrition Intervention Program utilizes specifically prepared materials, such as audio-visual slide-tape presentations, a Grocery Shopping Guide, pamphlets, and a Cook Book designed to aid the participant and his family in making informed choices of foods. Much time is spent on individualization of the Basic Eating Pattern so that cultural and ethnic attributes as well as personal preferences can be included. The concept that the improved choices of MRFIT will benefit both the participant and his family is a basic one. The participant is taught that food selection and eating habits are related to a myriad of social and cultural factors. Family eating patterns, foods prepared for holidays and special occasions, the work setting, television commercials and the reaction and influences of friends, family, and business associates compete with the participant's willingness to adopt a new eating style. Constant encouragement and assessment of progress in new eating behaviors are provided by the staff both to enhance the transfer of knowledge and skills and to reduce recidivism. Many of the particiants require sound authoritative nutritional information; the greatest obstacle in the way of dietary change is lack of motivation and conflicting priorities between health and the demands of daily living. A sub-group of particular interest is our Hispanic men. Although they are making progress in adapting their eating behaviors, cultural differences may act as deterrents.

All Intervention Staff have been trained by the nutritionists in the rationale and principles of the MRFIT eating pattern and have an active role in the dietary counseling directed toward risk factor reversal.

The baseline data for the Miami MRFIT Special Intervention Participants indicate that after one year progress has been made in approaching dietary goals.

2. Antihypertensive Efforts

Hypertension is the one risk factor for which medical treatment is given, utilizing a step-care protocol. The SI participant is considered hypertensive if he has a fifth phase diastolic reading of 90 mm Hg or greater on any two successive visits not more than a month apart. A participant is also considered hypertensive if he entered the program taking antihypertensive medication, or if he is placed on medication by a physician outside the MRFIT program at some time during the trial.

Blood pressure readings are taken after the participant has had a sitting rest period of at least five minutes. Four readings are taken in the sitting position, two on a standard Baumanometer and two on the Hawksley Random-Zero manometer which conceals the zero point until after the reading is taken. This is helpful in eliminating some elements of observer bias. All official readings are taken by certified technicians, whether nurses, counselors, physician or others. They are recertified for accuracy every six months using tape recordings of Korotkov sounds and double stethoscope checks.

Once confirmed as hypertensive, a participant who is 15% over ideal weight and has a diastolic pressure of less than 105 mm Hg may be placed on weight reduction and salt restriction for up to 16 weeks in an attempt to reduce blood pressure. If indicated, he may also be placed on our step-care drug regimen on order of a MRFIT physician. Hypertensive participants are seen at two week to four month intervals as the situation or protocol requires.

Table 25.2 summarizes the MRFIT antihypertensive drug protocol. The majority of the participants in the Miami Center, as in other MRFIT sites, are controlled on Step One or Step Two medications. The most commonly used combination is a diuretic and reserpine.

The day he is placed on drugs, the participant's diastolic pressure goal is determined to be 89 mm Hg, or 10 mm Hg below the level observed at the confirmation visit, whichever is lower. If a hypertensive participant has blood pressure readings below goal for several months, he may be placed in a step-down program. If the pressure returns to a level above

TABLE 25.2. MRFIT ANTIHYPERTENSIVE MEDICATION PROTOCOL

Step	Medication Category	Drug
One:	Diuretic	Chlorthalidone 50–100 mg q.d. or hydrochlorothiazide 50–100 mg q.d. (If persistent hypokalemia exists the following are substituted or added)
		Spironolactone 50–100 mg q.d.
		Triamterene 100–200 mg q.d.
Two:	Add Anti-adrenergic	Reserpine (0.1–0.25) or if not tolerated
		Methyldopa 500–2000 mg q.d.
		Propanolol 40–480 mg q.d.
Three:	Add vasodilator	Hydralazine 30–200 mg q.d.
Four:	Add Anti-adrenergic	Guanethidine 10–200 mg q.d.

Additional drugs provided when needed are:

1. 10% KCL elixir
2. Probenecid 500 mg tabs or Allopurinol 100 mg tabs
3. Digoxin 0.25 mg tabs

goal for two successive visits, however, he is placed back on the last dose of medication that controlled his pressure. When possible, it is preferred that a participant lower blood pressure by weight loss and salt restriction rather than by medication as we are seeking a lifestyle approach to preventive medicine. The participant's private physician may wish to prescribe antihypertensive medication and wish not to have us treat his patient for hypertension. In these instances we provide the drug if we have it, but do not try to divide the responsibility for the hypertension treatment. We do, however, continue to monitor the participant's progress.

A baseline blood pressure value was established for each participant. This was taken from the average of the second and the third screen diastolic blood pressures. The mean baseline national value of all MRFIT men was 91.0 mm Hg diastolic, and 90.2 mm Hg at the Miami Center. At one year the mean value in the SI group nationally was 84.6 and at two years, 82.5. At the Miami MRFIT the mean was 84.3 mm Hg at one year and 82.5 mm Hg at two years.

PRELIMINARY RESULTS AND SUMMARY

Figure 25.1 depicts a comparison of the typical U.S. diet with the MRFIT recommended eating pattern. The MRFIT pattern represents a 58% reduction in dietary cholesterol, 19% decrease in total calories from fat, 56% decrease in saturated fat and 233% increase in polyunsaturated dietary fat.

Figure 25.2 indicates that MRFIT men at baseline exhibited differences in eating patterns compared to the "typical" American diet pattern, as per Figure 25.1. Our MRFIT men at baseline reported an intake of 461 mg of dietary cholesterol, 38% of total calories from fat, 14% of calories from saturated fat and 6% from polyunsaturated fats. These figures represent a pattern closer to the MRFIT recommendation than are those of the typical American diet.

Figure 25.2 also shows the Miami Center's progress in approaching the MRFIT dietary goals at 12 months. The Miami participants decreased their dietary cholesterol from 461 mg to 298 mg. Reduction to MRFIT goals of 35% of total calories from lipids was achieved. Saturated fat calories have been reduced from 13.6% to 10.7%, and those from polyunsaturated sources increased from 6.4% to 8%.

Figure 25.3 indicates our experience in risk factor reduction up to the second year of intervention. A decrease in mean serum cholesterol from a baseline of 255 mg/dl to 236 mg/dl has been achieved. From a mean diastolic blood pressure of 90.2 mm Hg, the Miami MRFIT participants showed a decrease to 82.5 mm Hg. Regarding our smoking experience, 35.5% reported not smoking by the end of the second year of intervention.

While substantial progress has been made in the SI group, the data cannot at this time include usual care men. It is also inappropriate to report clinical end point data prior to the conclusion of the experiment at all centers.

We are, however, encouraged that a project of this magnitude and complexity has been successfully initiated and continued to its third year of operation. The staff of the Miami MRFIT, in concert with all the centers, is dedicated to fulfilling the intervention goal of the national program. It is our challenge to determine whether the control of coronary heart disease risk factors will contribute significantly to decreasing the incidence of myocardial infarction—the paramount clinical and public health problem of our time.

ACKNOWLEDGMENTS

Acknowledgement is given to the following for their essential contribution to the operation of the Miami Center: Frank Batista, Julio Benezra, Reva Berlin, Dolores Bramson, Rolando Gomez, Hollis Jackson, Joan Kaye, Martha Padron, Eleanor Parenio, Walter Smith, Joyce Weddle, Morris Gilbert, M.D., Hugh Gilmore, M.D., Scheffel Wright, M.D., and Richard Morgan, M.D., M.P.H.

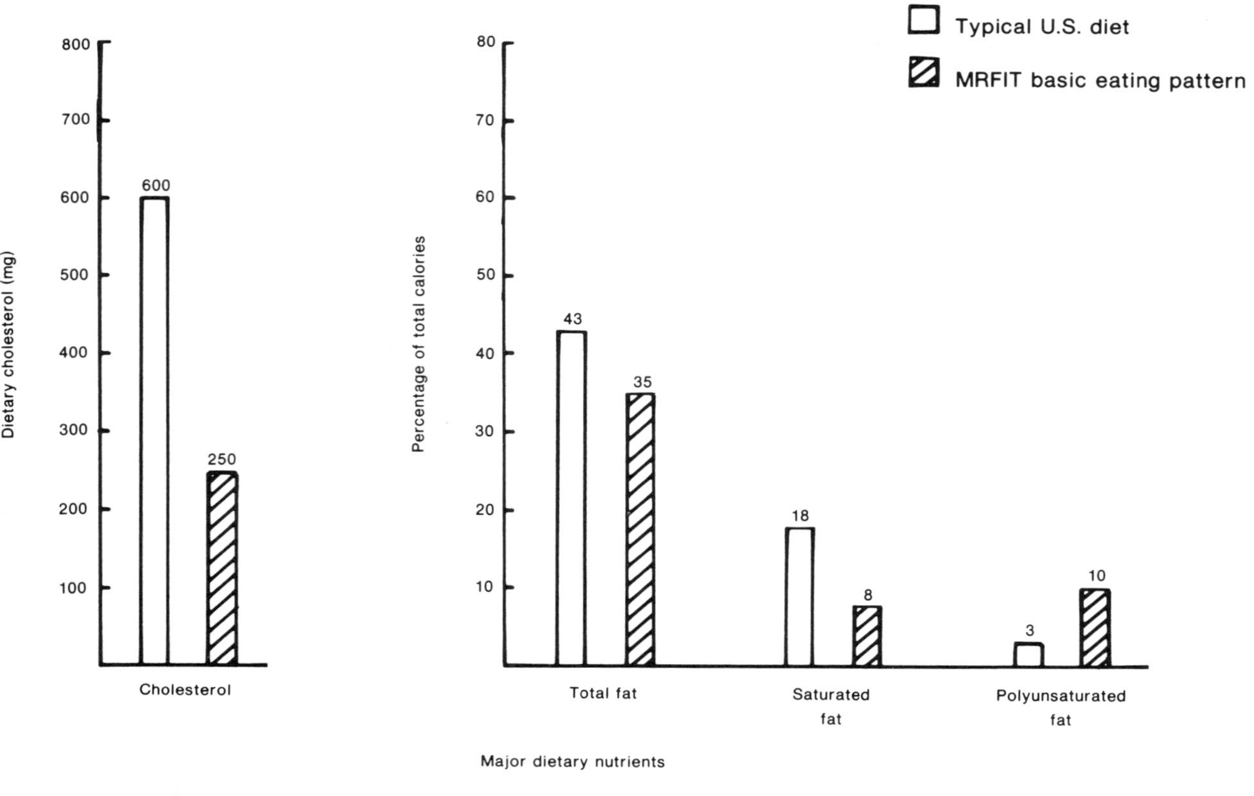

FIG. 25.1. COMPARISON OF THE TYPICAL U.S. DIET WITH MRFIT'S RECOMMENDED EATING PATTERN

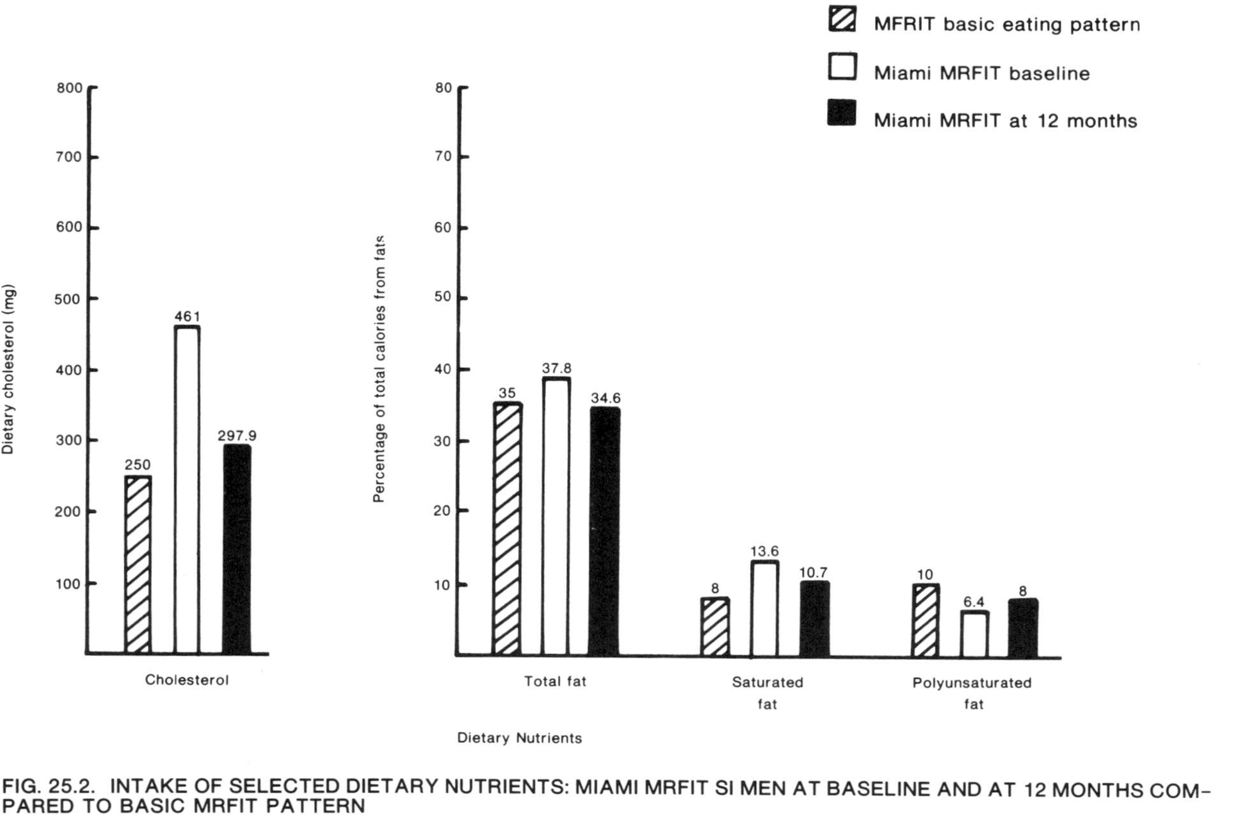

FIG. 25.2. INTAKE OF SELECTED DIETARY NUTRIENTS: MIAMI MRFIT SI MEN AT BASELINE AND AT 12 MONTHS COMPARED TO BASIC MRFIT PATTERN

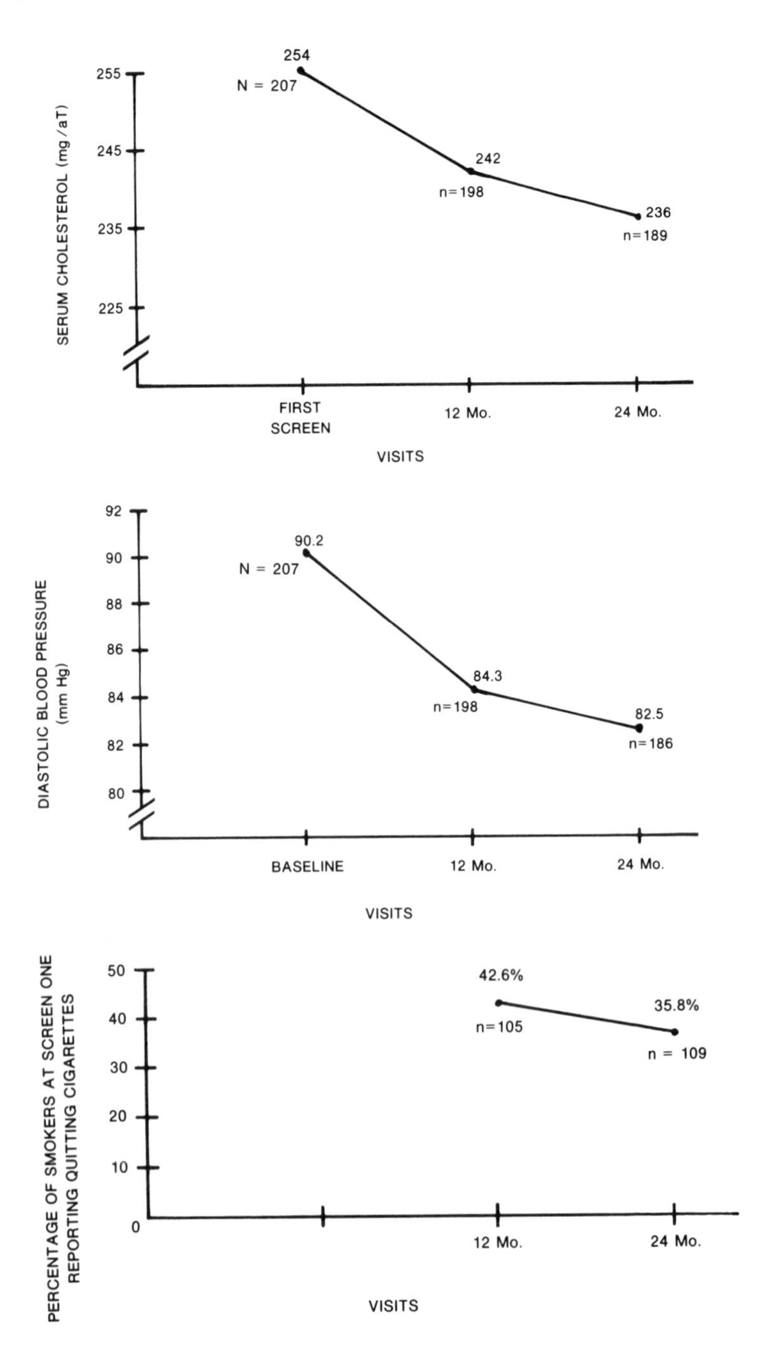

FIG. 25.3. DECREASE IN RISK FACTOR STATUS OF MIAMI MRFIT PARTICIPANTS DURING TWO YEARS OF INTERVENTION

REFERENCES

1. ARTERIOSCLEROSIS: A Report by the National Heart and Lung Institute Task Force on Arteriosclerosis. U.S. Department of Health, Education and Welfare publication No. (NIH) 72-137, June 1971.
2. PRIMARY PREVENTION OF THE ATHEROSCLEROTIC DISEASES, Report of Inter-Society Commission for Heart Disease Resources, Circulation 42:55–95, 1970.
3. MULTIPLE RISK FACTOR INTERVENTION TRIAL (MRFIT): A National Study of Primary Prevention of Coronary Heart Disease, JAMA Vol. 235 Bi, 8, p. 825–827, Feb. 23, 1976.
4. KANNEL, W.B., and GORDON, T.: The Framingham Study—An Epidemiological Investigation of Cardiovascular Disease, Section 27, May 1971, U.S. Government Printing Office.
5. MRFIT PUBLIC ANNUAL REPORT—1975–1976 U.S. Department of Health, Education and Welfare. Public Health Service, National Institute of Health.
6. JENKINS, C.D.; ROSENMAN, R.H.; and FRIEDMAN, M.: Development of an Objective Psychological Test for Determination of the Coronary-Prone Behavior Pattern in Employed Men, J. Chronic. Dis., 20: 371–379, 1967.
7. FINCHER, L., and RAUSCHERT, M.: Diets of Men, Women and Children in the United States, Nutrition Program News U.S. Department of Agriculture, September–October, 1969.

26

THE ROLE OF NUTRITION IN THE MANAGEMENT OF DIABETES MELLITUS

John I. Malone, M.D.
Patricia M. Leapley, R.D.

Diabetes mellitus is a disorder of defective energy production. This is the result of ineffective cellular utilization of glucose—the major substrate for energy production. Abnormal glucose utilization (metabolism) causes secondary effects upon lipid and amino acid metabolism. These substances also serve as fuel for energy production.

Clinically, diabetes was first recognized as a condition where the affected individual became weak, the flesh melted away and large volumes of "honey urine" emanated. During the late 18th century it was recognized that the body was excreting large quantities of sugar in the urine. This led Rollo to decide that the process could be corrected by decreasing the source of the sugar, namely, carbohydrate[1]. He therefore outlined a diet low in carbohydrate and high in fat and protein. This was the major therapeutic approach until the late 1920s, when insulin became available for the treatment of diabetes mellitus.

The use of insulin made a dramatic improvement in the treatment of diabetes. It was observed that insulin not only decreased the sugar level in blood and urine, but also promoted weight gain and increased vigor in the patient. Thus diabetes is a disorder not only of excess glucose, but also poor glucose utilization, that is corrected by insulin.

Dr. Malone is Professor of Pediatrics and Co-Director of the Diabetes Center University of South Florida—College of Medicine.

Mrs. Leapley is the Diabetes Center Dietitian, University of South Florida—College of Medicine.

Treatment of diabetes with one or more injections of insulin, however, is not sufficient to return the metabolism to normal. The blood glucose may reach nondiabetic levels for some portion of time but complete normalcy does not occur. Evaluation of other aspects of metabolism show that free fatty acids, triglycerides and cholesterol are also elevated in many insulin treated diabetics.

Exogenously administered insulin does not mimic the peak and valley physiologic insulin response to dietary stimuli. Insulin release is stimulated by pulses of glucose and amino acids entering the portal system following the ingestion of food[2]. The circulating level of insulin then returns to base line levels within 60 minutes of the initial stimuli. It is impossible to reproduce this type of insulin response with the treatment technique presently available. One therapeutic approach has been dietary. The knowledge that circulating insulin levels increase during the first 30 minutes following injection has led to the idea of taking insulin 30 minutes prior to the ingestion of a meal. This approach works best with multiple doses of rapid acting insulin timed to precede each feeding. This is presently not practical for most patients.

The preceding discussion is based on the assumption that the glucose concentration in the body fluids is the primary result of food consumption. This overlooks the fact that the adult human can maintain a normal blood glucose concentration when totally deprived of calories for weeks and in the case of obese subjects for months[3]. The blood glucose level is maintained by the action of the liver. During the immediate post-prandial period (4 to 8 hours) glucose is supplied by the breakdown of hepatic glycogen stores. Beyond this time glucose is produced in the liver from amino acids (gluconeogenesis). With prolonged fasting, alternate substrates (free fatty acids and ketone bodies) also are released which decrease glucose utilization and thereby help maintain an adequate level for brain metabolism. These metabolic responses to fasting occur because of decreased circulating insulin levels and increased levels of cortisol, epinephrine, growth hormone and glucagon. This unusual endocrine balance exists to some degree in most diabetics in the fed state. Therefore, in addition to the individual's food intake, a significant source of glucose, fatty acids and possibly ketone bodies is endogenous.

Another factor influencing the level of glucose is muscular activity. Increased muscular work results in greater glucose utilization in the face of unchanged insulin levels. This is a phenomenon noted in exercising nondiabetics and begins to occur an hour after the completion of the exercise[4]. It is, therefore, important to remember that there are other important factors that influence the level of glucose in addition to the food consumed. The importance of each of these factors depends on the type of diabetes.

TYPES OF DIABETES

A classification of diabetes mellitus has been developed by an international workgroup sponsored by the National Diabetes Data Group, National Institute of Health and approved by the American Diabetes Association. Two major categories have been designated: (1) Insulin dependent (2) Noninsulin dependent.

Insulin dependent diabetes is characterized by endogenous insulin deficiency and the tendency to develop ketosis, or ketoacidosis. This type of diabetes occurs most commonly during childhood and was previously termed "juvenile onset" diabetes. Insulin dependent diabetes may occur at any age and requires insulin administration for survival. These individuals have the greatest degree of endocrine imbalance and therefore the greatest production of endogenous glucose and ketone bodies. Since most of these individuals are young they also have the greatest variation of physical activity, which makes prediction of daily glucose utilization very difficult.

Noninsulin dependent diabetes is characterized by the presence of inadequate amounts of insulin to maintain normal glucose metabolism. These people make insulin. Seventy percent of these individuals are obese. A majority of these patients have enough insulin resistance caused by their obesity that weight reduction would lead to normal glucose metabolism. Most of these people produce little endogenous glucose and do have the level of blood glucose significantly influenced by their dietary intake.

Diabetes and pregnancy seems to be a special circumstance. The pregnant woman can be either insulin dependent or noninsulin dependent. She may not fit either of these categories but only manifest hyperglycemia during pregnancy (gestational diabetes). During the first trimester the severity of diabetes lessens and the sensitivity to insulin seems to increase[5]. This may be due to inhibition of anterior pituitary function or increased glucose utilization by the fetus. During the second and third trimester, the severity of the diabetes increases. This is thought to be due in large part to a hormone *chorionic somato mammatropin* (HPL) produced by the placenta. This is produced in larger quantities by the diabetic placenta which is larger than the nondiabetic placenta. It is also postulated that the placenta produces enzymes that destroy insulin. Thus factors other than dietary intake influence the blood glucose levels during pregnancy.

NUTRITIONAL GUIDELINES:

The nutritional management of people with diabetes is, therefore, much more complex than balancing dietary intake and insulin dosage. The following are general guidelines:

1. Teach the individual to eat a large variety of foods within a plan to provide balanced nutrition.
2. Balance control of diabetes against maintenance of normal body weight and normal growth, i.e.
   a. Poor control and poor growth and/or weight may require increased insulin and the same or increased calories
   b. Good control and poor growth and/or weight may require increased insulin and increased calories
   c. Poor control and normal growth and/or weight may require insulin dose unchanged, and decreased calories
   d. Good control and normal growth and/or weight
      Success!
3. Provide ideal nutrition for the pregnant woman or lactating mother and control the diabetes with insulin. It is more physiologic to increase insulin than to decrease calories during pregnancy.
4. Modify the diet as required to avoid hypercholesterolemia and hypertriglyceridemia. Blood levels should be monitored on a regular basis.
5. Encourage the patient to understand that nutritional planning is part of the treatment of diabetes.

SPECIFIC CONSIDERATIONS FOR NUTRITIONAL MANAGEMENT OF DIFFERENT TYPES OF DIABETES MELLITUS

Insulin Dependent Diabetes

As discussed previously in Chapter 11, the nutritional problems of children differ from those of adults. The nutrients must provide energy for physical activity. This varies on a daily basis and depends on school, social activities, TV programs and the weather. Energy expenditure varies with age during the first years of life as the child increases physical abilities and decreases the proportion of time spent sleeping.

Energy and nutritional requirements are also directly related to physical growth. Growth rate is not constant throughout childhood. The highest rate of increase occurs during the first two years of life, with another spurt in adolescence. The age at which increased energy is required for the adolescent growth spurt is variable and occurs between 10 and 18 years of age. An indicator of sufficient caloric intake and utilization in a healthy child is the rate of growth and weight gain. However, at insufficient levels of energy intake a child may maintain normal growth rates by a reduction of physical activity as an adaptive mechanism. This dysfunction is more difficult to assess than growth failure, as discussed earlier.

Casual observations of normal nondiabetic children suggest that quantity and quality of dietary intake vary widely from day to day. More objective quantitation of the food consumption of children confirms that impression[6]. Children provided the opportunity to self-select their diet demonstrated variable daily intake. Certain foods are consumed in excessive quantities while others are refused. The long term quality and quantity of food ingested, however, are appropriate. This suggests that constant caloric intake on a day to day basis may not be optimal for normal growth. It is more likely, however, that the individual child has an effective innate indicator of the quantity and quality of required calories. This indicator, by definition, is more physiologic than external calculated regulation of calories.

This is not to suggest that the growing child should not have his diet planned. The great attachment of children to television viewing and the coincident exposure to the highly desirable claims for high-calorie, low-quality food demands counter-education and regulation of the eating habits of children. A problem of equal importance is the present practice of continual snacking which is encouraged by and while watching television. In short, food ingestion is a major activity in many families unrelated to nutritional need. The physiologic directors of eating habits are being overridden by social and commercial influences.

Coronary heart disease is a major cause of death in both the diabetic and nondiabetic population. Two factors suggested as leading to an increased risk of coronary heart disease are hypertension and hypercholesterolemia[7]. There is much recent interest in the influence of childhood diets upon these factors (see p. 134).

Communities that have a high salt intake tend to have high average blood pressure[8]. Experimental evidence in rats indicates that animals have more hypertension in adult life if subjected to high sodium intake during infancy[9]. Although there is no direct evidence in humans that high salt intake predisposes to later hypertension, it seems logical to limit the use of salt in children at risk for hypertension. Children with diabetes are at an increased risk for both hypertension and coronary heart disease. Accordingly, these families are advised to avoid excess salt in their diet.

Hypercholesterolemia is also associated with increased risk for myocardial infarction. Hypercholesterolemia occurs in association with diabetes mellitus. A low cholesterol diet is the first step in correcting hypercholesterolemia[10]. This diet features avoidance of egg yolk, fatty meats and the use of skimmed milk (1% fat) and low cholesterol margarine. Early reports of using low cholesterol feedings to prevent hypercholesterolemia in infants with familial hypercholesterolemia suggest that dietary modification is beneficial[11].

Long term benefits from such a diet have not been determined. Dietary planning to avoid hypercholesterolemia in children with diabetes, however, seems judicious at this time. Thus, dietary and nutritional counseling is appropriate for the well being of all children. It is of particular importance for children who have diabetes, a dysfunction in normal energy metabolism that prevents physiologic compensation for poor eating habits.

Since children with diabetes have the same energy requirements for normal growth and development as nondiabetic children, the preceding discussion should serve as a model for action. When caloric intake must be varied from day to day the best regulator is the child's appetite center. No defect has been demonstrated in this function in children with diabetes. Meal planning and supervision must be employed, however, to allow this center to function optimally without interference from the continuous external advice to consume food products for reasons other than physiologic need.

Specific guidelines used in our clinic to help families and their children with diabetes are provided in the form of "A Managed Diet."

A MANAGED DIET

Meals

We restate here for emphasis the management of diets for children, described earlier in Chapter 11.

> Meals should contain a variety of foods necessary to provide the nutritional requirements for normal growth and development. Information required for this can be provided by a registered dietitian who may use the Exchange Lists for Meal Planning[12] as a guide. Major goals during the educational process are the utilization of a large variety of foods, an understanding of appropriate portion sizes and avoiding the concept of "safe" and "bad" foods. It is possible to consume too much of any food. All food items may be taken at appropriate times. Those foods with high sugar content while deficient in other nutritional value are appropriate at times of high energy needs. Thus, they should only be used at times of unusual energy expenditure (physical exertion) or the treatment of hypoglycemia, (see page 134).

NONINSULIN DEPENDENT DIABETES

Many of the specifics outlined for the insulin dependent diabetic apply to this group as well. Since most of these individuals are no longer actively growing, caloric control and consistency is important. There are a variety of formulas that provide reasonable estimates of caloric requirements for an average patient of a given age, sex and body build[14,15].

There is great individual variation in energy expenditure which often makes the ideal calculated caloric intake inappropriate for the individual in question. It therefore is important to obtain an accurate account of a patient's usual caloric intake during a one week interval. This information coupled with the individual's height and weight provide the information required for the dietary prescription. The goal of diet therapy is to determine the number of calories required to maintain ideal body weight. Knowledge of the patient's glycemic control (hemoglobin A_{1C}) and fasting levels of cholesterol and triglycerides are also helpful for prescribing the diet plan. Once the plan is organized time must be spent on nutrition education. A minimum of 10 hours is usually required before an individual fully understands the exchange system, menu planning, food preparation, nutrition labeling, alcohol intake, eating away from home, the role of exercise and behavior modification techniques to cope with obesity. Food models in the clinic and scales to weigh food at home are important to teach portion size. Many people who believe that they are following the prescribed diet without the desired results consume the correct foods in larger portions. Weekly and monthly follow up programs are important for the serious patient to reinforce the initial dietary concepts and solve new problems as they arise.

SPECIAL ISSUES

The Exchange System

This is a system which categorizes foods into groups. The foods in each group have approximately equivalent composition in terms of calories and proportions of carbohydrate, fat and protein. The Exchange System allows, if the correct portion size is used, the substitution of a variety of foods with approximately equivalent composition. This permits the use of a variety of foods while maintaining consistency of intake from day to day.

Exchange Lists are the groups of food used in the exchange system. The latest revision of the exchange lists[16] include milk, vegetable, fruit, bread, meat and fat exchanges. Any food within a particular list may be substituted for an equivalent amount of any other food in that list. This allows consistency of calories and nutrients while allowing a wide variety of food choices. The lists also emphasize foods low in cholesterol and saturated fats and relatively high in polyunsaturated fats.

Fiber

High fiber diets have attracted the attention of those interested in the management of diabetes mellitus. High fiber diets composed of commonly available foods have been accompanied by improved glycemic control, lowered serum cholesterol, elevated HDL-cholesterol and lower fasting serum triglycerides[17]. Long term side effects such as mineral depletion have been anticipated but thus far have not been observed. Increases in plant fiber can be achieved by using unrefined or minimally processed foods. It appears that some adults would benefit by having a higher percentage of the complex carbohydrate in their diet in the form of fiber rich material. Since the mechanism of the high fiber diet is not clearly understood, the safety and effectiveness of this approach in growing children is not certain.

Sweeteners

People have sought low calorie sweeteners to replace sugar in the diet. Realizing that the nutritional value of sucrose is low, non-nutritive substances such as cyclamates and saccharin have been acceptable substitutes.

Cyclamate is 30 times as sweet as sucrose. It has no associated aftertaste and had wide usage during the 1960s. It was withdrawn from general availability in 1969, after being found to be carcinogenic in animals[18].

Saccharin has been used for over 100 years. It is 350 times as sweet as sucrose but leaves a bitter aftertaste that has limited its wide-spread use. After cyclamate was removed from the market, the use of saccharin increased as the sweetening agent used in the many food products developed with cyclamate. The report that saccharin also has potential carcinogenicity has caused great turmoil among those interested in no-calorie sweeteners[19].

Non-glucose carbohydrate nutritive sweeteners are now receiving increased interest[20]. Fructose, sorbitol and xylitol are being used as nutritive sweeteners. Fructose has some advantage over glucose for use by individuals who have diabetes. Insulin is not required for the transport of fructose inside cells for metabolism. This sugar does contain the same number of calories as glucose and can be converted to glucose by the cell. Sorbitol and xylitol are poorly absorbed from the gastrointestinal tract, thus they have low caloric impact. Because they are not absorbed, sorbitol and xylitol may produce a dose-dependent osmotic diarrhea. It must be remembered when recommending the use of any of the nutritive sugar substitutes that per weight of agent absorbed they contain the same number of calories as glucose.

Alcoholic Beverages

Alcoholic beverages may be used by people who have diabetes with the approval of their physician. Alcohol contains calories (7 calories/gram) and does not require insulin for cellular utilization. Most alcoholic beverages contain considerable amounts of carbohydrate (beer and wine) or are mixed with sugar-containing beverages. These substances should be calculated as part of the daily meal plan or exchanged for other foods in the basic meal plan. One or two alcoholic drinks per day is an absolute maximum since this substance tends to cause hypoglycemia, the symptoms of which mimic drunkenness. This could result in unrecognized hypoglycemia with unfortunate consequences.

CONCLUSION

Nutritional planning is an important aspect of the treatment of diabetes. This should not be left to chance. It is important, however, that the physician and dietitian understand the different types of diabetes that the patient may have. This must be integrated with the nutritional needs of the patient. The physician and dietitian must remember that a diabetic is *not* being counseled about a diabetic diet. Rather, a human being with specific nutritional needs is being counseled who has, in addition to the usual problems of non-diabetics, a need to control the level of glucose in the blood.

REFERENCES

1. MARBLE, A. Current Concepts in Diabetes *in*: Joslin's Diabetes Mellitus; 11th Edition, A. Marble; P. White; R.F. Bradley, and L.P. Krall; Pg. 1–9 Philadelphia; Lea and Febiger; 1971.
2. CURRY, D.L.; BENETT, L.L.; and GRODSKY, G.M.; Dynamics of Insulin Secretion by the Perfused Rat Pancreas. Endocrinology 83: 572, 1968.
3. CAHILL, G.F., JR; Starvation in Man; New England Journal of Medicine 282: 668–675; 1970.
4. LARSSON, Y.A.; STERKY, G.G.; EKERGREN, K.E.; and MOLLER, T.G.; Physical Fitness and the Influence of Training in Diabetic Adolescent Girls. Diabetes 11: 109–116; 1962.
5. MINTZ, D.; SYKLER, J.; CHEZ, R.; Diabetes in Pregnancy—A Clinical Review. Diabetes Care 1: 49–63; 1978.
6. DAVIS, C. Feeding After the First Year; *In* J. Brennemann (Ed): Practice of Pediatrics. Hagerstown, Md., W.F. Prior Co., Inc. 1957, Vol. 1, Chapter 30.
7. LEVY, R.I. and RIFKIND, B.M.; Diagnosis and Management of Hyperlipoproteinemia in Infants and Children, American Journal Cardiol. 31: 547; 1973.
8. BURMAN, D.; Nutrition in Early Childhood *in* Textbook of Pediatric Nutrition, Churchill Livingstone, London and New York, 1976, Pg. 46.
9. DAHL, L.K; Salt and Hypertension; American Journal Clin. Nutrition 25: 231, 1972.

10. LEVY, R.I.; BONNELL, M., and ERNST, N.D.; Dietary Management of Hyperlipoproteinemia, Journal American Diet. Assoc. 58: 406, 1971.
11. GLUECK, C.J.; HECKMAN, F., SCHOENFELD, M., et al: Neonatal Familial Type II Hyperlipoproteinemia: Cord Blood Cholesterol in 1,800 Births, Metabolism 20: 597, 1971.
12. EXCHANGE LISTS FOR MEAL PLANNING: New York and Chicago: American Diabetes Association and American Dietetic Association, 1977.
13. KNOWLES, H.C. JR.; GUEST, G.M.; LAMPE, J.; *et al*: Course of Juvenile Diabetes Treated with Unmeasured Diet, Diabetes 14: 239–273, 1965.
14. A GUIDE FOR PROFESSIONAL EFFECTIVE APPLICATION OF EXCHANGE LISTS FOR MEAL PLANNING, New York and Chicago. American Diabetic Association and American Dietetic Association, 1977.
15. SELECT COMMITTEE ON NUTRITION AND DIETARY GOALS FOR THE UNITED STATES. 2nd Edition, Dec 1977, Washington, D.C. Government Printing Office No: 052-070-04376-8.
16. EXCHANGE LISTS FOR MEAL PLANNING: New York and Chicago: American Diabetes Association and American Dietetic Association, 1976.
17. ANDERSON, J.W.; MIDGLEY, W.R.; and WEDMAN, B. Fiber and Diabetes. Diabetes Care 2: 369–379, 1979.
18. EGEBERG, R.B. and STEINFELD, J.L. Report to the Secretary of HEW from the Medical Advisory Group on Cyclamates. Journal American Medical Association 211: 1358–1361, 1970.
19. KALTHOFF, R.K. and LEVIN, M.E. The Saccharin Controversy. Diabetes Care Vol. I: 211–222, 1978.
20. BRUNZELL, J.D. Use of Fructose, Xylitol, or Sorbitol As a Sweetener in Diabetes Mellitus. Diabetes Care Vol. I: 223–230, 1978.

27

NUTRITIONAL ANEMIAS

Richard R. Streiff, M.D.

INTRODUCTION

Nutritional anemias are usually gratifying to diagnose and to treat from the point of view of the patient as well as the physician. If the diagnosis is correct the patient will, in most cases, respond quickly and completely to inexpensive and harmless medication. If it were not for the fact that a number of fairly common problems masquerade as nutritional anemias and do not respond to the therapy, this discussion on diagnosis could be abbreviated.

In defining anemias of nutritional origin one has to consider them as a state in which the red blood cell count or hemoglobin level is lower than normal due to a deficiency of one necessary nutrient. In order for the anemia to be truly classified as nutritional, the lack of a single nutrient must produce anemia and this condition must respond specifically to the replacement with this missing nutrient.[49] A great number of deficiency anemias have been described in the literature but only three truly satisfy the strict criteria mentioned above. These are iron, vitamin B_{12} and folic acid deficiency anemia. Some of the anemias described to be secondary to protein deficiency, riboflavin deficiency, and vitamin E deficiency cannot really be considered true nutritional anemias because they are either caused by mixed deficiencies or associated with general malnutrition and cannot be cured by the addition of one identifiable nutrient.[26,19,46,4,41,50] In many cases several nutrients must be combined to cause anemias of this group to respond completely and appropriately. Anemias due to deficiencies of iron, folate and vitamin B_{12} are common. There are many more mild to moderate deficiencies than severe cases of anemia, but all of these deficiencies are significant enough to be a health problem world-

Dr. Streiff is Professor of Medicine, Veterans Administration Medical Center, and Department of Medicine, University of Florida, Gainesville.

wide. Many more people are affected by these nutritional anemias in poverty-stricken areas than in the more affluent areas of the world, but this does not mean that the physician can downplay the importance of nutritional problems even in the most affluent societies. The etiologies of deficiency anemias can be broken down into several categories: (1) abnormal or insufficient diet; (2) increased utilization of the nutrient; (3) increased nutrient losses; (4) malabsorption of the nutrient; and (5) interruption of the nutrient's metabolism or destruction by toxic agents or drugs.[7,25]

The impact and frequency of nutritional anemias on the total population and on several specific population groups have been fairly extensively studied by the World Health Organization (WHO), the Committee on Maternal Nutrition and several other groups.[48,49,52] These reports can be helpful and informative. The Committee on Maternal Nutrition[52] noted that the nutritional stress imposed by pregnancy in some cases causes a rather severe nutritional anemia with folic acid deficiency, iron deficiency or both. A much larger group of basically well-fed women developed significant moderate deficiencies during pregnancy or lactation and needed specific nutritional supplementation. Children in the active phase of growth require increased amounts of vitamins and nutrients on a weight basis when compared to adults, and in nutritionally deprived areas, anemia based on nutritional problems is quite prevalent. The extent of nutritional anemia problems in children, though recognized, has not been sufficiently studied to give us a complete picture.

FOLIC ACID DEFICIENCY ANEMIA

In well-developed and generally affluent countries such as the United States, frank and severe folic acid deficiency anemia might be said to be only the tip of the iceberg as far as folic deficiencies are concerned, since many people have subclinical or moderate deficiencies significant enough to cause health problems but mild enough to escape easy detection. The present adverse economic climate with the high cost of food will undoubtedly cause an increase in nutritional problems, and particularly anemias, among the elderly as well as pregnant women and children living on limited incomes.[27,7]

Folate deficiency can be diagnosed by several means: a serum folate level, a red cell folate level or both of these in conjunction with morphologic changes in the peripheral blood smear and/or the bone marrow aspirate or biopsy. If the serum folate level by itself is used as a diagnostic criterion, the incidence of folate deficiency found in any group will be higher than if a frank megaloblastic anemia with a low red blood cell folate is used for diagnosis. The serum folate level is very labile and falls quickly in the face of decreased folic acid intake, while the red blood cell folate level, a good measure of tissue folate stores, decreases much more slowly and is generally found to be low at the time a frank and significant folic acid deficiency anemia occurs. The frequency of folate deficiency reported by different studies must be considered in the light of the definition of deficiency and the method used in measuring the deficiency. A study done using only serum folic acid levels would give a falsely high incidence of folate deficiency, while another investigation using frank megaloblastic anemia or red cell folic levels may give a somewhat low incidence of folate deficiency.

The two groups of people who are at the highest risk for folate deficiency in North America are (1) alcoholics and (2) pregnant and lactating women. Pregnant and lactating women, particularly in low income areas, have approximately 30% deficiency rate as measured by red blood cell folic levels. This group of patients can, in most cases, be easily reached by therapeutic and corrective measures and they also tend to cooperate quite well in nutrition improvement programs. Efforts to give additional nutritional support to alcoholic patients have been met with less success, as one would probably predict.[51,25] It has been suggested that folate be added to some of the alcoholic beverages most commonly ingested by hardcore intercity alcoholics in order to decrease their folate deficiency rate. This suggestion has run into regulatory and philosophical complications and probably will not be instituted for some time, if ever.

Symptoms and Diagnosis of Folate Deficiency

The most common symptom of severe folic acid deficiency is directly related to the anemia itself, which usually causes some fatigue and decrease in exercise tolerance, occasional dizziness and related symptoms.[7] Other associated problems which occur more or less frequently are sore or smooth tongue, diarrhea, hyperpigmentation, abdominal cramps and weight loss. Most of these latter symptoms occur in less than 50% of the patients. Neuropathy associated with folate deficiency has been reported in a very few cases, but an absolute cause and effect relationship has not been established.[32,34] This symptom is traditionally associated with vitamin B_{12} deficiency and not folic acid deficiency.

The diagnostic approach for folic acid deficiency involves the usual appropriate history and physical examination with emphasis on dietary history. Laboratory tests should first include a complete blood count with a differential and calculation of a mean corpuscular volume (MCV). Most blood counts are now done by electronic particle counters which give very accurate mean corpuscular volume measurements, and these are most helpful in alerting the physician that a macrocytosis is present. A thorough review of the blood smear, searching for hypersegmented polymorphonuclear cells and the measurement of both serum and red cell folate levels as well as serum B_{12} levels, should be done in patients whom you strongly suspect of having the folic acid deficiency. The patient with folic deficiency anemia will have macroovalocytosis with an MCV usually over 110, but this will vary depending upon the severity of the deficiency.[36] Other problems, such as vitamin B_{12} deficiency, liver disease, etc., can also cause macrocytosis. Hypersegmentation of the polymorphonuclear cells is a usual feature in both folate and vitamin B_{12} deficiency.[7,25,42] An average lobe count of the polymorphonuclear cells greater than 3.5 is considered to be hypersegmentation; or one cell with seven or more distinct lobes is considered highly significant.[23] It is important to measure a serum vitamin B_{12} level along with the red cell folate level in order to interpret low red blood cell folate levels.[7] Red cell folate levels are very low in significant folate deficiency as well as in vitamin B_{12} deficiency. The latter finding is due to the fact that vitamin B_{12} deficiency causes a relative metabolic block to the uptake of folate by red cells in the bone marrow, giving a low red blood cell folate level.[16] Therefore, a patient with a low red blood cell folate level and a normal serum vitamin B_{12} level undoubtedly has a tissue folic acid deficiency, and if he has a macrocytic anemia this is then a folic acid anemia.[16]

The peripheral blood smear makes it possible for the physician to suspect a megaloblastic anemia secondary to either folate or vitamin B_{12} deficiency early in its development. This point is well-illustrated in the clinical experiments done by Herbert in 1962[23], in which he demonstrated that hypersegmentation and macroovalocytosis appeared as many as six or more weeks before a definite nutritional anemia developed in experimentally-induced folic acid deficiency.[23]

Folate Metabolism

Folic acid is found in the natural state in both vegetables and meats. The original source for folic acid is usually from plants or vegetables. Most naturally occurring folic acid is found in large molecular forms called polyglutamic folic acid. This form of folic acid has to be digested or broken down to a smaller more easily absorbable form of folic acid called monoglutamic folic acid.[5] This digestion or transformation takes place in the small intestine in the presence of specific enzymes.[5,31] The availability of food folate of both the large and small molecular forms varies greatly from one food product to the next.[40] The preparation or cooking of the food can also affect the content of folic acid greatly since folic acid is heat labile and is easily broken down or destroyed by cooking.[24] Some patients who have serious malabsorption problems for a number of nutrients also have similar problems with absorbing folic acids and a few patients appear to have a fairly specific malabsorption for folic acid.[7,25] Other nutrients, toxins or drugs can markedly decrease the absorption of folic acid in the small intestine. Some foods such as glucose can enhance folic acid absorption.[21] It is important to realize that even though our diet contains considerable amounts of folic acid, absorption problems and the destruction of folic acid in the foods make considerably smaller amounts of folate available to the body for utilization.[11]

Once the folic acid is absorbed and enters the serum its main metabolic work is one of transfer of one carbon fragment, primarily in the synthesis of DNA.[16] For this reason, the lack of folic acid causes a decrease in DNA production and the usual morphologic findings of megaloblastic anemia.[7,16] The biochemistry of folic acid and vitamin B_{12} are closely related. Therefore deficiencies in one of these vitamins often causes changes or abnormalities in the levels of chemistry of the other. It is for this reason that there are many similarities in the morphology and symptoms of vitamin B_{12} and folic acid deficiency.[7,25,16]

Therapy

After diagnosing a folic acid deficiency anemia it is important to emphasize to the patient that his diet, if it was deficient, should be changed to a more appropriate diet containing uncooked vegetables such as salads, tomatoes, etc. He should drink orange juice or other citrus juices, since they are also good sources of folic acid, and eat a well-balanced diet.[7] Patients who have malabsorption or hyperutilization problems should receive folic acid supplementation; in most cases 1 mg of folic acid once a day will be sufficient since the minimum daily requirement for folic acid is approximately 100 micrograms per day. It must be emphasized to patients who have a continuing problem of malabsorption that they will need to take folic acid for an indefinite period of time or forever. Patients who have a deficiency based on inappropriate or inadequate diet should take folic acid supplementation only until their anemia has cleared, and they should then be encouraged to maintain a more adequate diet. Follow-up clinic visits are necessary to make sure that the patient's anemia has responded completely.

VITAMIN B_{12} DEFICIENCY

Vitamin B_{12} deficiency is a fairly common deficiency in North America.[25] There are several reasons for becoming vitamin B_{12} deficient and the sum of all these etiologies makes this a fairly common occurrence. As mentioned in the section on folic acid, there are many similarities between the two deficiencies; but it is very important to clearly separate vitamin B_{12} from folic acid deficiency because the treatments are different and treatment with the wrong vitamin can, in the case of vitamin B_{12} deficiency, cause significant and long-lasting problems for the patient.[25,7]

The etiology of vitamin B_{12} deficiency can be (1) inadequate diet; (2) malabsorption of the inherited or acquired variety involving the stomach or the small intestine, specifically the ileum; (3) increased utilization for requirements and (4) miscellaneous rare etiologies.[7]

There are very few cases of vitamin B_{12} deficiency found in North American due to inadequate diet because meat is almost the exclusive source of vitamin B_{12} and is highly prized as a part of the usual American diet.[27] Most vegetarians will eat cheese or milk or animal protein rather than red meat and get adequate B_{12} from these other sources of animal protein. Very few vegetarians eat no animal products. Vegetable and plant products do not contain vitamin B_{12} with the exception of a few obscure seaweeds or algae. The daily requirement of vitamin B_{12} is 1 microgram and the body stores of B_{12} are sufficient in most cases for three to five or more years, so a person who is on a strict vegetarian diet for some time will show no ill effects until his body stores are depleted.

The most common and most significant cause of vitamin B_{12} deficiency is that of classical pernicious anemia.[7] This disease is most common in people over 50 or 55 years of age and is characterized by gastric secretion lacking in intrinsic factor which is necessary for the absorption of vitamin B_{12}.[7,25] The incidence of pernicious anemia in North America is said to be approximately 1 per 1,000. Since it is much more common in the older population,[25] areas of Florida do have a much higher incidence and can approach a frequency as high as 1 for every 400 to 500 people over the age of 55 to 60. Pernicious anemia has a significant hereditary component and this makes it appropriate to investigate a family more closely after one member has been shown to have pernicious anemia.[7] A congenital deficiency of intrinsic factor secretion has been noted in some forty or more cases in the literature. This is important since it occurs in infants and is significant during the first year of life, at which time therapy must be started and continued life long.[7] The typical gastric atrophy found in classical pernicious anemia is not found in the congenital lack of intrinsic factor; in fact, these patients have completely normal gastric mucosa but are unable to secrete intrinsic factor.

In most cases, patients who have had total or partial gastrectomies are left with little or no mucosa able to secrete intrinsic factor; thus they malabsorb vitamin B_{12} and become deficient. It is important to consider the possibility of B_{12} malabsorption shortly after their operation and test them for B_{12} absorption by way of a Schilling test. If this test is abnormal it is necessary to begin the patient on monthly-replacement vitamin B_{12} to prevent deficiency.[7]

Vitamin B_{12} is absorbed in the terminal ileum in the presence of intrinsic factor. If the patient has severe malabsorption, celiac disease, or tropical sprue involving the ileum, significant malabsorption can occur in spite of normal intrinsic factor levels. Small intestinal blind loops on the basis of surgical intervention or naturally occurring blind loops can be the basis of significant vitamin B_{12} malabsorption due to the large amount of bacteria in the stagnant loop of the small intestine. Patients with pancreatitis have been shown to malabsorb vitamin B_{12} in a significant number of cases. However, only a small percentage of these patients develop B_{12} malabsorption of a severity which will cause megaloblastic anemia.[44,45]

There have been a number of drugs associated with vitamin B_{12} malabsorption. Some of these are relatively common medications such as neomycin, colchicine, slow-release potassium chloride, ethanol, and p-aminosalicylic acid (PAS).[47,22,43,37,30] In most cases these drugs are not continued for long periods of time to cause serious vitamin B_{12} malabsorption but it is necessary to be aware that they can cause problems. It is interesting to note that it has been reported that extremely high doses of vitamin C at the level of 1 to 2 grams per day have been implicated in vitamin B_{12} deficiency. The mechanism appears to be one of destruction of the vitamin B_{12} by high doses of vitamin C in the GI tract. This could be a possible cause of vitamin B_{12} deficiency in patients taking large doses of vitamin C for protracted periods.[25] There have been a few cases of vitamin B_{12} deficiency described in patients who appear to have increased requirements for the vitamin. These are usually pregnant women, or patients with hemolytic anemias and thyrotoxicosis.[26,27] It is quite uncommon to see vitamin B_{12} deficiency on the base of hyper-utilization since the vitamin B_{12} stores are sufficient for many years, but this is a recognized cause of vitamin B_{12} deficiency.

Clinical Symptoms and Diagnosis

The patient with typical vitamin B_{12} deficiency anemia very frequently exhibits a hematocrit in the low 20's or upper teens.[7] Actually it is not rare to find a patient who presents feeling fairly well with a hematocrit of less than 10. The reason that the patients tolerate hematocrits this low is the fact that the anemia occurred very gradually and they acclimate themselves to the low hematocrit. Another common presentation is a patient complaining primarily of neuropathies of the feet and hands. Generally they describe it as numbness and tingling or they have difficulty walking, buttoning clothes, picking up cups, etc. These neurologic findings are almost always present in vitamin B_{12} deficiency to a greater or lesser degree and this is basically never found in folic acid deficiency. Vitamin B_{12} deficient patients frequently complain of sore tongue, weakness, rapidly graying hair and memory loss.[7]

Diagnosis of vitamin B_{12} deficiency should start with a history and physical emphasizing possible family history of B_{12} deficiency or pernicious anemia and the progression of fatigue, neuropathy or memory loss. A complete blood count with a blood smear and measurement of the mean corpuscular volume (MCV) will show a macroovalocytosis and an MCV of generally over 110 or 115[36]; hypersegmentation will also be present and in many cases a depressed white blood count and platelet count will be noted.[7,25] At this point you can confirm the diagnosis of Vitamin B_{12} deficiency by measuring the serum B_{12} level.[7,13,25] In order to pinpoint the etiology of the deficiency, a gastric analysis for free acid, intrinsic factor and a Schilling test will help diagnose the type and origin of the malabsorption. It is important to definitely separate vitamin B_{12} deficiency from folic acid deficiency because of the different therapy involved and because vitamin B_{12} deficient patients need monthly B_{12} injections for the rest of their lives and the folic acid deficient patients only need folic acid for a short period of time, accompanied by improved diet.[7]

Therapy

After specifically diagnosing vitamin B_{12} deficiency it is important to clearly discuss the diagnosis and its importance with the patient and emphasize that the vitamin deficiency cannot be corrected by oral vitamins (and that parenteral vitamin B_{12} therapy on a monthly basis will be necessary indefinitely). Subcutaneous injections of 1000 micrograms (1 mg) of vitamin B_{12} once a month is more than adequate for vitamin B_{12} deficient patients.[39] I find it helpful to train the patients to give their own B_{12} injections on a monthly basis and follow them with an office visit every six months to make sure that they are taking their injections faithfully.

IRON DEFICIENCY ANEMIA

Iron deficiency anemia is the most common nutritional anemia. In most instances, the basis of this anemia in adults is due to iron loss in the form of blood loss, and in children, particularly younger children, insufficient intake plus blood loss is the most common cause. The incidence of iron deficiency varies widely. It is much more prevalent in developing countries than in the developed countries of Europe and North America. Women are much more prone to iron deficiency than men, because of the significant iron cost of pregnancy and blood loss during menstruation. Incidence of iron deficiency in women varies between 10 and 25% in Great Britain, Sweden and North America. In developing countries such as Africa and Asia a 30 to 50% iron deficiency rate is not uncommon in women.[20] Iron deficiency rates of 5 to 20% have been estimated in developed countries and 30% in developing countries in the tropical areas.[38] The incidence of iron deficiency in children is less well documented; studies have shown that between 25 to 35% of children in developing countries between ages of 1 and 13 years have iron deficiency.[20]

Symptoms and Diagnosis

The symptoms of iron deficiency anemia are quite variable among patients with moderate to severe anemia. These are usually weakness, palpitations and dizziness common to any anemic state and are usually found in patients with a hemoglobin level of less than 10 grams. Patients also complain of sore tongue and mouth, listlessness and generalized fatigue.

Diagnosis of iron deficiency anemia starts with a history and physical examination with emphasis on possible sites of blood loss such as GI bleeding, increased menstrual bleeding, hookworm infestation, frequent pregnancies, etc. A complete blood count with a differential and blood smear examination and the mean corpuscular volume determination is very helpful. The red blood cells in a typical iron deficient patient are small and pale. A mean corpuscular volume under 75 is very suspect of iron deficiency or possible thalassemia. A stool examination for occult blood is necessary and many times this has to be repeated. The determination of serum iron and iron binding capacity are important to separate iron deficiency from other hypochromic anemias such as thalassemia. The serum iron and iron binding capacity will vary somewhat depending upon the method of the determination but usually a saturation of less than 10% is diagnostic of iron deficiency. In cases of iron deficiency, the serum iron decreases while the serum iron binding capacity increases, and in many cases the serum iron binding capacity will be as high as 400 to 450 with a serum iron of 15 or less.

Once the diagnosis of iron deficiency has been made, it is important to determine the cause for the deficiency, particularly in cases of blood loss, because this can be and often is the presenting symptom in patients who have ulcer disease or GI malignancies. Treatment for the patients with iron deficiency anemia does not need to be delayed during the diagnostic examination to determine the cause of the blood loss, but an absolute cause does need to be found and should not be deferred because the patient is feeling better following treatment.

Iron Therapy

Iron therapy should not be started before definite evidence is obtained that the patient is indeed iron deficient. Patients who have thalassemia minor and those with sideroblastic anemias frequently have blood smears which look identical to those of patients who have iron deficiency. Iron therapy in these cases is contraindicated. Oral iron therapy in most cases is the therapy of choice. Ferrous sulfate is the most commonly used iron preparation and is the one that is tolerated by patients as well as any other iron preparation.[3,6,17] In many instances, ferrous sulfate is mixed in a pill form with ascorbic acid or a similar reducing agent. The absorption of oral iron is significantly better when it is not taken with a meal but gastrointestinal symptoms caused by the iron are more likely to be greater if not taken with food.[2] The patients who tolerate oral iron therapy on an empty stomach should be encouraged to continue; if they have GI distress, iron taken with meals is also acceptable.[3] Ferrous sulfate tablets contain approximately 60 mg of elemental iron and the usual dose is 3 to 4 times a day. The most common causes for a failure to respond to oral iron are: (1) the patient is not cooperating and does not take the iron; (2) the patient has continuing blood loss which is greater than the iron therapy can correct; (3) the patient has a significant malabsorption syndrome; and (4) incorrect diagnosis, the patient's hypochromic anemia was actually secondary to infection or inflammatory disease, malignancy, thalassemia or sideroblastic anemia. Parenteral iron therapy is a well-established therapeutic procedure and acceptable when oral therapy has been unsuccessful or there are specific contraindications to oral iron therapy. The basic indications for parenteral iron administration are: (1) a demonstrated intolerance to oral therapy or inability of the patient to cooperate with that form of therapy; (2) significant malabsorption rendering oral therapy unsuccessful; (3) gastrointestinal disease such as gastritis or ulcerative colitis, which may be exacerbated by the irritant effect of oral iron.

Parenteral iron therapy has been found to be helpful in many instances but there are side effects. Some of these can be rather devastating such as anaphylactic reactions. Most untoward reactions are less dramatic and may be limited to minor itching, or rashes.

REFERENCES

1. ALFREY, C.P., and LANE, M. 1970. The effect of riboflavin deficiency on erythropoiesis. Semin. Hematol. 3:49.
2. BRISE, H. and HALBERG, L. 1962. Iron absorption studies II. Absorbability of different iron compounds. Acta. Medica Scandinavica, 171, supplement 376.
3. BRISE, H. 1962. Iron absorption studies II. Influence of meals on iron absorption in oral iron therapy. Acta. Medica Scandinavica, 171, supplement 376.
4. BRUNSER, O., REID, A., MONCKEBERG, F., MACCIONI, A., and CONTRERAS, I. 1968. Jejunal mucosa in infant malnutrition. Am. J. Clin. Nutr. 21:876.
5. BUTTERWORTH, C.E., and KRUMDIECK, C.L. 1975. Intestinal absorption of folic acid monoglutamates and polyglutamates: A brief review of some recent developments. Br. J. Haematol. 31, supplement 111.
6. CALLENDER, S.T. 1969. Quick and slow-release iron: a double-blind trial with a single daily dose regimen. British Medical Journal, 4, 531.
7. CHANARIN, I. 1969. The Megaloblastic Anaemias. Davis, Philadelphia.
8. CHANARIN, I. 1976. Investigation and management of megaloblastic anemia. Clin. Haematol. 5:747.
9. CHANARIN, I., ENGLAND, J.M., and HOFFBRAND, A.V. 1973. Significance of large red blood cells. Br. J. Haematol. 25:351.
10. CHUNG, A.S., PEARSON, W.N., DARBY, W.J., MILLER, O.N., and GOLDSMITH, G.A. 1961. Folic acid, vitamin B_6, pantothenic acid, and vitamin B_{12} in human dietaries. Am. J. Clin. Nutr. 8:573.
11. COLMAN, N., BARKER, E.A., BARKER, M., GREEN, R., and METZ, J. 1975A. Prevention of folate deficiency by food fortification. IV. Identification of target groups in addition to pregnant females in an adult rural population. Am. J. Clin. Nutr. 28:471.
12. COLMAN, N., GREEN, R., and METZ, J. 1975B. Prevention of folate deficiency by food fortification. II. Absorption of folic acid from fortified staple foods. Am. J. Clin. Nutr. 28:459.
13. COOPER, B.A., and WHITEHEAD, V.M. 1978. Evidence that some patients with pernicious anemia are not recognized by radiodilution assay for cobalamin in serum. N. Engl. J. Med. 299:816.
14. CORDANO, A., PLACKO, R.P., and GRAHAM, G.G. 1966. Hypocupremia and neutropenia in copper deficiency. Blood 28:280.
15. CROFT, R.F., STREETER, A.M., and O'NEILL, B.J. 1974. Red cell indices in megaloblastosis and iron deficiency. Pathology 6:107.
16. DAS, K.C., and HERBERT, V. 1976B. Vitamin B_{12} folate interrelations. Clin. Haematol. 5:697.
17. ELWOOD, P.C., and WILLIAMS, G. 1970. A comparative trial of slow-release and conventional iron preparations. Practitioner 204:812.
18. ENGLAND, J.M., WALFORD, D.M., and WATERS, D.A.W. 1972. Reassessment of the reliability of the hematocrit. Br. J. Haematol. 23:247.

19. FINCH, C.A. 1975. Erythropoiesis in protein-calorie malnutrition, *in* Protein-Calorie Malnutrition. (R.E. Olson, ed.) pp 247. Academic Press, New York.
20. GARBY, L. and AREEKUL, S. 1973. Fish-sauce as a vehicle for iron supplementation in Thailand. A study of its production and consumption, effects of addition of iron salts, absorption of iron from enriched meals and effect on the packed red cell volume values of one year's consumption of enriched fish-sauce in a Thai village. To be published.
21. GERSON, C.D., COHEN, N., HEPNER, G.W., BROWN, N., HERBERT, V., and JANOWITZ, H.D. 1971. Folic acid absorption in man: Enhancing effect of glucose. Gastroenterology 61:224.
22. HEINIVAARA, O., and PALVA, I.P. 1964. Malabsorption of vitamin B_{12} during treatment with p-aminosalicylic acid. Acta. Med. Scandinavica. 175:469.
23. HERBERT, V. 1962. Experimental nutritional folate deficiency in man. Trans. Assoc. Am. Physicians 75:307.
24. HERBERT, V. 1963. A palatable diet for producing experimental folate deficiency in man. Am. J. Clin. Nutr. 12:17.
25. HERBERT, V. 1975. Megaloblastic anemias, *in* Textbook of Medicine, 14th ed. (P.B. Beeson and W. McDermott, eds.) pp 1404. Saunders, Philadelphia.
26. HERBERT, V. 1977. The blood in hypothyroidism, *in* The Thyroid. (S.C. Werner and S. H. Ingbar, ed.) Harper & Row, New York in press.
27. HERBERT, V. 1977. Anemias, *in* Nutritional Disorders of American Women (M. Winick, ed) pp 79, Wiley, New York.
28. HERBERT, V., and ZALUSKY, R. 1962. Interrelations of vitamin B_{12} and folate metabolism: Folic acid clearance studies. J. Clin. Invest. 41:1263.
29. HERBERT, V., COLMAN, N., SPIVACK, M., OCASIO, E., GHANTA, V., KIMMEL, K., BRENNER, L., FREUNDLICH, J., and SCOTT, J. 1975. Folic acid deficiency in the United States: Folate assays in a prenatal clinic. Am. J. Obstet. Gynecol. 123:175.
30. JACOBSON, E.D., CHODOS, R.B., and FALOON, W.W. 1960. An experimental malabsorption syndrome induced by neomycin. Am. J. Med. 28:524.
31. KRUMDIECK, C.L., and BAUGH, C.M. 1969. The solid phase synthesis of polyglutamates of folic acid. Biochemistry 8:1568.
32. MANZOOR, M., and RUNCIE, J. 1976. Folate-responsive neuropathy: Report of ten cases. Br. Med. J. 1:1176.
33. MOLLIN, D.L., BOOTH, C.C., and BAKER, S.J. 1957. The absorption of vitamin B_{12} in control subjects in Addisonian pernicious anemia and in the malabsorption syndrome. Br. J. Haematol. 3:412.
34. REYNOLDS, E.H. 1976. Neurologic aspects of folate and vitamin B_{12} metabolism. Clin. Haematol. 5:661.
35. SAMUELSSON, G., and SJOLIN, S. 1972. An epidemiological study of child health and nutrition in a northern Swedish country. Acta Pediatrica Scandinavica. 61, 63–72.

36. SILVER, H., and FRANKEL, S. 1971. Normal values for mean corpuscular volume as determined by the Model S Coulter Counter. Am. J. Clin. Pathol. 55:438.
37. SOLAKANNEL, S.J., PALVA, L.P., and TUKKUNEN, J.T. Malabsorption of vitamin B_{12} during treatment with slow-release potassium chloride. Acta Medica Scandinavica. 187:431.
38. SOOD, S.K., BANERJI, L., and RAMALINGASWAMI, V. 1968. Occurrence of nutritional anemias in tropical countries. *In* Occurrence, Causes and Prevention of Nutritional Anaemias, ed. Blix, G. Uppsala: Almqvist & Wiksells.
39. SULLIVAN, L.W., and HERBERT, V. 1965. Studies on the minimum daily requirement for vitamin B_{12}. N. Engl. J. Med. 272:340.
40. TAMURA, T., and STOKSTAD, E., L.R. 1973. The availability of food folate in man. Br. J. Haematol. 25:513.
41. TANDON, B.N., MAGOTRA, M.L., SARAYA, A.K., and RAMALINGASWAMI, V. 1968. Small intestine in protein malnutrition. Am. J. Clin. Nutr. 21:813.
42. TISMAN, G., and HERBERT, V. 1971. Inhibition by penicillamine of DNA synthesis by human bone marrow in vitro. Fed. Proc. 30:518.
43. TOSKES, P.P., and DEREN, J.J. 1972. Selective inhibition of vitamin B_{12} absorption by paraaminosalicylic acid. Gastroenterology 62:1232.
44. TOSKES, P.P., HANSELL, J., CERDA, J., and DEREN, J.J. 1971. Vitamin B_{12} malabsorption in chronic pancreatic insufficiency. Studies suggesting the presence of a pancreatic "intrinsic factor." N. Eng. J. Med. 284:627.
45. TOSKES, P.P., DEREN, J.J., and CONRAD, M.E. 1973. Trypsin-like nature of the pancreatic factor that corrects vitamin B_{12} malabsorption associated with pancreatic dysfunction. J. Clin. Invest. 52:1660.
46. VITERI, F.E., ALVARADO, J., LUTHRINGER, D.G., and WOOD, R.P. 1968. Hematological changes in protein calorie malnutrition. Vitamin Horm. 26:573.
47. WEBB, D.I., CHODOS, R.B., MAHAR, C.Q., and FALOON, W.W. 1968. Mechanism of vitamin B_{12} malabsorption in patients receiving colchicine. N. Engl. J. Med., 279:845.
48. WHO GROUP OF EXPERTS. 1972. Nutritional Anaemias. WHO Technical Report Ser. #503, Geneva.
49. WHO SCIENTIFIC GROUP 1968. Nutritional Anaemias. WHO Technical Report Ser. #405, Geneva.
50. WILLIAMS, M.L., SHOTT, R.J., O'NEAL, P.L., and OSKI, F. 1975. Role of dietary iron and fat on vitamin E deficiency anemia of infancy. N. Engl. J. Med. 292:887.
51. WU, A., CHANARIN, I., SLAVIN, G., and LEVI, A.J. 1975. Folate deficiency in the alcoholic—Its relationship to clinical and haematological abnormalities, liver disease and folate stores. Br. J. Haematol. 29:469.
52. COMMITTEE ON MATERNAL NUTRITION. 1970. Maternal Nutrition and the Course of Pregnancy, National Academy of Sciences, Washington, D.C.

28

NUTRITION IN RENAL FAILURE

Stephen I. Rifkin, M.D.

The uremic patient has multiple nutritional problems including those associated with dietary protein intake, fluid and electrolyte balance, phosphate retention, and acid-base disturbances. In the last two decades, enormous strides have been made in the care of these patients. A better understanding of the nutritional needs of the uremic patient has developed, and problem areas have been better defined. In addition, the advent of dialysis has generated an entirely new area for nutritional investigation. This review will describe the present status of nutritional therapy in dialyzed and undialyzed renal failure patients, including some recent advances in our understanding of protein metabolism and their influence on dietary therapy.

PRINCIPLES OF PROTEIN METABOLISM

An understanding of protein metabolism is of critical importance in the dietary management of renal failure patients. Protein is composed of amino acids. The amino acids can be divided into two types, essential and nonessential. The essential amino acids cannot be synthesized by the body and must be supplied by the diet. There are at least nine essential amino acids, including histidine, an amino acid that has only very recently been shown to be essential. They are found in predominance in eggs, milk, and meat. The nonessential amino acids can be synthesized by the body. They are found in predominance in vegetable protein. Proteins that are primarily composed of essential amino acids are called high

Dr. Rifkin is Assistant Professor, Division of Nephrology, Department of Internal Medicine, University of South Florida College of Medicine, Tampa, and Assistant Chief, Division of Nephrology, James A. Haley Veteran's Administration Hospital, Tampa.

biologic value protein and conversely, those composed primarily of nonessential amino acids are called low biologic value protein.

The kidney is the principal organ responsible for the elimination of the nitrogenous products of protein catabolism, with urinary loss of nitrogen accounting for approximately 70 per cent of dietary nitrogen intake, fecal loss for about 10 to 20 per cent, and skin loss for the remainder. There is an enterohepatic circulation of urea, the chief nitrogenous end-product of protein catabolism. Urea is acted upon by bacterial ureases in the gastrointestinal tract to form ammonia. The ammonia is picked up by the portal circulation and carried to the liver, where it may be used to resynthesize urea. It was thought until very recently that the large pool of urea nitrogen found in renal failure patients could be utilized in significant amounts to resynthesize amino acids, thereby decreasing effective protein catabolism and improving nitrogen balance. However, it has been clearly demonstrated that this is not the case. Urea degradation is not substantially increased in renal failure.[1] In addition, Varcoe[2] found that even though utilization of urea nitrogen for albumin synthesis is considerably higher in the renal failure patient than in normals, in absolute terms, the contribution of urea nitrogen to albumin synthesis in the uremic is of minor nutritional significance. He also demonstrated an additional stimulus for urea reutilization of protein restriction, but even on a 30 gram per day protein diet, the contribution of urea nitrogen to albumin synthesis in the uremic was only 3.1 per cent. Richards also demonstrated the stimulus of protein restriction and found that it was a more potent stimulus to urea reutilization than uremia.[3]

Protein turnover appears to be an adaptive process with lower turnover rates in patients with low protein intakes. This is true of normals and renal failure patients alike. The mechanism for the adaptation to varying levels of protein intake has not been delineated. Efficient protein utilization also requires an adequate energy intake. People with inadequate caloric intakes will tend to utilize nitrogen sources for energy needs.

The toxins of renal failure appear to be primary by-products of protein catabolism. They are an ill-defined group, with molecular weights generally thought to be between 500 and 1500 daltons. These compounds accumulate in renal insufficiency and, depending upon the severity of the disease, may reach levels which produce symptoms. Thus, reduction in protein catabolism will decrease the quantity of toxins that must be eliminated.

DIETARY PROTEIN THERAPY IN RENAL FAILURE

The goal of dietary protein therapy is to supply an optimum protein intake to produce positive nitrogen balance while at the same time minimizing the production of uremic toxins by minimizing protein catabolism. This is done by placing the patient on a restricted protein diet. Adaptation to the diet will occur, and protein turnover will decrease. The quantity and composition of the diet will vary, depending upon the degree of renal dysfunction and the type of nitrogen source utilized. Recommended protein intakes at different levels of renal insufficiency range widely, with initial restriction to 50 grams per day recommended by various authors at glomerular filtration rates of from 20–30 cc per minute[4] to 7–10 cc per minute.[5] Intakes of 18–20 grams per day are recommended for glomerular filtration rates of 3–5 cc per minute. To these figures, one must add as replacement the daily urinary protein loss. Below approximately 2–3 cc per minute, standard protein restriction is inadequate to control uremic toxicity, and more severe restriction will result in malnutrition. The protein composition of this type of restricted diet is generally either high biologic value proteins or essential amino acids, or a mixture of the two.

An alternate diet pioneered by Walser[6] utilizes ketoacids. They are keto analogues of essential amino acids and lack the alpha-amino nitrogen of the amino acids. The treatment is based on the amination of the analogues by transamination from nonessential amino acids. Ketoacid analogues of all the essential amino acids are not available, so a combination of ketoacid analogues and essential amino acids is used in the diet. The ketoacid diet appears extremely efficient and effective in maintaining nutritional balance, while at the same time substantially reducing urea nitrogen levels. It also seems to have a direct and prolonged effect on protein turnover, the mechanism of which is not understood.[7] Keto analogues as a dietary supplement in the treatment of chronic renal failure are now marketed in several European countries, and clinical investigation of their utility continues. The major advantage would seem to be an ability to alleviate symptoms of uremia in patients unresponsive to other diets because of the severity of their renal insufficiency.

An additional requirement for nitrogen balance is adequate caloric intake. Otherwise, the efficiency of nitrogen utilization is significantly diminished. This may not be an easy task, particularly in children who tend to be anorexic. Caloric supplements such as Cal-Power may need to be utilized. A caloric intake of 3,000 kcal has been recommended for a working adult. Vitamin supplementation must also be undertaken as the protein restricted diets are all vitamin deficient.

UNRESOLVED ISSUES

Lest one feel that this field has been thoroughly explored and is entirely understood, I would like to point out some problem areas: (1)

The question of which amino acids are essential in the uremic is not absolutely clear, and the dietary requirements of specific essential amino acids have not been established in renal failure. There are abnormalities of amino acid metabolism in uremia. The amino acid chromatogram is abnormal.[8] The ratio of tyrosine to phenylalanine is abnormal.[9] The metabolism of hydroxyproline is slowed in patients with renal insufficiency.[10] A limited capacity of the uremic to synthesize a particular amino acid may exist and, in special circumstances, may make the amino acid functionally essential. The kidney's ability to metabolize amino acids in uremia may be compromised, and the clearance of amino acids has been shown to vary with renal function.[11] (2) The question of what type of protein composition is best has not been settled. Recent data suggest that a combination of essential and nonessential amino acids results in a better nutritional status than essential amino acids alone.[12] The metabolic cost of synthesizing the nonessential amino acids is not clear. Utilization of high biologic value protein sources for dietary protein may provide such a mixture. (3) The possibility of improving renal function with use of ketoacid diets has been raised but has not been proven.[13] (4) Finally, the dietary need for protein may vary with the severity of renal failure, age, sex, and nutritional status of the patients, so that a careful evaluation of each patient to insure that the patient is in nutritional balance is necessary. This is particularly critical in growing children.

PROTEIN INTAKE IN ACUTE RENAL FAILURE

In 1973, Abel[14] reported that the use of a parenteral solution for nutrition containing essential amino acids and glucose resulted in a decreased mortality as compared with a control group of patients in acute renal failure given glucose alone. There was the suggestion that the group receiving the "renal failure" solution had a shorter period of uremia, and that this might be the factor primarily responsible for increased survival. Toback[15] has provided some recent experimental data that expand this observation. He found that intravenous amino acid infusions to rats in acute renal failure decreased the level of renal functional insufficiency and enhanced phospholipid biosynthesis for new membrane formation in renal cortical cells. Thus, provision of an adequate nutritional intake, including protein, appears to be beneficial to patients with acute renal failure. There are a variety of products available to fulfill this goal, depending on whether the oral or parenteral route is used and whether the patient is on dialysis. These include Nephramine, a parenteral hyperalimentation solution containing essential amino acids and glucose, and Amin-Aid, an oral preparation of essential amino acids and a nonprotein source for calories.

DIETARY THERAPY IN DIALYSIS

The hemodialysis patient has substantially different dietary requirements than the undialyzed uremic. Amino acids are lost during dialysis. If a glucose bath is used, amino acid losses have been estimated to be approximately 1–2 grams per hour of dialysis, and 20–30 per cent of losses are essential amino acids. If a glucose-free bath is used, amino acid losses are 50 per cent higher. 20–50 grams of glucose are removed per six-hour dialysis using a glucose-free bath and approximately 4 grams per hour of glucose are added to the patient if a glucose bath is used.[16] In addition, abnormalities of protein metabolism are present in the dialysis patient.

It seems clear that the dialysis patient needs and can effectively utilize larger quantities of protein than the undialyzed uremic. A protein intake of between 0.8–1.25 grams/kilogram/day has been recommended. The maximum amount of protein that the patient can ingest without developing signs or symptoms of uremia appears to be a reasonable goal. Studies of the benefit of essential amino acid supplementation in patients on maintenance hemodialysis have been conflicting. Adults receiving 60–100 grams of protein per day had an improvement in their amino acid chromatogram,[17] but children on unrestricted protein intakes had no benefit.[18]

Recent research has demonstrated that most dialysis patients have a Type IV hyperlipoproteinemia with elevated plasma triglyceride levels, elevated very low density lipoproteins, decreased high density lipoprotein cholesterol, and normal plasma cholesterol levels.[19] This seems to be due to a defect in lipoprotein lipase activity. Since it appears that low levels of high density lipoprotein cholesterol are a significant cardiac risk factor, the Type IV hyperlipoproteinemia represents a potentially substantial problem in the dialysis population. Sanfelippo[20] has shown that a diet in which carbohydrate represented only 35 per cent of the total daily calories is effective in lowering fasting triglyceride levels in dialysis patients. Fasting triglyceride levels have also been responsive to clofibrate. The dosage of this drug must be substantially reduced in the dialysis population to prevent the occurrence of myotoxicity. Plasma levels must be monitored, and lower than usual levels have to be maintained to prevent the occurrence of toxicity.[21]

Peritoneal dialysis is an alternate modality of dialysis therapy that is becoming increasingly common. This method involves the repetitive instillation and removal of glucose-containing solutions from the peritoneal cavity for approximately 12 hours, three to four times per week. Patients on peritoneal dialysis have somewhat different protein requirements from hemodialysis patients. Protein losses due to peritoneal membrane permeability vary considerably with each patient but in general are greater than that found in hemodialysis. The presence of peritonitis may substantially increase losses. Protein intakes of 1.2–1.5 grams per kilogram per day have been recommended,[22] and protein malnutrition does not seem to be a problem if an adequate amount is consumed. Additional caloric and protein intake may be necessary during times of stress and infection such as peritonitis.

ELECTROLYTE AND ACID-BASE STATUS

It is extremely important for the renal failure patient to remain normovolemic. Dehydration may increase the degree of renal insufficiency, producing uremic symptoms. Overhydration may contribute to hypertension and congestive heart failure. The patient's volume status is primarily determined by his kidney's ability to handle sodium appropriately. This ability must be determined on an individual basis. Some patients, particularly those with predominant tubular disease, may be salt-wasters and require large amounts of sodium in order to prevent depletion. Other patients may handle sodium loads poorly and rapidly develop edema. As end-stage renal disease develops, even the salt-wasters tend to convert to salt retainers and experience the resultant problems of overhydration. In order to prevent or ameliorate these problems the daily urinary sodium excretion should be measured when the patient is either normovolemic or minimally edematous, and this amount of sodium should be given in the diet. Sodium intakes between 2 and 10 or more grams per day may be required. If the patient is unable to comply with the degree of sodium restriction necessary to maintain him edema free, diuretics may be useful. The loop diuretics in large amounts are effective down to glomerular filtration rates (GFR's) of about 5 cc per minute. Additionally, the use of diuretics may allow the patient to ingest enough sodium to make an otherwise unpalatable diet acceptable. The hemodialysis and peritoneal dialysis patients are usually restricted to about 2 grams of sodium per day. The average American diet contains large amounts of sodium, and a substantial effort must be made by the patient to comply with a 2 gm/day or less sodium restriction.

In general, renal failure patients handle potassium loads well until late in the course of their disease.[23] As end-stage renal disease occurs, a potassium restricted diet to levels of 40 to 60 meq per day will be required. High potassium foods include nuts, chocolate, bananas, dates, raisins, baked potatoes, and french fried potatoes.

In addition to electrolyte imbalances, acid-base disturbances may also occur in the renal failure patient. These patients may develop metabolic acidosis due to the presence of either renal tubular acidosis or the inability of the kidney to excrete fixed acids. Correction of this acidosis requires the addition of base generally through the administration of sodium bicarbonate. Care must be taken when treating with sodium bicarbonate as large sodium loads may be ingested, producing volume overload.

PHOSPHORUS

With the onset of renal insufficiency, a tendency towards phosphate retention occurs. This causes hypocalcemia which in turn stimulates increased parathyroid activity. Elevated parathormone increases renal clearance of phosphate, resulting initially in normal phosphorus and calcium levels, along with an elevated parathormone level. When the GFR reaches approximately 20–25 cc per minute overt phosphate retention occurs in spite of the increase in phosphate clearance caused by the elevated parathormone level. The secondary hyperparathyroidism that occurs as the result of phosphate retention and abnormalities of vitamin D metabolism found in uremics may result in bone dissolution and metastatic calcifications. In addition, there is some recent experimental data in rats that suggest that hyperphosphatemia has a deleterious effect on renal function, perhaps by causing precipitation of calcium phosphate in the kidney, and that control of hyperphosphatemia may prevent this deterioration.[24]

Dietary restriction of phosphorus results in an unpalatable and generally unacceptable diet. The mainstay of therapy is aluminum hydroxide. This compound binds phosphate in the gastrointestinal tract, preventing systemic absorption, thereby lowering serum phosphate levels. There is some controversy over the potential toxicity of aluminum in the uremic patient, but the evidence is mostly circumstantial and, where strongest, points to absorption of aluminum from dialysate water in the hemodialysis process, rather than absorption of large amounts of aluminum from the GI tract.

STATUS OF DIALYSIS VS. DIET

In the United States, dialytic therapy is preferred to rigorous nutritional restriction in the severely uremic patient. Dialysis allows for a much more palatable and varied diet. A good nutritional state is much more easily maintained, the patient's dietary life-style is much less compromised, and patient compliance is not nearly as crucial, as occasional indiscretions can be compensated for by vigorous dialysis. However, in patients who are not deemed dialysis candidates, or if dialysis is not available, dietary therapy can be effective treatment. Diets utilizing high biologic value proteins and/or essential amino acids may relieve uremic symptoms down to glomerular filtration rates of 2.5−5 cc per minute. Ketoacid diets may be of benefit in uremics with even lower GFR's, but patient compliance with these diets is extremely difficult to achieve without enormous inputs from the medical team. These types of protein restriction, combined with adequate caloric intakes, careful monitoring of electrolyte intake and acid-base balance, vitamin supplementation, and phosphate control, can produce a substantial prolongation of worthwhile existence.

REFERENCES

1. RICHARDS, P.: Nitrogen-Recycling in Uremia: A Reappraisal. Clin. Neph., 3:166, 1975.
2. VARCOE, R., HALLIDAY, D., CARSON, E.R., *et al*: Efficiency of Utilization of Urea Nitrogen for Albumin Synthesis by Chronically Uraemic and Normal Man. Clin. Sci. and Mol. Med., 48:379, 1975.
3. RICHARDS, P., BROWN, C.L., HOUGHTON, B.J., WRONG, O.M.: The Incorporation of Ammonia Nitrogen Into Albumin in Man: The Effects of Diet, Uremia, and Growth Hormone. Clin. Neph. 3:172, 1975.
4. BURTON, B.T.: Current Concepts of Nutrition and Diet in Diseases of the Kidney. J. Amer. Diet. Assoc. 65:623, 1974.
5. BERLYNE, G.M.: Dietary Treatment of Chronic Renal Failure, *in* Strategy in Renal Failure. Edited by E. Friedman. John Wiley and Sons, Inc., 1978.
6. WALSER, M., COULTER, A.W., DIGHE, S., CRANTZ, F.R.: The Effect of Keto-Analogues of Essential Amino Acids in Severe Chronic Uremia. J. Clin. Invest., 52:678, 1973.
7. SAPIR, D.G., OWEN, O.E., POZEFSKY, T., WALSER, M.: Nitrogen Sparing Induced by a Mixture of Essential Amino Acids Given Chiefly as Their Keto-Analogues During Prolonged Starvation in Obese Subjects. J. Clin. Invest. 54: 974, 1974.
8. KOPPLE, J.D.: Abnormal Amino Acid and Protein Metabolism in Uremia. Kid. Int. 14:340, 1979.
9. JONES, M.R., KOPPLE, J.D., SWENDSEID, M.E.: Phenylalanine Metabolism in Uremia and Normal Man. Kid. Int., 14:169, 1978.
10. HART, W., VAN DEN HAMER, C.J.A., VAN DER SLUYS VEER, J.: The Use of Hydroxy-DL-Proline $2^{14}C$ in the Investigation of Hydroxyproline Metabolism in Normal Subjects and in Patients with Renal Insufficiency. Clin. Neph., 6:379, 1976.
11. BETTS, P.R., GREEN, A.: Plasma and Urine Amino Acid Concentrations in Children with Chronic Renal Insufficiency. Nephron, 18:132, 1977.
12. PENNISI, A.J., WANG, M., KOPPLE, J.D.: Effects of Protein and Amino Acid Diets in Chronically Uremic and Control Rats. Kid. Int., 13:472, 1978.
13. WALSER, M.: Ketoacids in the Treatment of Uremia. Clin. Neph. 3:180, 1975.

14. ABEL, R.M., BECK, C.H., JR., ABBOTT, W.M., *et al*: Improved Survival From Acute Renal Failure After Treatment with Intravenous Essential L-Amino Acids and Glucose. NEJM, 288:695, 1973.
15. TOBACK, F.G.: Amino Acid Enhancement of Renal Regeneration After Acute Tubular Necrosis. Kid. Int., 12:193, 1977.
16. QUARTO DI PALO, F., BUCCIANTI, G., VALENTI, G.F., *et al*: Nutritive Hemodialysis in Renal Failure. Dial. and Trans. 7:457, 1978.
17. PHILLIPS, M.E, HARVARD, J., HOWARD, J.P.: Oral Essential Amino Acid Supplementation in Patients on Maintenance Hemodialysis. Clin. Neph., 9:241, 1978.
18. COUNAHAN, R., EL-BISHTI, M., CHANTLER, C.: Oral Essential Amino Acids in Children on Regular Hemodialysis. Clin. Neph., 9:11, 1978.
19. RAPOPORT, J., AVIRAM, M., CHAIMOVITZ, C., BROOK, J.G.: Defective High-Density Lipoprotein Composition in Patients on Chronic Hemodialysis, NEJM, 299:1326, 1978.
20. SANFELIPPO, M.L., SWENSON, R.S., REAVEN, G.M.: Response of Plasma Triglycerides to Dietary Change in Patients on Hemodialysis. Kid. Int., 14:180, 1978.
21. DIGUILIO, S., BOULU, R., DRÜCKE, T., *et al*: Clofibrate Treatment of Hyperlipidemia in Chronic Renal Failure. Clin. Neph., 8:504, 1977.
22. BLUMENKRANTZ, M.J., ROBERTS, C.E., CARD, B., *et al*: Nutritional Management of the Adult Patient Undergoing Peritoneal Dialysis. J. of the Amer. Diet. Assoc., 73:251, 1978.
23. VAN YPERSELE DE STRIHOU, C.: Potassium Homeostasis in Renal Failure. Kid. Int., 11:491, 1977.
24. IBELS, L.S., ALFREY, A.C., HAUT, L., HUFFER, W.: Preservation of Function in Experimental Renal Disease by Dietary Restriction of Phosphate. NEJM, 298:122, 1978.

29

NUTRITION AND FOOD SELECTION

Lewis A. Barness, M.D.

From the beginning of history, attempts have been made to define "normal nutrition." Once basic caloric needs were satisfied, man has attempted to use nutrition as a tool to attain perfect health and longevity. Periodically, a perfect diet or a perfect system appears, which, with a holistic approach, attempts to allay disease and debility. When each diet or system falls short of its goals, disillusion affects not only the diet or system used but also casts umbrage on better founded nutritional principles.

Nutrition is concerned with the production of food (agriculture, ichthyology, food science), availability (politics, economics), selection (sociology, culture, psychology), utilization (physiology, biochemistry) and prevention and treatment of disease (medicine). At present, we know only that food must be consumed and absorbed and that it must supply all essential nutrients in sufficient but not excessive quantities. Essential nutrients include protein, carbohydrate, fat, vitamins, minerals, and water. Calories are supplied by protein, carbohydrate and fat. While proportions of these may vary daily, calories consumed must equal calories utilized lest weight and energy vary daily. Sufficient water must be consumed daily to maintain body functions. Minerals and vitamins can be stored in the body for variable times. U.S. Recommended Dietary Allowances (Chapter 13, this volume) are revised periodically on the basis of available information. Allowances are made for age, sex, and physiological state, are designed to meet the needs of most people, and include

Dr. Barness is Chairman of Pediatrics, University of South Florida College of Medicine, 12901 North 30th Street, Tampa, Florida.

averages which, if consumed daily, would satisfy these requirements. Sources of these nutrients are not stated. (See Table 29.1).

Until and if more specific information becomes available, prudence suggests the use of varied sources of nutrients. Not only is variety likely to supply all known nutrients and even as yet undiscovered essentials, but also variety is important to provide psychological encouragement to good eating habits. With wider recognition of toxicants, both natural and man-added in some foods, variety also helps to dilute specific toxicants consumed.

Before the era of extensive food processing, all essential nutrients could be obtained from a diet consisting largely of 4 sources. These became the "basic four", a still useful concept which recommended one or two servings from high quality protein, dairy, vegetable-fruit, and bread-cereal sources.

Utilization of food requires absorption and metabolism. Fats are digested and absorbed in the small intestine after being transformed into an emulsion by peristalsis. After these droplets are hydrolyzed by lipases and bile salts to form micelles, they are absorbed through the brush border of the intestine, combined with cholesterol and protein to form chylomicrons and transported through the lymphatics into the circulation. Fatty acids with fewer than 12 carbon atoms, medium chain triglycerides, are absorbed directly through the brush border attached to albumin. Approximately 95% of ingested fat is utilizable as energy. Fat is also used in fat-soluble vitamin absorption, taste, membrane formation and stability. Essential fatty acids, found mainly in vegetable oils, are needed also for prostaglandin formation, cellular stability, and other functions.

Carbohydrate digestion begins in the mouth and proceeds through the stomach and small intestine. Starches are broken down to simple sugars by the action of enzymes and appropriate pH changes. Monosaccharides are attached to carrier proteins and absorbed into the blood stream. This transport mechanism requires sodium ion. Approximately 95% of ingested carbohydrate is also utilizable as energy.

Protein hydrolysis occurs in the stomach and upper intestine. Enzymes split the proteins into peptides and amino acids and are absorbed through the brush border, requiring energy. After absorption protein metabolism, including formation of new proteins, ammonia and urea, also requires energy so that net energy available from food proteins is about 75%. While protein is an inefficient energy source, it is critical for the formation of enzymes, hormones, serum proteins, cellular integrity and many other functions.

Studies in animals and humans are used to measure the ability of ingested proteins to form needed protein components. By comparing

TABLE 29.1. RECOMMENDED DIETARY ALLOWANCES, REVISED 1980[a]. FOOD AND NUTRITION BOARD, NATIONAL ACADEMY OF SCIENCES–NATIONAL RESEARCH COUNCIL

Designed for the maintenance of good nutrition of practically all healthy people in the U.S.A.

							Fat-Soluble Vitamins			Water-Soluble Vitamins		
Category	Age (Years)	Weight (kg)	Weight (lb)	Height (cm)	Height (in.)	Protein (g)	Vitamin A (μg R.E.) [b]	Vitamin D (μg) [c]	Vitamin E (mg α T.E.) [d]	Vitamin C (mg)	Thiamin (mg)	Riboflavin (mg)
Infants	0.0–0.5	6	13	60	24	kg × 2.2	420	10	3	35	0.3	0.4
	0.5–1.0	9	20	71	28	kg × 2.0	400	10	4	35	0.5	0.6
Children	1–3	13	29	90	35	23	400	10	5	45	0.7	0.8
	4–6	20	44	112	44	30	500	10	6	45	0.9	1.0
	7–10	28	62	132	52	34	700	10	7	45	1.2	1.4
Males	11–14	45	99	157	62	45	1000	10	8	50	1.4	1.6
	15–18	66	145	176	69	56	1000	10	10	60	1.4	1.7
	19–22	70	154	177	70	56	1000	7.5	10	60	1.5	1.7
	23–50	70	154	178	70	56	1000	5	10	60	1.4	1.6
	51+	70	154	178	70	56	1000	5	10	60	1.2	1.4
Females	11–14	46	101	157	62	46	800	10	8	50	1.1	1.3
	15–18	55	120	163	64	46	800	10	8	60	1.1	1.3
	19–22	55	120	163	64	44	800	7.5	8	60	1.1	1.3
	23–50	55	120	163	64	44	800	5	8	60	1.0	1.2
	51+	55	120	163	64	44	800	5	8	60	1.0	1.2
Pregnant						+30	+200	+5	+2	+20	+0.4	+0.3
Lactating						+20	+400	+5	+3	+40	+0.5	+0.5

[a] The allowances are intended to provide for individual variations among most normal persons as they live in the United States under usual environmental stresses. Diets should be based on a variety of common foods in order to provide other nutrients for which human requirements have been less well defined.
[b] Retinol equivalents: 1 retinol equivalent=1 μg retinol or 6 μg β-carotene.
[c] As cholecalciferol: 10 μg cholecalciferol=400 I.U. vitamin D.
[d] α-tocopherol equivalents: 1 mg d-α-tocopherol=1 α T.E.
[e] 1 N.E. (niacin equivalent)=1 mg niacin or 60 mg dietary tryptophan.
[f] The folacin allowances refer to dietary sources as determined by *Lactobacillus casei* assay after treatment with enzymes ("conjugases") to make polyglutamyl forms of the vitamin available to the test organism.

ESTIMATED SAFE AND ADEQUATE DAILY DIETARY INTAKES OF ADDITIONAL SELECTED VITAMINS AND MINERALS[a]

		Vitamins			Trace Elements[b]	
Category	Age (Years)	Vitamin K (μg)	Biotin (mg)	Pantothenic Acid (mg)	Copper (mg)	Manganese (mg)
Infants	0–0.5	12	35	2	0.5–0.7	0.5–0.7
	0.5–1	10–20	50	3	0.7–1.0	0.7–1.0
Children and Adolescents	1–3	15–30	65	3	1.0–1.5	1.0–1.5
	4–6	20–40	85	3–4	1.5–2.0	1.5–2.0
	7–10	30–60	120	4–5	2.0–2.5	2.0–3.0
	11+	50–100	100–200	4–7	2.0–3.0	2.5–5.0
Adults		70–140	100–200	4–7	2.0–3.0	2.5–5.0

Source: from Recommended Dietary Allowances, Revised 1980. Food and Nutrition Board, National Academy of Sciences-National Research Council, Washington, D.C.

[a] Because there is less information on which to base allowances, these figures are not given in the main table of the RDA and are provided here in the form of ranges of recommended intakes.

Water-Soluble Vitamins				Minerals					
Niacin (mg N.E.)[e]	Vitamin B_6 (mg)	Folacin[f] (μg)	Vitamin B_{12} (μg)	Calcium (mg)	Phosphorus (mg)	Magnesium (mg)	Iron (mg)	Zinc (mg)	Iodine (μg)
6	0.3	30	0.5[g]	360	240	50	10	3	40
8	0.6	45	1.5	540	360	70	15	5	50
9	0.9	100	2.0	800	800	150	15	10	70
11	1.3	200	2.5	800	800	200	10	10	90
16	1.6	300	3.0	800	800	250	10	10	120
18	1.8	400	3.0	1200	1200	350	18	15	150
18	2.0	400	3.0	1200	1200	400	18	15	150
19	2.2	400	3.0	800	800	350	10	15	150
18	2.2	400	3.0	800	800	350	10	15	150
16	2.2	400	3.0	800	800	350	10	15	150
15	1.8	400	3.0	1200	1200	300	18	15	150
14	2.0	400	3.0	1200	1200	300	18	15	150
14	2.0	400	3.0	800	800	300	18	15	150
13	2.0	400	3.0	800	800	300	18	15	150
13	2.0	400	3.0	800	800	300	10	15	150
+2	+0.6	+400	+1.0	+400	+400	+150	[h]	+5	+25
+5	+0.5	+100	+1.0	+400	+400	+150	[h]	+10	+50

[g] The RDA for vitamin B_{12} in infants is based on average concentration of the vitamin in human milk. The allowances after weaning are based on energy intake (as recommended by the American Academy of Pediatrics) and consideration of other factors, such as intestinal absorption.

[h] The increased requirement during pregnancy cannot be met by the iron content of habitual American diets or by the existing iron stores of many women; therefore, the use of 30 to 60 mg supplemental iron is recommended. Iron needs during lactation are not substantially different from those of non-pregnant women, but continued supplementation of the mother for 2 to 3 months after parturition is advisable in order to replenish stores depleted by pregnancy.

Trace Elements[b]				Electrolytes		
Fluoride (mg)	Chromium (mg)	Selenium (mg)	Molybdenum (mg)	Sodium (mg)	Potassium (mg)	Chloride (mg)
0.1–0.5	0.01–0.04	0.01–0.04	0.03–0.06	115–350	350–925	275–700
0.2–1.0	0.02–0.06	0.03–0.06	0.04–0.08	250–750	425–1275	400–1200
0.5–1.5	0.02–0.08	0.02–0.08	0.05–0.1	325–975	550–1650	500–1500
1.0–2.5	0.03–0.12	0.03–0.12	0.06–0.15	450–1350	775–2325	700–2100
1.5–2.5	0.05–0.2	0.05–0.2	0.1–0.3	600–1800	1000–3000	925–2775
1.5–2.5	0.05–0.2	0.05–0.2	0.15–0.5	900–2700	1525–4575	1400–4200
1.5–4.0	0.05–0.2	0.05–0.2	0.15–0.5	1100–3300	1875–5625	1700–5100

[b] Since the toxic levels for many trace elements may be only several times usual intakes, the upper levels for the trace elements given in this table should not be habitually exceeded.

various proteins, biological values of proteins are determined. Biological values are closely related to absorbability of proteins and the content and balance of essential amino acids. For human use, the essential amino acids in eggs and meat appear best balanced and these sources provide protein of highest biological values. Vegetables and cereals individually may be deficient in one or more essential amino acids but mixtures of these same foods frequently provide the necessary balance. If essential amino acids remain unbalanced they are largely excreted.

Though discussed separately, the absorption of one group of substances facilitates or inhibits the absorption of another group. For example, fat absorption facilitates mineral absorption, particularly calcium, and fat malabsorption is accompanied by increased excretion of protein and carbohydrate. Similarly, the metabolic pathways of carbohydrate, protein, fat, minerals and vitamins are interrelated.[1]

With changing life styles and changes in food preparation, attempts have been made to define dietary practices to meet stated goals. Senator McGovern's Select Committee listed 7 goals which have, because of their implications, received controversial attention. Those goals are:

1. To avoid overweight, consume only as much energy (calories) as is expended; if overweight, decrease energy intake and increase energy expenditure.
2. Increase the consumption of complex carbohydrates and "naturally occurring" sugars from about 28 percent of energy intake to about 48 percent of energy intake.
3. Reduce the consumption of refined and processed sugars by about 45 percent to account for about 10 percent of total energy intake.
4. Reduce overall fat consumption from approximately 40 percent to about 30 percent of energy intake.
5. Reduce saturated fat consumption to account for about 10 percent of total energy intake; and balance that with poly-unsaturated and mono-unsaturated fats, which should account for about 10 percent of energy intake each.
6. Reduce cholesterol consumption to about 300 mg. a day.
7. Limit the intake of sodium by reducing the intake of salt to about 5 grams a day.

The goals suggest the following change in food selection and preparation:

1. Increase consumption of fruits and vegetables and whole grains.
2. Decrease consumption of refined and other processed sugars and foods high in such sugars.

3. Decrease consumption of foods high in total fat, and partially replace saturated fats, whether obtained from animal or vegetable sources, with poly-unsaturated fats.
4. Decrease consumption of animal fat, and choose meats, poultry and fish which will reduce saturated fat intake.
5. Except for young children, substitute low-fat milk for whole milk, and low-fat dairy products for high-fat dairy products.
6. Decrease consumption of butterfat, eggs and other high cholesterol sources. Some consideration should be given to easing the cholesterol goal for pre-menopausal women, young children and the elderly in order to obtain the nutritional benefits of eggs in the diet.
7. Decrease consumption of salt and foods high in salt content.

Concerns have been expressed that the data base for these goals is far from established, that failure to accomplish these goals would lead to general disillusionment, that massive changes in the food supply would be needed, that certain desirable states such as the elimination of iron deficiency, the wider adoption of breast feeding, the elimination of dental caries, and guaranteed adequate nutrition for the pregnant woman are not addressed, and other concerns. Nonetheless, publication of these goals has served to focus on the possibility that nutritional changes could affect the health status of the community.

While individual needs and desires will continue to modify diets, the physician must be prepared to recognize deficiencies or excesses which may occur with certain diets. Vegetarian diets require variety, lack of all animal sources may lead to vitamin B_{12} deficiency. High fiber diets, while usually beneficial, may inhibit essential mineral absorption. Megavitamins are not only expensive and usually useless but may cause specific toxicity. Reducing diets frequently cause loss of body protein rather than body fat, and may also be accompanied by dehydration and put undue strain on kidneys. "Natural" foods may contain as many toxins or contaminants as commercially grown foods. Good nutrition can be obtained by eating only sufficient total calories to maintain desired weight, with free use of fresh vegetables, whole grains, beans, lean meat, fish, poultry and limited snack foods which consist largely of sugar, salt and fat.

REFERENCE

ANDERSON, C.E. Energy and Metabolism. Chapter 2, p. 10 in Nutritional Support of Medical Practice, Ed. H.A. Schneider, C.E. Anderson and D.B. Coursin. Harper and Row, Hagertown 1977.

30

NUTRITIONAL ASPECTS OF OBESITY

George A. Bray, M.D.

INTRODUCTION

Obesity is a common problem in all affluent societies. Estimates of the number of overweight individuals in the United States vary from 10 to 50 million, depending upon the criteria used. Using 20% above desirable weight as the index of obesity, recent prevalence data for this country show that 24% of the women and 14% of men aged 18 to 74 are overweight[1]. These numbers indicate that at least 16.3 million American women and 8.5 million American men are significantly overweight. The importance of these data lies in the associated medical and social risks and the current social setting which says that "thin is in".

One of the Dietary Goals presented in the document prepared by the Senate Select Committee on Nutrition and Human Needs clearly states the basic philosophy for prevention and treatment of obesity.

"To avoid overweight, one should consume only as much energy as is expended. If overweight, decrease energy intake and increase expenditure."[2]

The difficulty comes in putting this sound dietary advice into practice. Anyone who has tried knows how difficult it can be to translate this recommendation into action. Since treatment is so often difficult prevention would be preferable. In no field is the old adage that "an ounce of prevention is worth a pound of cure" more apt than in obesity. As yet, however, we don't know how to prevent obesity, nor can we accurately identify obese individuals before they become obese. The best we can do

Dr. Bray is Professor, Department of Medicine, UCLA School of Medicine, Harbor-UCLA Medical Center, Torrance, California.

is to identify families where both parents are fat, but even then not more than 80% of the children will be obese[3].

Vanity is probably the major reason why individuals attempt to lose weight. In our society excess weight is considered by many to be socially undesirable, particularly among women. Associated medical problems are a second reason for seeking treatment for obesity and represent a particularly important motivation for middle-aged men. At the time of his first heart attack, the overweight man is advised to reduce his weight, and the pounds seem to "melt off". Weight reduction is also indicated for individuals with diabetes mellitus, osteoarthritis, hypertriglyceridemia (Type IV and V), and in problems of vascular insufficiency. Whatever the reason, a high degree of motivation is needed to achieve and maintain weight loss with any form of therapy. One of the primary responsibilities for any person who is involved in treating or advising obese people is to motivate the person to provide continuing sympathetic understanding for difficulties which they may experience when trying to lose weight.

The appropriate treatment for obesity depends on the risk associated with the degree of excess weight. This can in turn be expressed by using the body mass index. The body mass index is measured as $Wt/(Ht)^4$. With weight measured in kg and height in meters the normal values range between 20 and 26. A nomogram for determining the body mass index (BMI) is shown in Figure 30.1[4].

A body mass index of 30 is equivalent to 30% overweight, a degree of excess weight that is associated with a 25 to 30% extra risk to life. People with a body mass index over 40 are at very high risk and may have up to 11 times the extra risk to life of people with normal weight. The risk to health of extra weight goes up along with the rise in body weight. Thus all treatments to be considered in dealing with obese patients should be evaluated in terms of the degree of obesity and its attendant risk.

LOW RISK TREATMENTS

Diet and Nutrition

There are four areas to be considered in the use of diet and nutritional education in treating obesity. These are: (1) selection of the desired degree of caloric restriction in relation to the person's total caloric needs; (2) the distribution of these calories between carbohydrate, protein, and fat to provide an adequate amount of all nutrients; (3) the frequency with which the foods are to be eaten; and (4) the situations in which food is ingested.

Over the past 70 years a voluminous literature has accumulated concerning metabolic requirements of human beings. These caloric needs can

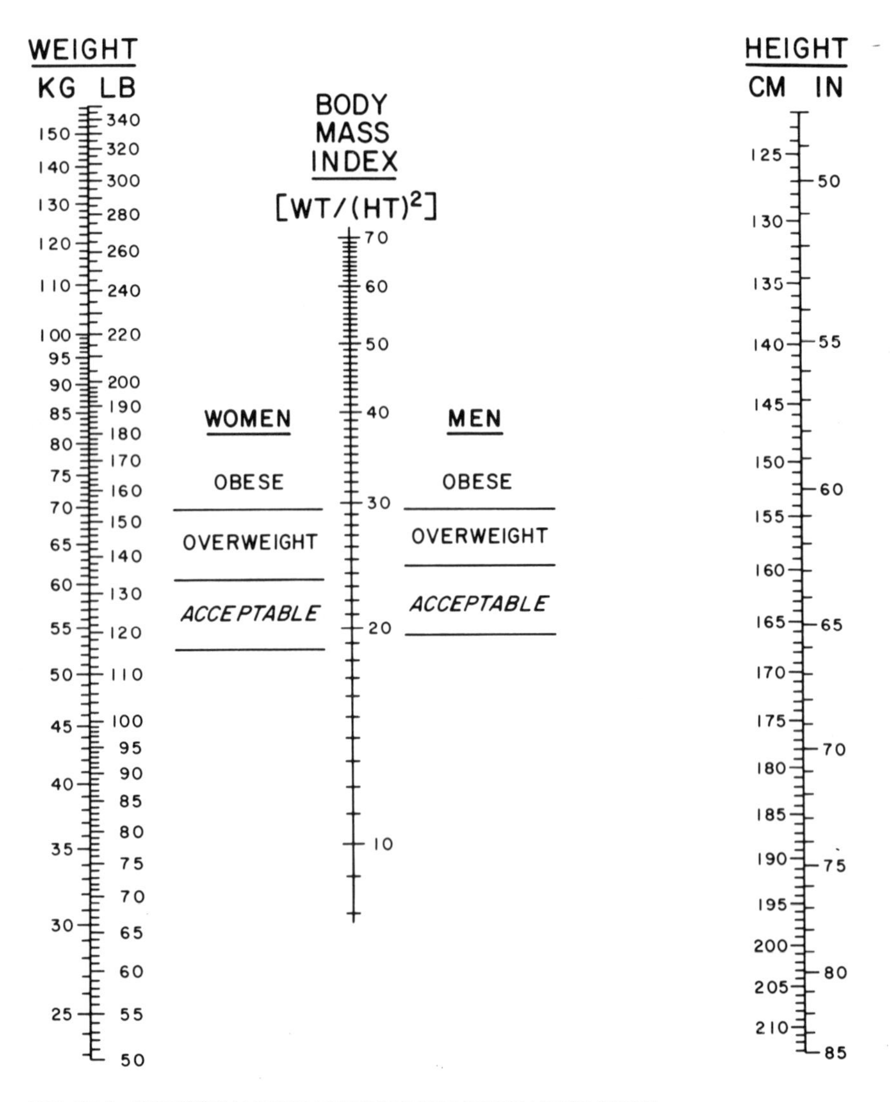

FIG. 30.1. NOMOGRAM FOR DETERMINING BODY MASS INDEX.
A straight edge is attached from the individual's weight on the left side to the point on the right hand line which corresponds to their height. The body mass index is the point at which this line connecting weight and height crosses the central vertical lines (Copyright George A. Bray, 1978. Reprinted with permission).

be divided into three components: the requirements for basal metabolism; heat loss due to the thermic effects of food; the energy needed for activity. Basal metabolic needs are slightly lower for women than for men. Basal needs include requirements for maintenance of normal cellular composition, for brain metabolism, for protein synthesis, for activity of smooth muscle, and for the reabsorption of solutes and water by the kidney. Table 30.1 shows the average levels of energy intake in relation to age (Recommended Dietary Allowances, 1979)[5].

TABLE 30.1. MEAN HEIGHTS AND WEIGHTS AND RECOMMENDED ENERGY INTAKE

Category	Age	Weight		Height		Energy Needs (with range)	
	(years)	(kg)	(lb)	(cm)	(in)	(kcal)	(MJ)
Infants	0.0–0.5	6	13	60	24	kg × 115 (95–145)	kg × .48
	0.5–1.0	9	20	71	28	kg × 105 (80–135)	kg × .44
Children	1–3	13	29	90	35	1300 (900–1800)	5.5
	4–6	20	44	112	44	1700 (1300–2300)	7.1
	7–10	28	62	132	52	2400 (1650–3300)	10.1
Males	11–14	45	99	157	62	2700 (2000–3700)	11.3
	15–18	66	145	176	69	2800 (2100–3900)	11.8
	19–22	70	154	177	70	2900 (2500–3300)	12.2
	23–50	70	154	178	70	2700 (2300–3100)	11.3
	51–75	70	154	178	70	2400 (2000–2800)	10.1
	76+	70	154	178	70	2050 (1650–2450)	8.6
Females	11–14	46	101	157	62	2200 (1500–3000)	9.2
	15–18	55	120	163	64	2100 (1200–3000)	8.8
	19–22	55	120	163	64	2100 (1700–2500)	8.8
	23–50	55	120	163	64	2000 (1600–2400)	8.4
	51–75	55	120	163	64	1800 (1400–2200)	7.6
	76+	55	120	163	64	1600 (1200–2000)	6.7
Pregnancy						+ 300	
Lactation						+ 500	

The data in this table have been assembled from the observed median heights and weights of children shown in Table 1, together with desirable weights for adults given in Table 2 for the mean heights of men (70 inches) and women (64 inches) between the ages of 18 and 34 years as surveyed in the U.S. population (HEW/NCHS data).

The energy allowances for the young adults are for men and women doing light work. The allowances for the two older age groups represent mean energy needs over these age spans, allowing for a 2% decrease in basal (resting) metabolic rate per decade and a reduction in activity of 200 kcal/day for men and women between 51 and 75 years, 500 kcal for men over 75 years and 400 kcal for women over 75 (see text). The customary range of daily energy output is shown for adults in parentheses, and is based on a variation in energy needs of ± 400 kcal at any one age (see text and Garrow, 1978), emphasizing the wide range of energy intakes appropriate for any group of people.

Energy allowances for children through age 18 are based on median energy intakes of children these ages followed in longitudinal growth studies. The values in parentheses are 10th and 90th percentiles of energy intake, to indicate the range of energy consumption among children of these ages (see text).

From: Recommended Dietary Allowances, Revised 1980, Food and Nutrition Board, National Academy of Sciences-National Research Council, Washington, D.C.

These energy requirements need to be modified in relation to physical activity. For the average American 20 to 30 years of age, the basal metabolic rate is approximately two-thirds of the total daily need; with advancing years total energy needs decrease more than basal metabolism. A woman aged 15 to 18 years who is 5 ft. 4 in. tall and weighs 120 lbs. would require approximately 2,100 calories per day for normal levels of activity. By contrast, a woman 6 ft. tall weighing 145 lbs. would need 2,800 calories. By age 60, these figures would fall to approximately 1,800 calories per day for the shorter woman and just over 2,200 calories per day for the taller one. For men the figures are somewhat higher. A 5 ft. 9 in. tall man weighing 176 lbs. would require 2,800 calories per day. The corresponding figures for men aged 51 to 75 are 2,400.

After assessing the person's daily caloric needs, the next goal is to provide a reasonable caloric deficit. The caloric deficit is the difference between calories required to maintain weight and the calories in a diet. If a caloric deficit of 1,000 calories is maintained, a loss of approximately 7,000 calories will result each week. Since a pound of fat tissue contains approximately 3,500 calories, a 1,000 calorie deficit each day will produce a two pound loss of fat each week from stores to provide the calories needed for metabolism and activity. In grossly obese people with larger caloric requirements, severe calorie restriction may be unacceptable and realistically unattainable. It is usually best to restrict calories by no more than 500 to 1,000 per day below maintenance levels. Occasionally, however, exceptions to this rule will be necessary. A three-day meal plan for a 1,200 calorie diet is presented in Table 30.2. For most people this will provide about a 500 cal/day deficit.

With adherence to any diet, two phases of weight loss are observed. The first is and reflects primarily the loss of fluids as the body adjusts to

TABLE 30.2. SUGGESTED MENU PLANS

Breakfast	Breakfast	Breakfast
Orange juice, ½ cup Egg, cooked or poached, 1 Toasted roll, ½ Beverage	Strawberries, 1 cup Corn flakes, ⅔ cup Skim milk, 1 cup Beverage	Grapefruit sections, ½ cup Cottage cheese, 3 oz. Toast, 1 slice Beverage
Lunch	Lunch	Lunch
Sardine Sandwich sardines, 2 oz. bread, 2 slices Cottage cheese, 3 oz. with mixed green vegetables Peach, 1 Beverage	Cottage cheese and chives, 3 oz. Celery hearts Whole wheat bread, 2 slices Apple, 1 Beverage	Tomato stuffed with shrimp, seafood cocktail sauce, 4 oz. Green bean salad, vinegar dressing Roll, 1 Plums, raw, 3 Beverage
Dinner	Dinner	Dinner
Tomato juice, 8 oz. Ham steak, 4 oz. Brussel sprouts, ½ cup Mixed green salad with lemon or vinegar dressing Grapefruit, ½ Beverage	Salmon, broiled or poached, 6 oz. Baked potato Broiled tomato Tossed green salad with spiced vinegar dressing Cantaloupe, ½ Beverage	Broiled chicken, 4 oz. Steamed carrots, ½ cup Romaine lettuce, lemon dressing Pineapple, 1 slice Beverage
Snack	Snack	Snack
Skim milk, 2 cups	Skim milk, 1 cup Berries, ½ cup	Skim milk, 2 cups Puffed wheat, ⅔ cup Orange, 1

utilizing its stored fat. After some days excess fluid is depleted and subsequent weight loss is slower. After the first one to three weeks on any diet, many people become distressed with the slowness of weight loss. Many may experience feelings of depression[6]. This frustration is compounded by the tendency of some individuals to adapt to caloric restriction by decreasing energy expenditure. If this happens, the prescribed diet will produce a smaller weight loss than anticipated, leading to even greater exasperation on the part of the patient. Reassurance and understanding are most important at this time.

New diets frequently appear in popular magazines and in book form. This suggests that none of them is ideal; if there were an ideal diet, there would be no need for continued appearance of new ones. A critique of some of these diets was published recently[7]. The low carbohydrate, high fat diet is a frequently recurring theme. It has been propounded intermittently for over one hundred years. This program raises the question of whether an imbalanced diet in one or other of its major nutrients is more beneficial in producing weight loss than a diet which is balanced in all components. Research has provided discordant data on this question. From the results shown in two careful studies, the answer would appear to be "no"[8,9]. Patients were hospitalized and the fraction of calories provided as fat, carbohydrate, and proteins was varied over a wide range. After the initial phase of weight loss due to the excretion of water, changes in the distribution of calories between carbohydrates, fat, and protein had no influence on the rate at which further weight was lost[10]. Other studies have suggested that a very low carbohydrate diet may increase the rate at which body fat is catabolized[11]. A diet with 30 grams of carbohydrate per day seemed to cause more weight loss than diets with 60 or 104 grams of carbohydrate but which were otherwise identical in composition and number of calories. The results of this study require confirmation before it can be fully accepted. The long-term consequences to health of a low carbohydrate diet are still open to question, particularly for pregnant women, individuals with kidney disease and in diabetics.

The frequency with which food is ingested may also be important in weight control. The rate of weight loss is not changed by the frequency with which food is eaten. However, in normal college age males, the frequency of feedings did not have a significant influence on carbohydrate tolerance and on the level of cholesterol. When these men were fed either a weight-maintaining or a weight-reducing diet in one meal, they showed impairment in glucose tolerance and higher levels of plasma cholesterol compared to the same diet fed in three or six feedings. These data would suggest that it is wise to eat three or more meals per day as plasma cholesterol will be significantly lower and glucose tolerance improved[12].

How effective are diets in the treatment of obese patients? A summary of the results of dietary treatments for obesity was published in 1959 by Stunkard and McLaren-Hume and marked a watershed in this field[13]. On average only 5% of people who entered diet clinics lost 40 lbs. and 25% lost 20 lbs. There was a considerable difference between clinics in the percentage of people who were successful. That is, some people are more successful than others in losing weight and the clinical setting seems to influence the results. This implies that behavioral factors which might be termed "motivation" play a central role in the success of any treatment. A more recent review comparing diet with other studies is shown in Figure 30.2[14]. The nine studies included here used diet alone accompanied by other therapies.

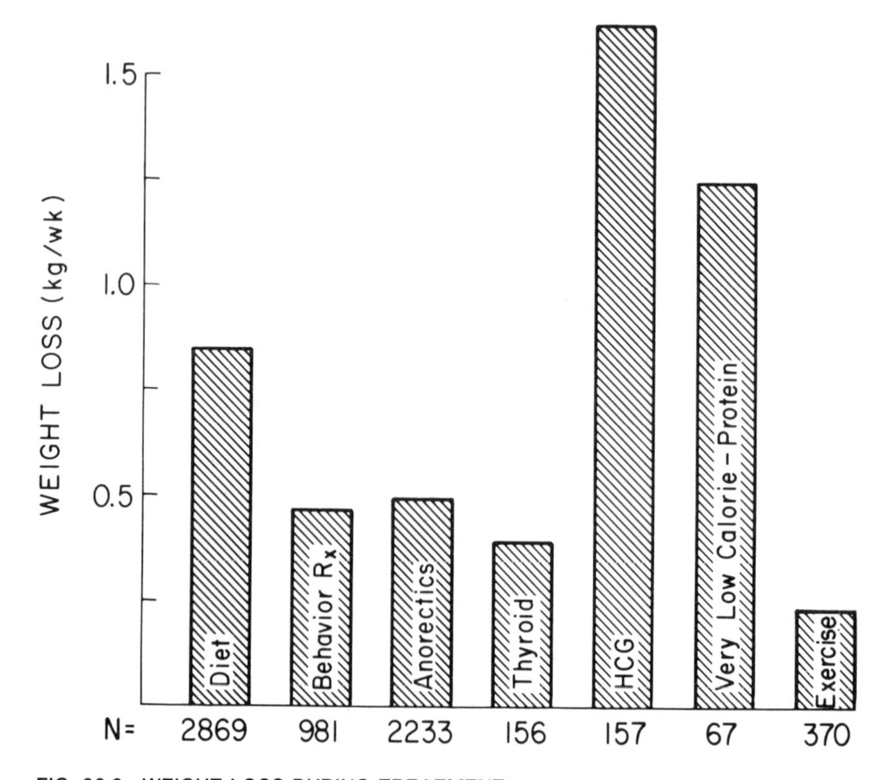

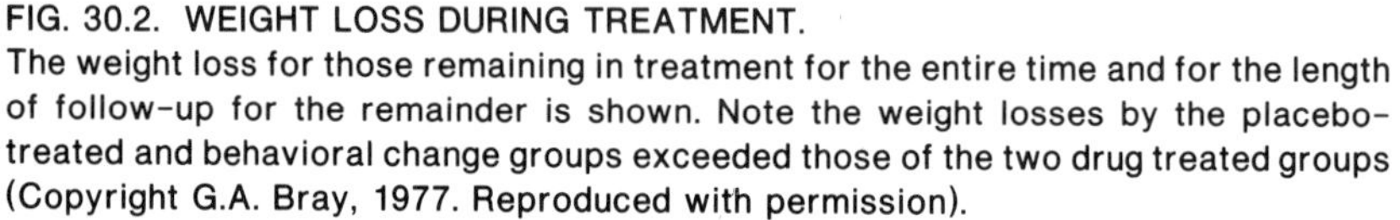
FIG. 30.2. WEIGHT LOSS DURING TREATMENT.
The weight loss for those remaining in treatment for the entire time and for the length of follow-up for the remainder is shown. Note the weight losses by the placebo-treated and behavioral change groups exceeded those of the two drug treated groups (Copyright G.A. Bray, 1977. Reproduced with permission).

Programs for Behavioral Change of Eating

During the past decade a series of techniques have been developed for helping overweight subjects gain more control over the environmental situation in which they eat. By analyzing eating behaviors it is sometimes possible to make important changes in the way people eat food. These can be described under 3 headings: 1) Antecedents of Eating; 2) Behavior of Eating; and 3) Consequences of Eating. These are the ABCs of behavioral change in eating. Details are available elsewhere[15-17] but the basic procedures are similar. To evaluate the antecedents of eating patients are instructed to record the foods they eat and where they eat them. In succeeding weeks they keep additional records of when they eat, with whom they eat, the places they eat, and the activities associated with eating as well as the foods they like and dislike. This provides an assessment of the factors in the environment which trigger or cue eating (Antecedents). This can be done step wise using a card like the one shown in Figure 30.3 for recording calories[18]. From an analysis of these various records suggestions for changing and controlling eating behavior can be made.

DAILY CALORIE MONITOR		CALORIES	©BRAY 1976
FOOD EATEN	DAY	LIQUID	SOLID

FIG. 30.3. FORM FOR RECORDING CALORIES.
With the use of a calorie guide patients are instructed to record the caloric value for liquid and solid foods which they eat. At the end of the week the totals for each day under the two categories are summarized to give a picture of the entire caloric intake for the week.

In another exercise patients are instructed to record how frequently they eat, how rapidly they eat, and whom they eat with (Behavior of Eating). With this information it is possible to suggest other changes in eating behavior. For example, patients are encouraged to eat on smaller plates which will reduce the amount of food taken in one sitting. They are also encouraged to cook only one serving at a time. If they want more food they have to go back and cook it. Serving dishes are not put on the table.

Finally, the patients are helped to understand the consequences of their behavior and develop rewards for successful change. There has to be an important reason if you are to change your eating behavior successfully. Obese people need to set up some system of rewards to accomplish this. There are a number of technique for rewards. One is with money which is paid back for success. There are others like new clothes, a vacation, etc. that work as well.

The problem of helping patients count calories has occupied the attention of the Harbor-UCLA Clinic for several years. A recording form on which we have patients write down their foods and caloric values is shown in Figure 30.3. We supplement this monitor with a description of how to use the nutritional information available on the labels of many foods[18]. The caloric (energy) content of a serving size is available for patient use. They only have to weigh or measure the foods. Recently we have developed a glass calibrated to show the caloric values of various beverages as a technique for continuous monitoring and feedback. The markings on the glass were drawn to provide an estimate of the caloric value for given foods or beverages (Figure 30.4). Every time a liquid is poured into the Calorie Glass^{R} ** the caloric value is immediately visible. This provides a continuous feedback about the caloric value of foods or liquids being ingested. For example skim milk has ⅔ the calories of whole milk and this difference is registered every time milk is poured into the Calorie Glass^{R}. Caloric values of various juices are also provided showing that tomato juice is much lower in calories than most other juices.

The first successful use of behavior therapy for treatment of obesity was published by Stuart in 1967[19]. The striking weight losses in 8 of the 11 patients in this report set off a wave of excitement about the possible uses of behavioral approaches to treat obesity. A recent review that has critically compared the results of behavioral and pharmacologic approaches to the treatment of obesity has dampened the enthusiasm for behavioral techniques[14] (Figure 30.2.) The mean rate of weight loss was 0.47 kg/wk among the 981 patients treated with behavioral techniques and published between 1967 and 1977. This compares with an average

---

**Calorie Glass^{R} and Calorie Cup^{R} from Diet Way Products, P.O. Box 5122, Sherman Oaks, CA.

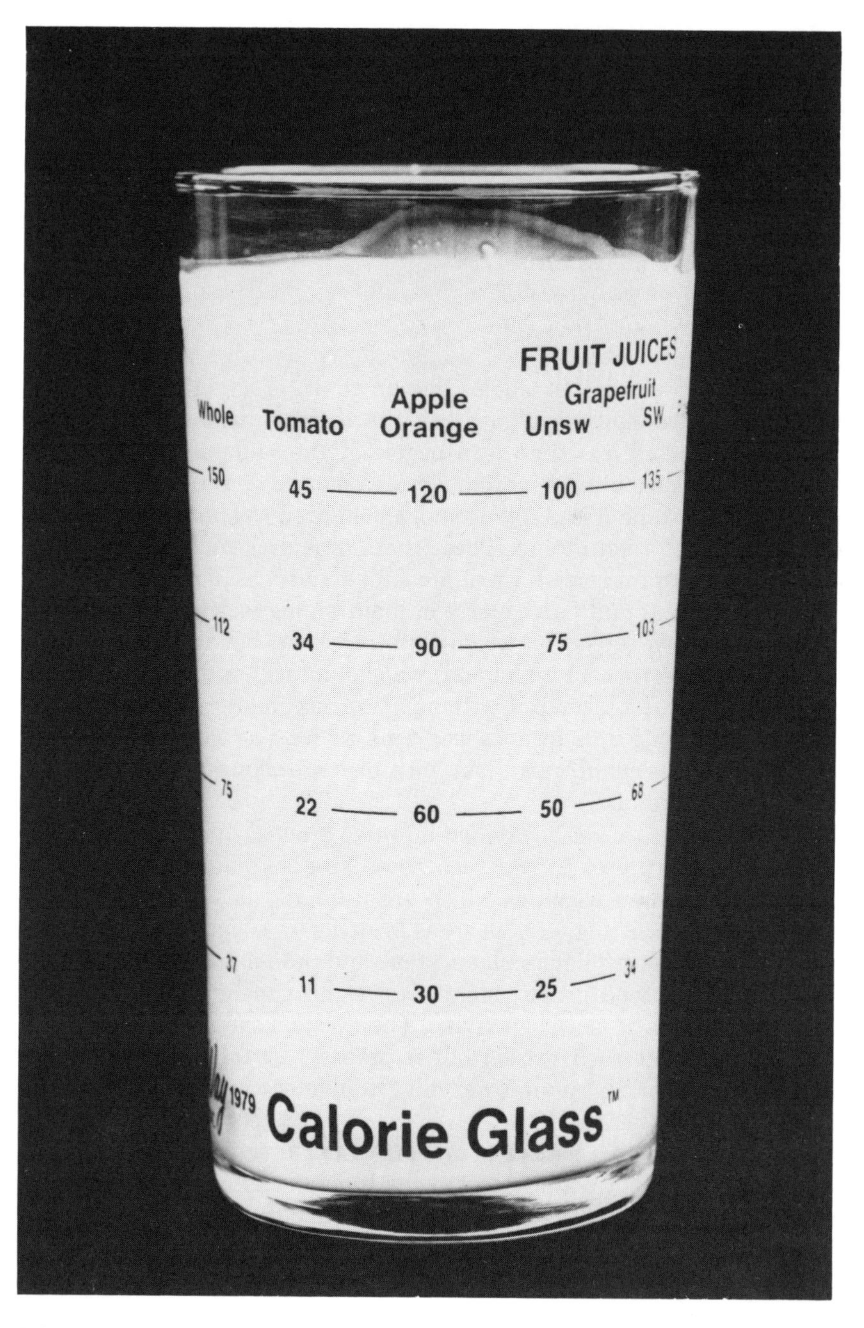

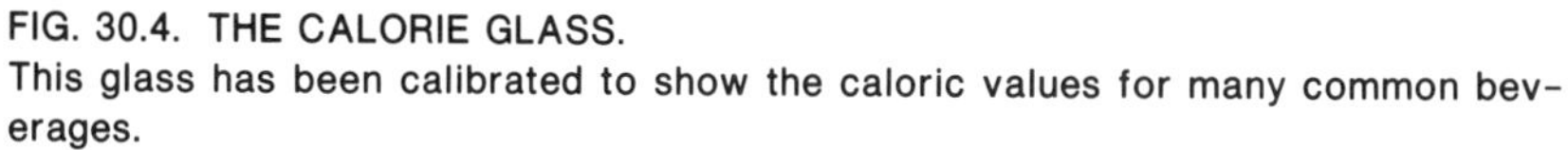
FIG. 30.4. THE CALORIE GLASS.
This glass has been calibrated to show the caloric values for many common beverages.

rate of weight loss of 0.50 kg/wk in 2233 patients treated with appetite suppressants where data was published over the same decade. In one long term study both nutritional and behavioral change groups were followed for five years. The optimistic early results for the patients in the behavioral program appeared to erode and with the passage of time the differences were essentially the same. Nontheless some patients obviously benefited more than others, and some clinical settings appear to provide a better milieu for success.

Exercise

Obese subjects, whether adolescent or adult, are relatively inactive. When using pedometers to measure the distance walked, overweight individuals walked less than lean people of the same age, sex, and occupation. Using time-lapse motion pictures showed obese adolescents in a summer camp to be less active than lean children[20]. This inactivity may in turn increase food intake. These facts provide strong arguments to support the need for some form of physical activity as part of any weight reducing program and particularly in maintaining weight loss.

The effects of exercise on weight loss are clear, but its practical usefulness is less certain. In individuals who voluntarily increase their energy expenditure (i.e. exercise) without a corresponding increase in food intake, extra weight is lost. In a recent review, however, the rate of weight loss was significantly less with exercise alone than with other therapies (Figure 30.2)[14].

Physical activities can be divided into two groups: those which involve aerobic expenditure of energy such as walking, bicycling, swimming, or running; and those activities which are primarily isotonic such as calisthenics, weight lifting, etc. There is evidence to suggest that the optimal effects on the cardiovascular system, and probably the optimal state for maintaining food intake and body weight, can be achieved by relatively low levels of aerobic activity. The exertion should raise the pulse rate somewhat at each session but if properly performed need not be longer than 15 or 20 minutes per day. Equivalent units of exercise are shown in Table 30.3[21].

The importance of the rate at which various activities are performed should also be noted. Walking fast expends more energy than walking the same distance slowly. That is, walking one mile at three miles per hour will take more energy than walking one mile at a rate of one or two miles per hour. The underlying mechanism for this effect may be related to the inefficiency of moving the legs more rapidly. Whatever the exact explanation may be, however, it seems important to undertake walking, as well as all other activities, at a pace which is sufficiently rapid to provide

TABLE 30.3. EQUIVALENT UNITS OF EXERCISE

Walking	3 mi
Bicycling	3 mi
Running	1½ mi
Swimming	800 y
Playing	36 holes of golf

the cardiovascular system with the beneficial effects of increasing pulse rate and cardiac output, as well as providing maximum caloric utilization by performing work at a comfortable and moderately rapid pace.

DRUG THERAPY

Thyroid

Thyroid hormone has been widely used in the treatment of obesity. In 1964 Gordon and his colleagues[22] published a treatment program in which they hospitalized patients for a 48 h fast, then put them on a 1320 calorie diet accompanied by doses of triiodothyronine (T_3), which were increased up to a maximum of 125μg/d, and injections of a mercurial diuretic. A reevaluation of this program including 2 control groups, one of which received neither T_3 nor mercurial diuretic, has been published[3]. The patients treated with the total program lost more weight expressed either in absolute terms or relative to body weight. The other two groups lost more slowly. In Table 30.4 the rate of weight loss is expressed in kg/wk for patients treated with the total program and for the placebo group who received no T_3 or mercurial diuretic (Group C). The weight loss was 1.47kg/wk for the T_3 treated patients and 1.05kg/wk for the placebo treated group.

The use of T_3 for treatment of obesity has also been carried out with outpatients including a controlled double-blind trial of T_3 and placebo published from our laboratory[23]. The design was a crossover with two treatment periods of four weeks each with two weeks on no medication in between. The triiodothyronine (225μg/dl) was given either before or after the placebo. Thus all subjects received both placebo and T_3. Weight loss with triiodothyronine averaged 0.98kg/wk (Table 30.2). During the treatment with placebo the patients actually gained 0.78kg/wk. These subjects weighed an average of 30 to 40 kg more than did those treated in the hospital. The smaller weight loss in the outpatient group indicate that they were not adhering to the diet as well as the hospitalized patients and, thus, use of T_3 was not as effective as with in inpatients.

Appetite Suppressants

Table 30.5 lists some of the appetite suppressant drugs currently on the market. All of them are derived from phenethylamine except mazindol.

TABLE 30.4. WEIGHT LOSS BY PATIENTS PARTICIPATING IN HOSPITAL AND OUT-PATIENT STUDIES OF TREATMENTS FOR OBESITY

Treatment	Dose of Drug	Diet kcal/d	Study Design	Duration d.	N	B-W(kg)	Weight Loss (kg/wk)			
							Treatment	N	B-W(kg)	Placebo
Hospital										
Triiodothyronine	125μg/d	1320	Parallel	28	6	105	1.60	6	109	1.15
Outpatient										
Triiodothronine	225μg/d	1000	Crossover	28	12	146	.98			.78
Study 1 Mazindol	1mg tid	1000	Parallel	84	10	105	.42	9	118	.51
Diethylpropion	25mg tid				10	112	.26	4	114	.52
Study 2 Mazindol (hGH)	2mg/d	1000	Parallel	49	24	94	.63	12	92	.65
Human Chorionic Gonadotropin	125u/d	550	Parallel	42	18	80	1.47	14	80	1.35
Acupuncture		None	Crossover	21	24	66	0.17			0.0

TABLE 30.5. ANORECTIC AGENTS CURRENTLY EMPLOYED FOR THE TREATMENT OF OBESITY IN THE UNITED STATES

Generic Name	Proprietary Name	DEA Schedule[a]
d,1-Amphetamine	Benzedrine and others	II
Methamphetamine	Desoxyn and others	II
Phenmetrazine	Preludin	II
Phendimetrazine	Plegine	III
Benzphetamine	Didrex	III
Chlorphentermine	Pre-Sate	III
Clortermine	Voranil	III
Mazindol	Sanorex	III
Fenfluramine	Pondimin	IV
Diethylpropion	Tenuate, Tepanil	IV
Pentermine	Fastin, Ionamin (resin)	IV
Phenylpropanolamine	Many	Over the counter

[a]Drug Enforcement Administration: The schedules of the Controlled Substances Act are numbered in order of decreasing potential for abuse; drugs in Schedule II (amphetamine, methamphetamine and phenmetrazine) are the most restricted.

Phenylpropanolamine (PPA) is the only member of this group available without a prescription. The oldest of the prescription drugs is dextroamphetamine. However, this drug is associated with significant central excitatory effects and with numerous cases of addiction. Chemical modifications of the clinically available compounds has produced considerable variation in the central excitatory effects, but left the appetite suppressant effect intact.

The evidence supporting effectiveness of the appetite suppressants has been reviewed by Scoville[24] and by Sullivan and Comai[25]. In the review of applications submitted to the FDA, Scoville reported that drug-treated patients lost an average 0.51 lb/wk (0.22 kg/wk) more than the placebo-treated control groups.

During the past decade three new appetite suppressing drugs have been marketed: Fenfluramine (Pondimin[R]); mazindol (Sanorex[R]); and clortermine (Voranil[R]). Studies with one of these drugs has increased our knowledge of the interaction of this drug and a program of behavioral change. In the first clinical trial we examined a behavioral program, a placebo and two appetite suppressing drugs[26]. All patients were given a 1000-calorie diet and there were no changes for participating in this study. There were two goals. The first was to evaluate predictive factors that might identify prospectively those patients who were going to be successful during the course of the program. Second, we wanted to compare behavioral treatment with drug treatment in terms of weight loss and duration of attendance at the clinic. A total of 120 patients were started on the program. The two appetite suppressants were mazindol (Sanorex[R]) and diethylpropion. Figure 30.5 shows the number of patients remaining in the clinic with time after starting the study. The drop-out rates were essentially identical for the 4 treatments with about half of the patients still in treatment after 8 weeks.

Before beginning the specific treatment, each patient completed a variety of pencil and paper tests. The tests included measures of self-esteem, social acceptance, locus of control, responsiveness to stimuli, attitudes toward weight loss and knowledge about nutrition. Success was related to social conformity and a desire for social acceptance. Locus of control and self-esteem were not related to success. Individuals who believed that poor eating habits caused their obesity also tended to be more successful. Finally, success was more likely in those who were less responsive to environmental cues[27].

Weight loss for the full 14 weeks and for all patients at the time where they dropped out of the program are shown in Figure 30.6. Patients in the behavioral program and the placebo groups lost weight as well as, or better than, those in the drug-treated groups. These findings strengthened our interest in behavioral change. The success of the placebo-treated groups also intrigued us. On the other hand, the high drop-out rate was discouraging because it probably reflected failure for the people who dropped out.

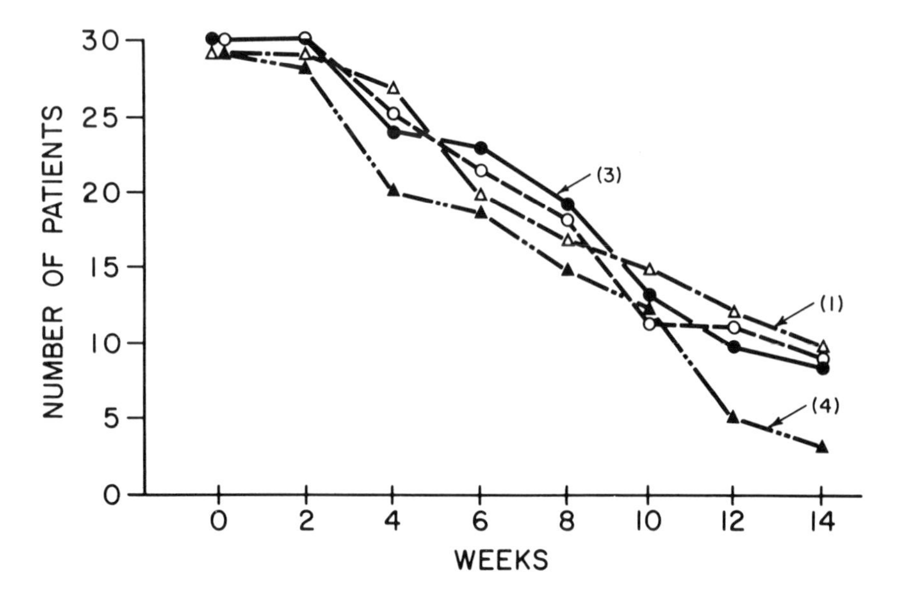

FIG. 30.5. DROP-OUT RATE FROM CLINIC DURING TREATMENT. The number of patients remaining in treatment each two weeks is shown for the mazindol (Δ), diethylpropion (o), placebo (•), and behavioral change (4) groups. (Reproduced from Reference 26 with permission).

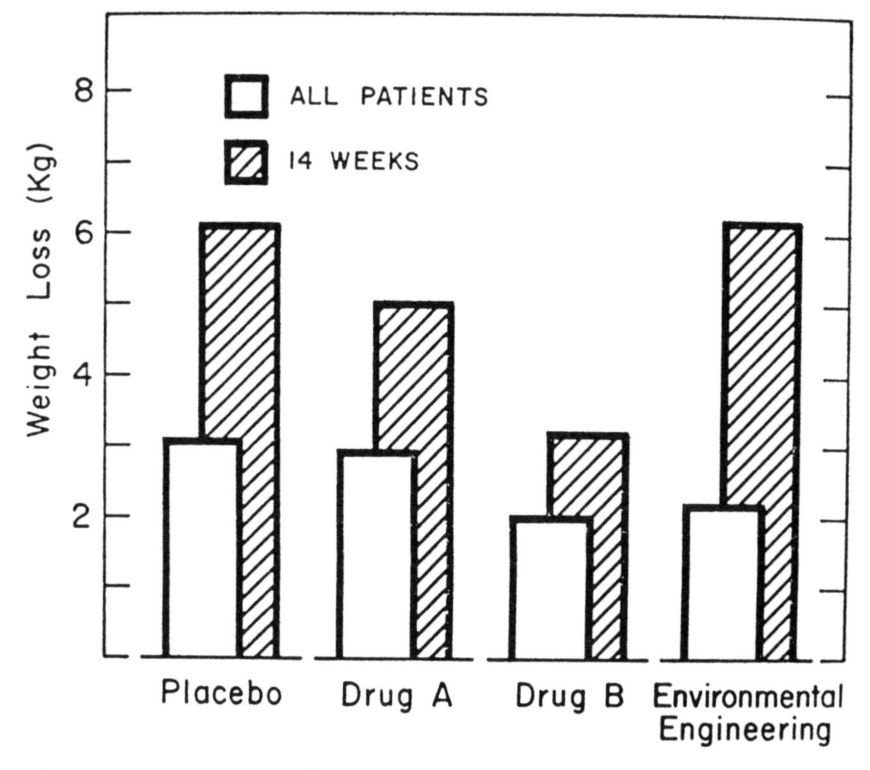

FIG. 30.6. RATES OF WEIGHT LOSS DURING TREATMENT WITH VARIOUS APPROACHES.
The data for the bars on the left were obtained from Reference 14, those on the right from the paper by Genuth in Advances in Obesity Research, (G.A. Bray, ed.). (Copyright G.A. Bray, 1979. Reprinted with permission).

A second study compared appetite suppressing drugs with behavioral change therapy. In this sophisticated study each treatment group had 12 patients, 4 on placebo and 8 on drug. There were 5 replicates of this basic grouping, so that each replicate of 12 patients was assigned to one of 5 therapists. The use of 5 different therapists gave us a chance to address the question of whether physicians or non-physicians are better therapists[28]. Our study was also part of a five-hospital study using the same design. The data from the other four hospitals is shown on the left in Figure 30.6, the data from our clinic on the right. All patients in our clinic participated in a behavioral program designed collectively by the five therapists. This behavioral program made our study different from the four clinics, none of which had a behavioral program. In the other clinics, the drug-treated patients lost an average of 6 lbs. In our clinic the placebo-treated patients lost almost as much weight as the drug treated

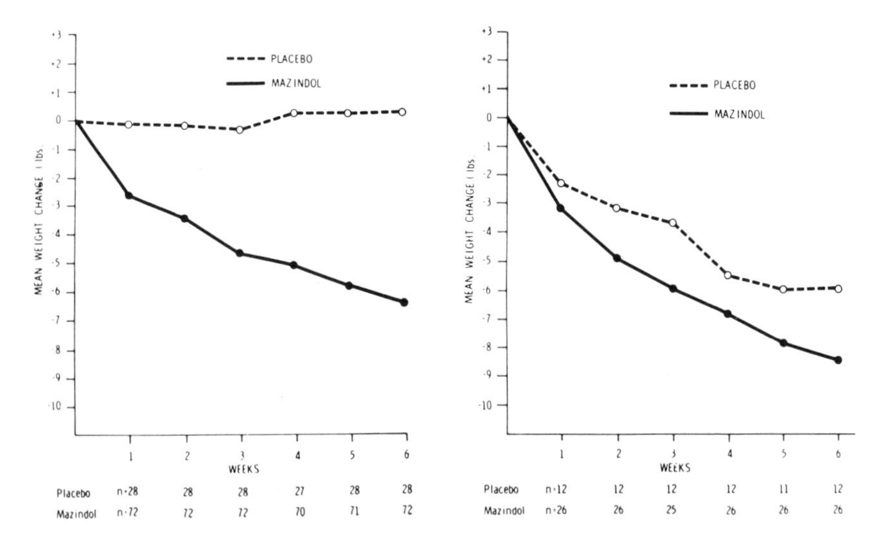

FIG. 30.7. WEIGHT LOSS DURING TREATMENT WITH MAZINDOL OR PLACEBO. The left hand panel shows the data on the four clinics in which the protocol was used without any behavioral program. The right hand panel shows the patients in our clinic who were treated with a behavioral program (footnote 1) and either placebo or drug. (Adapted from Mazindol data).

patients in the other four clinics. Calculations of weight loss show that drug treated patients in our clinic lost about .42 kg/wk and the placebo-treated group .28 kg/wk (Table 30.4). Thus the placebo group lost about 4 times as much weight as the placebo-treated group in the other clinics (Fig. 30.2).

Chorionic gonadotropin

In 1954 Simeons introduced the use of injections of human chorionic gonadotropin (hCG) into the treatment of obesity[29]. Several recent controlled trials of hCG and an appropriate placebo have been conducted to evaluate its effectiveness (Figure 30.2)[30]. All patients were given a balanced very low calorie diet (550 kcal/d). The two groups of patients treated with either placebo or hCG in our clinic lost weight at almost identical rates; those treated with hCG lost an average of 8.8 kg, the placebo-treated group 8.1 kg or 1.47 kg/wk for hCG-treated and 1.35 kg/wk for the placebo-treated groups. These rates of weight loss were above those for placebo-treated patients on the 1320 kcal/d diet in the hospital. Only a few dietary or behavioral studies show such rapid weight loss. To what is the placebo effect in the hCG study to be attributed?

There are two possibilities. The first is that the daily visit to the therapist's office to get the injection was a potent motivating factor. There is some evidence to support this idea. In a study where injections were given only 3 times a week or at home by the patient the weight loss was slower. A second possibility is there is some effect of injection per se but this seems less likely.

HIGH RISK TREATMENT

Starvation

Fasting or the zero calorie diet as an approach to treating obesity has been in use for over 20 years. In the early days of fasting, weight loss is predominately water[31]. As this early and rapid loss of water slows, the contribution to weight loss made by fat becomes a greater percentage of total weight loss. In the beginning of a fast, metabolism of fat accounts for only 20% of the weight lost, although providing almost all of the fuel for bodily functions. Gradually the weight lost from metabolism of fat rises to 70%. Against these benefits is the fact that there have been several deaths reported during total fasting. Thus total fasting has to be considered a hazardous approach to losing weight.

Very Low Calorie Protein Diets

One of the most popular recent diets has been the very low calorie high protein diet[32]. During total starvation weight loss occurs at a rate of about 1 pound per day, but because of many potential complications total starvation must be carried out in a hospital. The loss of protein during a total fast has been a troublesome problem until it was found that eating 50 to 100 g of protein each day could nearly completely prevent it. However, very low calorie diets (less than 800 kcal/d) containing only protein may be a hazardous form of treatment for obesity, since these diets have been associated with a significant number of deaths. Recently the Center for Disease Control has evaluated 59 individuals who died after or while using liquid protein diets to help them lose weight[32]. Fifteen of these deaths were in women who had no prior evidence of cardiovascular disease. This suggests that fasting or very low calorie diets composed of protein alone can be hazardous and that they are only appropriate for people who have high risk associated with their obesity.

Acupuncture

Acupuncture is derived from the Old Chinese art of inserting needles at special points on the body for relief of pain. It has been alleged that there is a feeding center which can be manipulated by acupuncture and that this center is located in the region of the ear. To test this possibility a group of obese patients were treated by acupuncture using small staples placed in the "active" or "inactive" sites in the ear[33]. Bilateral and unilateral active or inactive sites were used. No specific dietary prescription was used. The weight loss in the group receiving acupuncture was 24 grams per day; the placebo group lost no weight (Table 30.2). The variability among patients, however, made this difference statistically not significant. The conclusion of this study was that when acupuncture works it works because of adherence to the diet with which it is used; acupuncture alone was ineffective.

Jaw-wiring

Ingestion of solid food requires separation of the teeth and use of the teeth for mastication. Mandibular fixation, or wiring the jaws together, prevents ingestion of solid but not of liquid foods. The use of jaw-wiring to reduce the intake of solid foods has been reported by several groups of investigators. During the time when the jaws are wired together, there is a significant loss of weight[34]. In one study, 16 patients lost 20 kg (45 lbs) in the first five months. The problem however is that when the wires are taken off, they tend to regain this weight. Moreover, there are the potential risks to the dental structures as well as the hazard of aspiration. In the view of some, jaw-wiring is best reserved for rapid weight loss prior to some other form of surgical therapy. For these reasons jaw-wiring is put in the higher risk group of treatments.

Intestinal Bypass

Diets, exercise, behavioral change, and anorectic drugs have generally been unsuccessful for massively obese patients. The increased risk of obesity to the life of such patients has led many surgeons to perform operative procedures for obesity, including gastric and intestinal bypass operations. Two types of intestinal bypass have been used most widely[35]. The end-to-side operation attaches a segment of jejunum measuring approximately 14 inches from the ligament of Treitz to the side of the ileum four inches from the ileocecal valve. The end-to-end operation attaches the jejunum (14 inches) to the end of the ileum and anastomoses the defunctionalized ileal end to the colon. Weight loss with these operations ranges from 10 to 150 pounds the first year, depending on the length of bowel left in continuity. The mortality from this procedure runs up to 10% but averages overall about 3%. In addition, there are many short- and long-term complications, including liver failure, fluid and electrolyte imbalance, protein malnutrition, renal stones, and metabolic bone disease. For these reasons the intestinal bypass operations are now done less frequently than a few years ago.

Gastric Bypass

Gastric bypass procedures pose a viable alternative to the jejunoileal bypass. This procedure was pioneered by Mason and his colleagues who had become discouraged with some of the untoward results seen with small bowel bypass[36]. They tried several different procedures, including a gastric exclusion, a partial gastric exclusion and a total gastric transsection. Problems with hemorrhoids, rectal discomfort and diarrhea which were frequently observed in the patients with jejunoileal bypass, were not seen in patients with gastric bypass. Similarly, fatigue, lethargy and bloating were also not observed in the gastric bypass group. Of more interest was the fact that the late complications of liver disease, renal stones and polyarthritis which represent a major group of difficulties for patients undergoing jejunoileal bypass were uncommon in the individuals with a gastric bypass.

Vagotomy

The most recent surgical approach to obesity has been bilateral subdiaphragmatic truncal vagotomy. An experimental rationale for this procedure was reported. In animals with obesity produced by injury to the ventromedial hypothalamus, subdiaphragmatic vagotomy will reverse the obesity. In the initial report of three patients, vagotomy was followed by successful weight loss in all three individuals[37]. In a larger study from the same Swedish hospital a group of ten patients were reported, nine of whom lost weight satisfactorily following subdiaphragmatic truncal vagotomy. All of the patients were without feelings of hunger and experience no difficulty in losing weight after this operation intervention.

Comment

This review of treatment for obesity is intended to focus first on the individual who needs the treatment so that no one is subjected to unnecessary risks. After the appropriate evaluation has been completed to determine risks, the most appropriate therapies are those with the least risk. We prefer to offer patients the opportunity to participate in the choice of treatment which they will receive. Nutritional counselling, including low and very low calorie nutritionally balanced diets, are available to all individuals. In addition, the program for behavioral change which we have labelled ABC's is available for those who wish it. Since a behavioral program can be as effective as appetite suppressants we prefer to begin with the behavioral program. We also devote attention to helping patients understand the energy value of foods using any of the tools which are available, including nutrition labels, diet scales, handbooks of caloric values for foods, and the Caloric Glass. We also believe that attention should be paid to increasing the movement and activity of patients depending on their needs and abilities. Appetite suppressant drugs may also be useful following a program of intermittent usage. Various cognitive procedures such as assertiveness training and relaxation training may also be helpful. For those who are at high risk from their obesity or its attendant problems some of the risk treatments may be appropriate including very low calorie protein diets (often called protein sparing fasts), jaw-wiring, gastric or intestinal bypass. It is important to emphasize, however, that this latter group of treatments carry increased risk. Thus the decision to use them requires that the patient be fully informed of the extra risk and in this way participates in the treatment program.

REFERENCES

1. BRAY, G.A. Obesity in America (G.A. Bray, ed). Washington, D.C., DHEW Publ. No. (NIH) 79-359, 1979, p. 4.
2. UNITED STATES, SENATE COMMITTEE ON NUTRITION AND HUMAN NEEDS. Committee Print: Dietary Goals for the United States. 95th Congress, 1st session, 1977.
3. BRAY, G.A. The obese patient. Vol IX in the series: Major Problems in Internal Medicine, Philadelphia, W.B. Saunders Co., 1976.
4. BRAY, G.A. Definition, measurement, and classification of the syndromes of obesity. Int. J. Obesity 2:99–112, 1978.
5. RECOMMENDED DIETARY ALLOWANCES. National Academy of Sciences. Washington, D.C., 9th revised edition, 1979.
6. STUNKARD, A.J. and RUSH, J., Dieting and depression reexamined. A critical review of reports of untoward responses during weight reduction for obesity. Ann. Intern. Med. 81:526–533, 1974.
7. BERLAND, T. Diets '79 Everything you should know about the diets making news. Consumer Guide Magazine Health Quarterly, V. 223, Spring 1979.
8. PILKINGTON, T.R.E., GAINSBOROUGH, H., ROSENOER, V.M. and CAREY, M. Diet and weight reduction in the obese. Lancet 1:856, 1960.
9. KINSELL, L.W., GUNNING, B., MICHAELS, G.D., RICHARDSON, J., COX, S.E., and LEMON, C. Calories do count. Metabolism 13:195–204, 1964.
10. YANG, M.U., and VAN ITALLIE, T.B.: Composition of weight lost during short-term weight reduction. J. Clin. Invest. 58:722–730, 1976.

11. YOUNG, C.M., SCANLAN, S.S., IM, H.S. and LUTWAK, L. Effect on body composition and other parameters in obese young men of carbohydrate level of reduction diet. Am. J. Clin. Nutr. 24:290–296, 1971.
12. YOUNG, C.M., HUTTER, L.F., SCANLAN, S.S., RAND, C.E., LUTWAK, L. and SIMKA, V. Metabolic effects of meal frequency in normal young men. J. Amer. Diet Assoc. 61:391–398, 1972.
13. STUNKARD, A.J., and McLAREN-HUME, M. The results of treatment for obesity. Arch. Intern. Med. 103:79–85, 1959.
14. WING, R.R., and JEFFERY, R.W. Outpatient treatments of obesity: A comparison of methodology and clinical results. Int. J. Obesity 3:261–279, 1979.
15. STUART, R.B., and DAVIS, B. Slim chance in a fat world: Behavioral control of obesity. Champaign, Illinois, Research Press Co, 1972.
16. FERGUSON, J.M. Habits, Not Diets. Bull Publishing, Palo Alto, California, 1976.
17. JORDAN, H.A., LEVITZ, L.S., and KIMBRELL, G.M. Eating is Okay! A radical approach to successful weight loss. The behavioral-control diet explained in full. (edited by Steve Gelman) New York: Rawson Associated Publishers, Inc. 1976.
18. BRAY, G.A. Obesity. Disease-A-Month. XXVI (1):1–85, 1979.
19. STUART, R.B. Behavioral control over eating. Behav. Res. Ther. 5: 357–385, 1967.
20. BULLEN, B.A., REED, R.B., and MAYER, J. Physical activity of obese and nonobese adolescent girls appraised by motion picture sampling. Am. J. Clin. Nutr. 14:211–223, 1964.
21. BRAY, G.A. Clinical management of the obese adult. Postgrad. Med. 51:125–130, 1972.
22. GORDON, E.S., GOLDBERG, M., and CHOSY, G.J. A new concept in the treatment of obesity. JAMA 186:156–166, 1963.
23. BRAY, G.A., MELVIN, K.E.W., and CHOPRA, I.J. Effect of triiodothyronine on some metabolic responses of obese patients. Am. J. Clin. Nutr. 26:715–721, 1973.
24. SCOVILLE, B. Review of amphetamine-like drugs by the Food and Drug Administration: Clinical data and value judgments. In: Obesity in Perspective. A conference sponsored by the John E. Fogarty International Center for Advanced Study in the Health Sciences. Ed. G. A. Bray. DHEW Publ. No. (NIH) 75-708, 1976, pp. 441–443.
25. SULLIVAN, A.C., and COMAI, K. Pharmacological treatment of obesity. Int. J. Obesity 2:167–189, 1978.
26. DAHMS, W.T., MOLITCH, M., BRAY, G.A., GREENWAY, F.L., ATKINSON, R.L., and HAMILTON, K. Treatment of obesity: Cost-benefit assessment of behavioral therapy, placebo and two anorectic drugs. Am. J. Clin. Nutr. 31(3):774–778, 1978.
27. RODIN, J., BRAY, G.A., ATKINSON, R.L., DAHMS, W.T., GREENWAY, F.L., HAMILTON, K., and MOLITCH, M. Predictors of successful weight loss in an out-patient obesity clinic. Int. J. Obesity 1:40–48, 1977.

28. ATKINSON, R.L., GREENWAY, F.L., BRAY, G.A., DAHMS, W.T., MOLITCH, M.E., HAMILTON, K., and RODIN, J. Treatment of Obesity: Comparison of physician and nonphysician therapists using placebo and anorectic drugs in a double-blind trial. Int. J. Obesity 1:113–120, 1977.
29. SIMEONS, A.T.W. The action of chorionic gonadotropin in the obese. Lancet 2:946–947, 1954.
30. GREENWAY, F.L., and BRAY, G.A. Human chorionic gonadotropin (hCG) in the treatment of obesity: A critical assessment of the Simeons method. West. J. Med. 127:461–463, 1977.
31. DRENICK, E.J. Weight reduction by prolonged fasting. In: Obesity in Perspective. Fogarty International Center, Series on Preventive Medicine, (ed. G. A. Bray) DHEW Publ. No. (NIH) 75-708, 1976, pp. 341–360.
32. GENUTH, S.M., CASTRO, J.H., and VERTES, V. Weight reduction in obesity by outpatient semistarvation. JAMA 230:987–991, 1974.
33. MOK, M.S., VOINA, S. and BRAY, G.A. Treatment of obesity by acupuncture. Am. J. Clin. Nutr. 29:832–835, 1976.
34. RODGERS, S., GOSS, A., GOLDNEY, R., THOMAS, D., BURNET, R., PHILLIPS, P., KIMBER, C., and HARDING, P. Jaw wiring treatment of obesity. Lancet 1:1221–1223, 1977.
35. MASON, E.E., PRINTEN, K.J., BLOMMERS, T.J., and SCOTT, D.H. Gastric bypass for obesity after ten years experience. Int. J. Obesity 2: 197–206, 1978.
36. KRAL, J.G. Vagotomy for treatment of severe obesity. Lancet 1:307–309, 1978.

31

FACTS AND FICTIONS ABOUT MEGAVITAMIN THERAPY

Victor Herbert, M.D., J.D.

An American physician wrote, "Quackery kills a large number of U.S. citizens each year than all the diseases it pretends to cure." One might expect that this commentary of the times was written yesterday, but it wasn't. It appeared in an 1861 issue of *National Quarterly Review*. Today, we are still inundated with health misinformation, quackery, gimmicks, Laetriles, and the latest rage—vitamin megadoses.

What do we have to know in order to give our patients intelligent advice when they come to us with what they've read in the lay press or what they heard on a TV talk show? What we have to know is, what vitamins are, what they *can* do and what they *can't* do.

First, the definition of a vitamin. It's an organic molecule not made in the human body and required in small amounts to sustain normal metabolism. Notice that there are three exceptions to this definition. On adequate exposure to sunlight you can make vitamin D in your skin. Of course, D is really a hormone, but that's a different subject. The vitamin niacin can also be synthesized in humans to significant degree from the amino acid tryptophane, and intestinal bacteria make significant amounts of vitamin K. Crucial to the definition of a vitamin is that lack of it produces a specific deficiency syndrome, and supplying it cures that deficiency.

Dr. Herbert is Professor and Vice Chairman of Medicine, State University of New York, Downstate Medical Center, New York.

Vitamins can function in two ways—as vitamins and chemicals. The fat soluble vitamins function as regulators of specific metabolic activity; the water soluble vitamins function as coenzymes. The fact that they function as coenzymes is fundamental to understanding why the term megavitamin therapy is a misnomer by definition. The vitamin coenzymes come in from food, seek out the cells that need them, are taken into the cell, and combine with a protein already present. The protein is called an apoenzyme. The vitamin coenzyme coming in from outside attaches to the apoenzyme within the cell to form a holoenzyme (or enzyme, for short). It is this which serves the catalytic function that all coenzymes serve. So, it is not the vitamin by itself, but only when combined with its apoenzyme within the cell that it becomes capable of vitamin function. The quantity of apoenzyme any cell can make per unit time is limited, as is the capacity of any cell to make any other protein per unit time. That limited capacity is saturated at levels of vitamin roughly in the range of the recommended dietary allowance (RDA). Since the protein apoenzyme is saturated by a level of vitamin in the range of the RDA, it is obvious that any excess coming in cannot possibly serve a vitamin function. The concept of megavitamin therapy is predicated on total failure to understand the basic biochemical concept just stated.

Vitamins can also serve chemical functions. That is what they do when present in an excess over and above the amount that can saturate the apoenzyme. The excess will serve whatever function vitamins can perform as chemicals. The most classic example is the reduction action of vitamins C and E. Both can do harm as strong reducing agents when present in excess quantity. Vitamin C, being water soluble, will go to areas where the milieu is water, and E, being fat soluble, will go to areas where the milieu is fat. If there are excesses, they will present excessive reducing action in those areas.

NUTRITION—FACTS AND FALLACIES

The key to understanding good nutrition for the layman is very simple. The layman reads a lot of nutritional garbage in some monthly magazines and newspapers which confuses him into thinking that he has to know exactly what vitamin A does, and exactly what magnesium does, so on and so forth. This is all nonsense. The layman doesn't have to know the intricacies of the value of each specific nutrient any more than to be a good driver it's necessary to know how a carburetor functions. One doesn't need to know the machinery of a motor to be a good driver. Running the human machine, also, from a nutritional point of view, is very simple.

Many years ago, the U.S. Department of Agriculture decided the way to simplify nutrition for laymen was to break nutrition down into food groups. They divided the foods in terms of their nutrient content into seven groups. If you ate from those seven groups each day you were guaranteed good nutrition, assuming you didn't have disease, such as intestinal malabsorption. The seven food groups turned out to be a little hard for people to remember, so the USDA reduced it to four basic food groups. These are the basis of nutritional teaching now.[1] All you have to tell your patients, and all they have to know to understand the basics of getting good nutrition for themselves each day, is to take each day foods from the grain group, the milk group, the meat group, and the fruit and vegetable group. At the end of the day the patient should be able to look back and say, "In the course of this day I've had four portions from the grain group (and that includes cereals, breads, pastas, etc.), four portions from the fruit and vegetable group (including one fresh uncooked fruit or vegetable or fruit juice), two to four portions from the milk group (depending on whether it's a child or an adult or a pregnant woman), and two portions from the meat group (and that includes fish and fowl as well as meat)." That would automatically include adequate quantities of each of the vitamins and minerals that we know of (though it may be marginal in iron for women in the child-bearing years). Final rule: eat less calories to lose weight; eat more to gain.

That's the totality of what the layman needs to know about good nutrition. Instead he's bombarded with all kinds of ridiculous advice about "natural" foods and other things. There's a good article by Max Gunther, "The Worst Diet Advice . . . is the kind dispensed on many TV shows," that appeared in the January 11, 1975 *TV Guide*. *The Health Robbers* is another very important book because it is an attempt to tell people how to recognize and avoid health quackery of every description. It contains a chapter by Jean Mayer on obesity quackery, a chapter by William Masters on sex clinic quackery, and a chapter by neurologist Arthur Taub of Yale on quackupuncture. Each chapter is heavily factually documented but nevertheless written in so clear and lucid a way that you can give this reference to your patients as something they can read when they have a question about any dubious health claim. There are about six chapters dealing with the various forms of nutrition misinformation and quackery, including a chapter entitled The Confused (Nutrition) Crusaders, which deals with a number of people and their claims, including Adelle Davis, Carlton Fredericks, the Shute brothers with their vitamin E claims, Cheraskin's *New Hope for Incurable Diseases*, and Linus Pauling. You may recall that Adelle Davis took the position that if you followed her nutrition advice you would never get cancer. She doesn't give that advice anymore, since she died of cancer. *The Health Robbers* is so important that it was the first book ever reviewed by *Consumers Reports*.[2] I urge you to have a copy on your bookshelf. It's not widely available; you can get it from the publisher.[3] I must make a disclaimer at this point. Although I wrote a chapter (The Health Hustlers: How to Spot a Food Quack), neither I nor any of the other chapter authors get royalties. As indicated at the beginning of the book, the royalties go to the Lehigh Valley Committee Against Health Fraud, Inc., a major organization fighting quackery of all types in the health field. There's also a chapter by Tom Jukes[4] on the "organic" rip-off, pointing out the misinformation in natural food teachings, and noting the New York State public hearings on organic foods. The Director of the New York State Food Laboratory reported more products labeled "organic," and purchased at health food stores, contained pesticide residues than foods not labeled organic (30% vs 20%).

There is *no* need for added vitamins when eating a well-balanced diet. There are some who believe in "nutritional insurance," that is, taking a capsule a day containing the RDA of the major vitamins. I have no quarrel with that. I think it's totally unnecessary, but if it makes someone feel better he or she is only out a couple of cents a day, and not the greater amounts that one spends if one follows the advice of *Prevention Magazine* and the National Health Federation.

It's been alleged that megadoses of vitamins are harmless. This is *not* true. Generally speaking, the literature shows that at doses about 10 times the RDA, we start to see toxic effects. So, as a general rule, a megadose is 10 times the RDA or more. There's an increasing body of evidence of various forms of harm resulting from megadoses of various nutrients. Those of you who follow the *Annals of Internal Medicine* may recall the 1976 report that megadoses of vitamin C raise the urine uric acid level and may precipitate gout in people so predisposed. Another harm is that although most of us catabolize ascorbic acid (vitamin C) fairly rapidly past the oxalic acid stage and excrete it in our urine, some (possibly about one out of fifteen) have a congenital defect whereby they can't get ascorbate past the oxalic acid stage readily, and those people will have an increased susceptibility to oxalate kidney stones. When I talked on this subject at Columbia University it turned out that one of the medical students had just had an attack of renal colic due to a kidney stone after seven weeks of following his mother's advice to take a gram of C each morning prior to breakfast.

What are other undesirable side-effects of megadoses of C? Rebound scurvy is a particularly dangerous one when it occurs in a newborn. This was reported from Nova Scotia some years ago. The RDA for C is 45 mg a day (except for pregnant women in whom it's 60 and lactating women in whom it's 80). 450 mg of C a day would be a megadose. If a pregnant woman is taking a megadose of C, her body's machinery for destroying the C is speeded up in order to get rid of all that excess reducing capacity. That speeded up machinery will now destroy C, hypothetically, let's say,

10 times as fast as normal. The fetus acquires the same speeded up machinery to get rid of the transplacentally-passed ascorbate. Hence, the newborn is born with a C-destructive machinery 10 times normal, but is getting normal C from mother's milk, which it destroys with 10 times normal speed. Therefore, the newborn runs out of C and gets scurvy with dangerous life-threatening bleeding. This is clearly an undesirable side-effect. It has also been reported in adults who stop megadoses of C "cold turkey" rather than tapering off over a period of, let's say, about 10% a day or 20% every other day. In adults it's been reported to produce bleeding into the gums and skin, loosening of the teeth, roughening of the skin (i.e., the stigmata of scurvy).

VITAMIN C MEGADOSES—THUMBS DOWN

About 13% of American Blacks and even a larger percentage of Sephardic Jews, Orientals, and certain other ethnic groups have congenital glucose 6-phosphate dehydrogenase (G6-PD) deficiency, which is activated into hemolytic anemia by a strong reducing agent. In the March 1977 issue of *Blood* there is a paper describing the severe hemolysis produced by megadoses of C. In that article, the authors reflect on a patient who died from a megadose of C with its accompanying severe hemolysis. A similar phenomenom was reported from Montefiore Hospital in the Bronx in a patient with sickle cell disease. This is biochemically logical because it is reduced sickle hemoglobin which takes the sickle shape and clogs capillaries. If you give a megadose of C to a patient with SS hemoglobin you're going to convert his oxidized SS hemoglobin to reduced SS hemoglobin. It's going to take the sickle shape, and that patient can go into a severe sickle crisis.

Where else is mega-C dangerous? When diabetics check their urine, two of their favorite tests are the Testape® test and the Clinitest.® Megadoses of C cause the Testape test to be falsely negative and the Clinitest to be falsely positive. Now, if the patient doesn't know that and if he doesn't inform his physician, the physician won't know that the patient is getting false-positive or false-negative test results, and that patient runs the risk of either diabetic ketoacidosis or insulin shock. Also, it has recently been reported that the strong reducing action of megadoses of C causes tests for blood in the stool to be falsely negative. If you suspect a patient has a carcinoma of the colon and you do three stool guaiacs and they're all negative, it may be because the patient is one of the almost two million people in the United States taking megadoses of C. Your clinical suspicion of a carcinoma of the colon may be correct, but the negative stool tests may throw you off the track.

Where else is mega-C harmful? In our own research unit, we've been studying the effect of megadoses of C on vitamin B_{12} in food, in the bile, and in body stores. We found that mega-C, when added to a typical VA Hospital diet, could destroy 50% to 95% of the B_{12} in the diet. You can prevent the destruction of B_{12} by megadoses of C if you introduce the appropriate amount of iron, whose redox potential will antagonize the reducing action of C on the B_{12}. The same happens when you eat a meal. If the quantity of redox agents such as iron is appropriate, then a megadose of C will not harm the B_{12} in that meal. If it's not appropriate it may. We'll see where that dispute goes in the next year or two.

C AND THE COMMON COLD

It's been alleged that vitamin C prevents colds. As it happens there's absolutely no evidence for that. If you look in the 1974 Congressional Record you'll see a Chicago radio station colloquy between Linus Pauling and Victor Herbert in which Linus Pauling admits that there's no evidence that vitamin C *prevents* colds. However, he did then, and continues to hew to the line that C reduces the symptoms of colds by about a third. If you look at the *evidence* on the reduction of cold symptoms you'll find it's largely subjective.

This is an area where much trouble arises in informing the public about nutrition. The public is unable to tell the difference between anecdote and science. When Carlton Fredericks, for example, whose doctorate is not in nutrition, makes an allegation on the basis of anecdotal evidence that sugar is bad for you, or that megadoses of C are good for you, this to the layman is just as good evidence and just as important as scientific data in a medical journal. This is a fundamental flaw in the logic of the layman, and the fundamental difference between the layman and the trained scientist or trained physician who learns that anecdote is not reality. Reality is what you can objectively ascertain and not what somebody said. If you look at the objective data regarding vitamin C and the common cold, you'll find that in late 1976 in the *New England Journal of Medicine* the same group that two years earlier reported that megadoses of C reduced colds in Navajo children report that they were wrong the first time. When they did the study the proper way, with proper controls, they found out that megadoses of C *did not* reduce the symptoms of colds. Anderson's group in Canada divided over 2,000 patients into eight groups: six got megadoses of C and two got placebos. Guess which group had the least colds? One of the two placebo groups. So, there is really little evidence that C has any value versus colds. There is some slight evidence it may have a mild antihistaminic effect. If we take claim at its most favorable possibility, is it worthwhile to take a megadose of C 365 days a year, with the possible undesirable side-effects, in order to achieve a mild antihistaminic effect during the eight days out of the entire year that the average person has a cold? Anecdotal and testimonial evidence is as worthless in medicine as it is in law, where it is excluded from courts as hearsay (see my article citing the pertinent medical quackery cases in the November 18, 1977 issue of *Science*).

NO VALUE FOR SCHIZOPHRENIA

What about megavitamin therapy for schizophrenia? This is heavily pushed and *completely anecdotal.* There is no scientific study demonstrating that megavitamin therapy has any value in schizophrenia. If you want facts look at the official report of the American Psychiatric Association Task Force on Vitamin Therapy in Psychiatry. They convened a group of experts who went over the various reports of the proponents of megavitamin therapy and ascertained that they were all anecdotal. There was not a single scientific controlled study showing any value. That report was published in 1973, you can get a copy of it from the American Psychiatric Association in Washington, D.C. Linus Pauling was upset by the report and the American Journal of Psychiatry published his views on orthomolecular psychiatry in the November 1974 issue. I urge you to read not only this eloquent argument by a brilliant man, but also the three papers immediately following the Pauling paper, which completely devastate that argument.

What about the undesirable side-effects of the large doses of nicotinic acid and nicotinamide used by the promoters of orthomolecular psychiatry? These undesirable side-effects begin with frequent mild ones like flushing and itching, and go on to liver damage with hyperbilirubinemia and jaundice, and many other abnormalities, including severe dermatoses, elevated serum glucose and serum uric acid levels, and elevated concentrations in the serum of enzymes which arise from the liver (and are associated with liver damage), as well as peptic ulceration. As you may know, a large national study of the use of megadoses of niacin was completed which notes the chemical effect of lowering serum lipid levels on the survival of men who've had heart attacks.[5] This study showed absolutely no value with respect to mortality if one takes megadoses of niacin to lower serum lipid levels. What it did show was that the megadoses of niacin produced an increased frequency of cardiac arrhythmias, gastrointestinal problems, and abnormal blood chemistry findings.

We know that if you lower the serum level of lipid or vitamin or anything else, it does not necessarily mean that the tissue level is lowered. Therefore it does not necessarily have any clinical value. Clinical value is determined by what happens in the cells, not by what happens in the serum. If, for example, an agent lowers the serum lipid level by driving the lipid into the coronary arteries, that's not a good thing. Lowering the serum level by itself, unless you know what it means in terms of the tissue level and the intracellular level in the shock organs, may have no meaning or a bad meaning instead of a good one.

THE TRUTH ABOUT VITAMIN E

Let's turn now to vitamin E, so heavily touted as the sex tonic of the age. Is it true? As you can guess, it is not. Not much has been done yet to determine whether massive doses of E are toxic, but there is a fair amount of literature beginning to develop on it.[6] We're not even sure E is a vitamin. We know that its role in humans is in helping in the metabolism of polyunsaturated fatty acids (PUFA), and we know that premature infants may have a tendency to increased red cell hemolysis which can be corrected by adding vitamin E. Does that mean they have E deficiency? Hematologists know that when an anemia responds to a given nutrient or a given agent, it doesn't necessarily mean the patient was suffering from a deficiency of that agent. Just because pneumococcal pneumonia responds to penicillin doesn't mean it's due to penicillin deficiency. The fact that the hemolysis of premature infants responds to vitamin E turns out, in a study reported by Oski and his associates in the *New England Journal of Medicine,* to be due to the fact that premature infants invariably are given large amounts of iron supplement. This strong redox action of the iron in association with the PUFA in their diets brings about the weakening of the red cell membrane and increased susceptibility to hemolysis, especially *in vitro* in the presence of peroxide. Instead of adding a reducing agent such as E, simply reduce the amount of iron supplement in their diet. The problem goes away just as it does by giving them megadoses of E (or by itself by waiting three months).

The allegations of vitamin E as a sex vitamin go back to the original study in the early '20s which first isolated vitamin E. This was a study in rats in which all fat was extracted from the diet and most of the fat was put back, except one fraction. That fraction happened to be the one containing the subsequently isolated vitamin E. It was found that these rats became generally weak, suffering from generalized malaise and debility (including debility in sexual function), and when this fraction that was deleted was added back, they became normal again, including normal sexual function. That's the basis for the anecdotal allegations that vitamin E increases sexual potency in humans. It's almost impossible in the U.S. to get a vitamin E deficiency unless you're suffering from intestinal malabsorption, in which case your patients shouldn't be dosing themselves with megadoses of E to the exclusion of medical care. Even if you put a patient on a no-E diet, as Horwitt did for years, or even if you have a patient with generalized intestinal malabsorption (such that he's unable to absorb fats and therefore has reduced absorption of the fat soluble vitamins like E), after years of such a situation you don't see any clinical disease. All you see is an increased susceptibility of the red cells to hemolysis when exposed to H_2O_2 (hydrogen peroxide), and if you do a proctosigmoidoscopic exam you'll see some ceroid pigment in the colon.

What are the undesirable side-effects of megadoses of E? The ones reported so far include headaches, nausea, fatigue, dizziness, and blurred vision. Blurred vision is particularly interesting because E in large doses antagonizes vitamin A, and that may be the mechanism whereby the blurred vision occurs. The only report in the literature relating to human gonad function is that megadoses of E may *decrease* function, contrary to the allegations of the promoters of E that it *enhances* it. Megadoses of E also have undesirable effects in the skin and mucous membranes, including inflammation of the mouth, chapping of the lips, GI disturbances, muscle weakness, low blood sugar, increased bleeding tendencies, and degenerative changes.

It is interesting to note that one of the early advocates of vitamin E as a preventive of heart attacks recently had a heart attack himself and had a triple coronary bypass operation.

WHAT WE KNOW ABOUT B_{12}

There are vitamins whose toxicity in megadoses has not yet been clearly established, for example, vitamin B_{12}. There's been only one case so far of so-called allergy to vitamin B_{12} and we're not sure whether it's real or related to a preservative in the B_{12} preparation. B_{12} is, of course, a favorite "remedy." Because of its nice color, it looks potent and people think it's potent. The fact is, every objective study demonstrates that B_{12} is not an appetite stimulant and any such effect is that of a placebo. Contrary to the allegations that B_{12} helps various neurologic disorders, it has absolutely no value in any neurologic disorder other than that due to B_{12} deficiency, where a low serum B_{12} level gives you the diagnosis. There is one possible exception—tobacco amblyopia. Since some ophthalmologists insist that there's no such thing as tobacco amblyopia, it's hard to work out exactly what's going on there. B_{12} in the hydroxo form does bind cyanide, and it's been alleged that it's the cyanide in tobacco smoke that produces tobacco amblyopia (if, in fact, it does exist). There may be a rational tie here, because B_{12} in the hydroxocobalamin form will bind cyanide and will itself then be converted to cyanocobalamin. There are certain foods which are very high in cyanogens (cyanide generating substances), such as cassava in Africa, where huge populations all suffer from chronic cyanide poisoning because of the daily ingestion of cassava. It's been alleged that this type of poisoning can be reduced with injections of hydroxocobalamin.

THE LAETRILE FRAUD

It's interesting that a cyanogen right now is very popular in the U.S. That cyanogen is, of course, Laetrile, which is currently the most popular form of quackery in this country. This quack cure for cancer is promoted under the guise that it is a vitamin (B_{17}) which it is not. Vitamin B_{17} is a *trade name* created for it by its promoters; there is currently no law preventing promoters from trade-naming cyanide as vitamin B_{17}, or arsenic as vitamin B_{18}, for that matter. The *scientific* designation of a substance as a vitamin, on the other hand, requires that it conform to the dictionary definition of the word. It has been alleged (with no evidence) that it cures cancer by destroying cancer cells because of the cyanide it releases. Study of the cyanide released by Laetrile shows that the cyanide, as you would expect, diffuses throughout the body and does not home in on cancer cells or any other cells. If the dose used releases enough cyanide to be toxic to cells it will kill the host, as we know from a report in June 1977 from Buffalo, New York, of the ten month old girl who took her father's Laetrile pills and died of cyanide poisoning. Laetrile has been studied at many places and found to be fraudulent. The Merck Index says Laetrile (under its chemical name, amygdalin) is a poison which has been falsely promoted as a cancer cure since 1840. These facts have been in the Merck Index, available in every hospital and pharmacy in the country, since it was first published in 1889. Laetrile is a trade name for amygdalin. It is 2 parts glucose, 1 part benzaldehyde, 1 part cyanide, and no parts vitamin. There is also a synthetic Laetrile®, which is 1 part glucose, 1 part benzaldehyde, 1 part cyanide, no parts vitamin, and mutagenic by Ames test. Low grade cyanide poisoning occurs in nearly every patient taking Laetrile. See the Merck Index listing for "hydrogen cyanide" for the symptoms of low grade cyanide poisoning (nausea, vomiting, diarrhea, hypotension, progressively increasing weakness, etc.). Only one of these symptoms may appear at any one time.

We do know that if a cancer patient takes Laetrile instead of undergoing curative therapy, that patient will die. This has been reported in a number of diseases, particularly Hodgkin's, where we now know we can cure stages I through III. If a patient with stage I through III Hodgkin's is talked out of chemotherapy and radiation (which is now believed to be curative), and gets Laetrile instead, that patient will die of Hodgkin's—that death, in my view, is murder. There is precedent for calling it murder, and there is precedent for convicting such people of murder. Let me give you that precedent. It's on page 2 of the book, *The Health Robbers*, and it's the case of a little girl who had been scheduled for surgery to remove a tumor from her left eye. Her doctors thought cure was possible because the tumor had not spread. Shortly before the operation, in the hospital waiting room, her parents met a couple who told them how a chiropractor had cured their son's brain tumor without surgery. Mrs. Epping phoned the chiropractor and informed him of her daughter's diagnosis. Without ever seeing the child, the chiropractor replied, yes, he could help by chemically balancing her body. Elated by this promise, the parents removed their daughter from the hospital, refused the surgery which would have enucleated the eye (but saved the child), and the chiropractor treated her with vitamins and food supplements. (You should know that the promoters of Laetrile call it a food supplement, and they're trying to get a bill through Congress forbidding the FDA from asserting any authority over food supplements.) Despite the new treatment with food supplements, the tumor grew quickly, became tennis ball size, and pushed her eye out of its socket, so that there was no longer any hope that surgery could save her. She died within a few months. The Assistant DA for Los Angeles County was incensed and indicted the chiropractor for murder. He was convicted of second degree murder and sentenced to prison. I predict that we will see similar things happening to some of the promoters of Laetrile. Those who promote Laetrile point out that cyanocobalamin also contains cyanide; they neglect the fact that an average dose contains one million times as much cyanide as an average dose of cyanocobalamin.

Let's come back to the harmful effects of megadoses of some other nutrients. B_6 in megadoses used to be believed to be harmless, but now that megadoses are being used more frequently, there's evidence that large doses may produce liver disease. It's been established in rats and there is a study under way in humans.

Megadoses of folate also used to be considered harmless, but it's been established that large doses antagonize the protective effect of dilantin against convulsions in patients with epilepsy. Patients with epilepsy who take dilantin, and who've been free of convulsions for years because of the dilantin, can be thrown into convulsions with a megadose of folate. This was reported by Butterworth's group in the *American Journal of Clinical Nutrition.*

PANGAMIC ACID ("VITAMIN B_{15}")

According to both the American Food and Drug Administration and the Canadian Food and Drug Directorate, this substance has no known values for humans, and may be harmful. The FDA is pursuing a number of court actions against Pangamate purveyors.

VITAMIN C AND CANCER

It was reported in that eminent medical journal, *The National Enquirer*, that Linus Pauling and Cameron working at a great international medical research center in Scotland (which turns out to be a modest regional hospital in the Scottish Highlands) found that megadoses of vitamin C increase survival of terminal cancer patients four-fold. This was published in the *Proceedings of the National Academy of Science*, a prestigious journal. You have to realize, however, that the basic criterion for getting something published in this journal is to be a member of the Academy. In fact, what was being described, in my view and in the view of a number of cancer experts, is the placebo effect. The fact that these patients lived an average of eight months instead of an average of two months is simply due to the fact that the patients were in the hands of enthusiastic doctors who felt that they could help. This is true at every cancer center in the United States. Put a patient in Sloan-Kettering or in Roswell Park or in MD Anderson, and that patient is going to live longer. The hope of the patient, and the fact that the doctor is interested in the patient, makes a tremendous difference; this relates to the placebo effect[7], which we'll come back to in a moment. First, I want to refer you to a study on megadoses of C in cancer which goes the other way. This is a report in *Nature* in 1976 by a group at the University of Vancouver in British Columbia, who found that megadoses of C may have mutagenic effects and induce neoplasia.

THE PLACEBO EFFECT

Let's touch now on the placebo effect. This is very strong and very real. Lay persons do not usually understand that placebos not only work when the illness is just emotional, but also in remitting real symptoms of real disease. If the patient believes he will be helped, he often will. This is crucial to remember. If you go back to the famous World War II study of Beecher, the professor of anesthesiology at Harvard who devoted a great deal of his life to studying placebo therapy and to studying medical ethics, you'll recall that he observed with his associates that 68% of soldiers with severe battlefield injuries needed no morphine for pain relief, whereas 83% of civilians with the same type of injury did need morphine. This is the placebo effect. Beecher has stated that the placebo effect is a powerful therapeutic tool "on the average about one-half to two-thirds as powerful as morphine in the usual dose in relieving severe pain." If both the doctor and the patient believe something will relieve a symptom, it often will. Those of you who took psychosomatic medicine know from the statistics in that field that 80% of symptoms with which patients present when they first see a doctor will go away without treatment. Four out of five times, whatever you do or don't do, including what you add to or subtract from the patient's diet, is going to be associated with complete relief of the symptom even though in four out of five instances that symptom is going to go away with no treatment.

The possibility that placebo effect may be mediated by endorphin release deserves study, since any mind-body interaction in relation to pain may well involve these endogenous painkillers.

There's nothing wrong with giving a patient vitamin B_{12} or something else as a placebo, provided you know what you're doing, and provided you continue to observe the patient to ascertain whether there's some underlying disease causing the subjective complaint—and then deal with that underlying disease. Using placebo therapy without knowing what you're doing is quackery. Using placebo therapy when you know what you're doing and when you're observing the patient for real disease, is appropriate.

REFERENCES

1. ROBINSON, C.H., and LAWLER, M.R.: Normal and Therapeutic Nutrition, 15th ed. Macmillan Co., New York, 1977.
2. FEBRUARY, 1977, p. 67.
3. BARRETT, S., and KNIGHT, G. (Editors): The Health Robbers. George Stickley Inc., 210 West Washington Square, Philadelphia, Pa., 19106 ($10.50).
4. JUKES, T.: What You Can Tell Your Patients About "Organic" Foods, Medical Times, October 1975.
5. JAMA, January 29, 1974.
6. HERBERT: Letter to the Editor—Vitamin E Report, Nutr. Rev. 35:158, 1977.
7. MILLER, T.P.: Psychophysiologic Aspects of Cancer, Cancer 39:413–418, 1977.

32

NUTRITION REFERENCES FOR YOU AND YOUR PATIENT

Yank D. Coble, Jr., M.D.

Vast sums are being spent by the American public on "health food," nutrition supplements, diet books, diet foods, weight reduction gimmicks, and nutrition information. Publishers have observed, profitably, that nutrition leads on magazine covers sell "off the rack" even better than sex. Thus, it is not surprising that the food quackery beliefs and practices of today, and those who are profiteering from it, can be compared to the patent medicine craze of the last century.

For the most part, self-acclaimed authorities, faddists, and hucksters have been the disseminators of this nutrition misinformation that Rynearson so appropriately labeled as "hogwash." Unfortunately, some of our well intentioned but misguided media and even some of our colleagues as well are distributing the "hogwash." Even more unfortunate, it can be harmful to more than the consumer's pocketbook, as evidenced by the megavitamins, liquid protein, and other diet fads, which have resulted in disease and even death.

"What do you recommend I read about nutrition, Doctor?" is a familiar question. Obviously it is difficult for the general public today to choose the eminent nutrition author over the misinformer, both of whom may be featured side by side on the news stand. Thus the physician, with his understanding of the appeal of nutrition misinformation and recognizing its dangers, is in a position to provide appropriate authoritative and interesting nutrition information.

Consistent with the efforts of our FMA President, O. William Davenport, to concentrate our scientific activities in the field of nutrition this year, we have provided below a list of nutrition references that we hope

Dr. Coble is a Specialist in Endocrinology and Nutrition in practice in Jacksonville, Fla.

will be of use to you and your patients. To Drs. Lewis Barness, George Christakis, and Donald Macdonald and the other physicians and nutritionists who made recommendations and suggestions about this list, I wish to express my appreciation.

The first list contains general references on nutrition for your patient. **Recommended Dietary Allowances,** item #6, is a reference valuable to any physician's office but is also of interest to the more sophisticated patient wishing specific data on allowances of each individual nutrient. Reference #7, **Nutritive Value of American Foods**, is also a valuable document for physicians' offices but of particular value to the sophisticated layman who is interested in content of foods. Reference #8, the **Index of Nutrition Education Materials,** provides a large bibliography of authoritative and attractive nutrition materials.

The second list relates primarily to the area of food faddism, quackery, and nutrition misinformation. References #1, #2 and #3 are written for the general public. Reference #4 should be of particular interest to the physician.

The third list relates to the most frequently neglected but vital segment of nutritional, exercise.

The fourth list is applicable to a specific nutritional problem, obesity. The magnitude of this problem in the United States and the single generally accepted approach—good nutritional and exercise habits—justify specific references in this area.

The fifth list is directed to the physician or health professional.

I. GENERAL NUTRITIONAL REFERENCES

1. Eat OK—Feel OK: Food Facts & Your Health
   Frederick J. Stare, M.D. & Elizabeth M. Whelan, Sc.D.
   The Christopher Publishing House, North Quincy, Mass. 1978 ($9.75)

2. Let's Talk About Food
   Philip L. White, Sc.D. & Nancy Selvey, R.D.
   P.F.G., Inc., 545 Great Road, Littleton, Mass. 01460 1977 ($6.95 cloth; $5.00 paper)

3. Realities of Nutrition
   Ronald M. Deutsch
   Bull Publishing Company P.O. Box 208, Palo Alto, Calif. 94302, 1976 ($9.95)

4. Nutrition & Food Choices
   Kristen W. McNutt & David R. McNutt
   Science Research Associates
   1540 Pagemill Road, Palo Alto, Calif. 94304
   1978 ($12.95)

5. Nutrition Source Book
   National Dairy Council
   6300 N. River Road
   Rosemont, Ill. 60018, 1978
   (complimentary from publisher)

6. Recommended Dietary Allowances
   8th Revised Edition, 1974 Food and Nutrition Board
   National Academy of Sciences
   2101 Constitution Avenue
   Washington, D.C. 20418
   (9th edition planned for 1980)
   ($4.25 paper)

7. Nutritive Value of American Foods (Revised April 1977)
   United States Department of Agriculture
   Agriculture Research Service (For Sale by Superintendent of Documents, U.S. Gov't. Printing Office, Washington, D.C. 20402—Stock #001-00-03184-8) ($5.15)

8. Index of Nutrition Education Materials
   The Nutrition Foundation
   888 17th Street, N.W.
   Washington, D.C. 20006 ($8.75)

II. NUTRITION MISINFORMATION, FOOD FADDISM AND QUACKERY

1. New Nuts Among The Berries
   Ronald M. Deutsch
   Bull Publishing Company
   P.O. Box 208
   Palo Alto, Calif. 94302, 1977 ($8.95)

2. Panic In The Pantry
   Elizabeth M. Whelan, Sc.D. & Fredrick J. Stare, M.D.
   Atheneum, New York, New York
   Dist by: Book Warehouse, Inc., Vreeland Avenue
   Patterson, N.J. 07512, 1976 ($3.95 paper)

3. The Health Robbers: How To Protect Your Money & Your Life
   Stephen Barrett, M.D., Editor & Gilda Knight, Co-editor
   George F. Stickley Company, Publisher
   210 West Washington Square
   Philadelphia, Penn. 19106, 1976 ($10.50)

4. Nutrition Misinformation and Food Faddism
   D.M. Hegsted & Philip L. White, editors
   The Nutrition Foundation
   Office of Education
   888 17th Street, N.W.
   Washington, D.C. 20006, July 1974 ($2.50)

III. PHYSICAL FITNESS AND NUTRITION

1. The New Aerobics
   Kenneth H. Cooper, M.D.
   M. Evans & Company, Inc.
   New York, New York 1970
   Hardbound distributed by J. B. Lippincott Company,
   E. Washington Square
   Philadelphia, Penn. 19105 ($6.95)
   Paperback distributed by Bantam Books, Inc.,
   414 E. Golf Road, Desplaines, Illinois 60016 ($2.95)

2. Nutrition For Athletics
   The Nutrition Foundation
   Office of Education
   888 17th Street, N.W.
   Washington, D.C. 20006 ($3.00)

3. The President's Council on Physical Fitness & Sports
   (Information provided on request)
   C. Carson Conrad, Executive Director
   Washington, D.C. 20201

IV. OBESITY

1. Healthy Approach To Slimming (OPOO3)
   American Medical Association
   P.O. Box 821
   Monroe, Wisconsin 54566, 1978 ($1.00)

2. Slim Chance In A Fat World
   Richard B. Stuart & Barbara Davis
   Research Press Company
   Champaign, Ill. 1972 ($4.95)

3. Permanent Weight Control
   Michael J. Mahoney & Kathryn Mahoney
   W.W. Norton & Co., Inc.
   500 5th Avenue
   New York, New York 10036, 1976 ($7.95)

4. Obesity
   The Nutrition Foundation
   Office of Education
   888 17th Street, N.W.
   Washington, D.C. 20006 (complimentary)

5. Eating Is Okay!
   Henry A. Jordan, M.D.
   New American Library, Inc.
   1301 Avenue of the Americas
   New York, N.Y. 10019, 1978 ($1.50 paper)

V. NUTRITION REFERENCES FOR THE PHYSICIAN AND HEALTH PROFESSIONAL

1. Nutritional Support of Medical Practice
   Howard A. Schneider, Ph.D., Carl E. Anderson, Ph.D., & David B. Coursin, M.D.
   Harper & Row, Publishers
   2350 Virginia Avenue
   Hagerstown, Md. 21740, 1977 ($25.00)

2. Nutrition Reviews: Present Knowledge in Nutrition (4th edition)
   The Nutrition Foundation
   Office of Education
   888 17th Street, N.W.
   Washington, D.C. 20006, 1976 ($8.50)

3. Nutrition Reviews
   The Nutrition Foundation
   Office of Education
   888 17th Street, N.W.
   Washington, D.C. 20006
   (subscription $15.00 per year)

4. Drug-Induced Nutritional Deficiencies
   Daphne A. Roe, M.D.
   The AVI Publishing Company, Inc.
   250 Post Road E.
   Westport, Conn. 06880, 1976 ($21.00)

5. American Journal of Clinical Nutrition
   8650 Rockville Pike
   Bethesda, Maryland 20014 ($35.00 per year for non-members)

6. Journal of Parenteral & Enteral Nutrition
   The Williams & Wilkens Company
   428 East Preston Street
   Baltimore, Maryland 21202
   ($35.00 per year for non-members)

7. Nutrition Today
   Nutrition Today, Inc.
   703 Giddings Avenue
   P.O. Box 1829
   Annapolis, Md. 21401
   (bi-monthly publication, annual subscription $14.75)

8. Alcohol and the Diet
   Daphne A. Roe, M.D.
   The AVI Publishing Company, Inc.
   250 Post Road E.
   Westport, Conn. 06880 ($21.00)

33

NUTRITION QUIZ

Committee on Nutrition

Choose the **one** correct or most appropriate answer to the following questions by circling the letter:

1. **Nutrition can be defined as the science and art of**
   a) The use of food to promote health.
   b) How micronutrients work metabolically.
   c) How and why people eat the way they do.
   d) Many sciences such as agriculture, epidemiology, clinical medicine.
   e) All of the above.

2. **Chemicals in food are often looked at negatively. A hot steamy solution containing, among other things, caffeine, tannin, essential oils, butyl, isoamyl, phenyl ethyl, hexyl and benzyl alcohols, and geraniol describes which of the following beverages:**
   a) Coffee
   b) Tea
   c) Buttered rum
   d) Spiced wine
   e) Chocolate drink

3. **The function of mucus in the gastrointestinal tract is to provide the following role(s):**
   a) Emulsify food particles.
   b) Protect the epithelium.
   c) Buffer acids or alkalies.
   d) All of the above.
   e) (b) and (c)

4. **Which of the following statements accurately describes a micronutrient?**
   a) Essential in small amounts for human growth and welfare.
   b) Functions primarily at the cellular, molecular and enzymatic levels.
   c) Few known elements currently identified.
   d) (a) and (b)
   e) All of the above.

5. **Serum cholesterol can be effectively lowered by all of the following except:**
   a) Vitamin E
   b) Relatively high dietary intake of polyunsaturated fatty acids.
   c) Relatively low dietary intake of palmitic and stearic fatty acids.
   d) Cholestyramine.
   e) Weight loss in the obese.

6. **Which of the vitamin deficiencies may require medical emergency treatment?**
   a) Vitamin E
   b) Vitamin D
   c) Pantothenic acid
   d) Vitamin C
   e) Vitamin A

7. **Of the following, which can be considered to be related to decreased prevalence of colon cancer?**
   a) Milk
   b) Cereal grains
   c) Sugar Cane
   d) Tea
   e) Halvah

8. **Which is popularly believed to be effective in preventing coronary heart disease, but has yet to be proven?**
   a) Vitamin B_{15}
   b) Xanthine oxidase
   c) Vitamin E
   d) Vitamin A
   e) Pantothenic acid

9. **Regarding the prevalence of malnutrition in the U.S.,**
   a) The overall prevalence is 30%.
   b) There is no evidence that it exists.
   c) From 8–18% of low income groups have low or deficient serum vitamin levels.
   d) A negligible prevalence of signs and symptoms of vitamin deficiency exists.
   e) Iron deficiency is uncommon.

10. **Which of the following vitamins can cause severe toxicity and death?**
   a) Pantothenic acid and pyridoxal phosphate
   b) Vitamin A and Vitamin E
   c) Vitamin D and Vitamin A
   d) Vitamin D and Vitamin B_{12}
   e) None of the above

11. **Which of the following are effective in decreasing elevated serum triglyceride levels?**
   a) Decrease in dietary alcohol and administration of clofibrate.
   b) Decrease in monounsaturated lipids and oligosaccharides.
   c) Increase in polyunsaturated fatty acids and Vitamin C.
   d) Decrease in protein and lipids.
   e) None of the above.

12. **The approximate prevalence of serum cholesterol levels 260 mg/dl or above in U.S. men (age 35–56) is**
   a) 20%
   b) 30%
   c) 10%
   d) 50%
   e) 15%

13. **The Framingham Study findings revealed the following except**
   a) A serum cholesterol level of 260 mg/dl is associated with a 6-fold risk of coronary heart disease.
   b) Elevated serum cholesterol, hypertension and smoking are the prime risk factors of coronary heart disease.
   c) High salt intake is related to hypertension.
   d) Obesity is related to sudden death.
   e) Sedentary individuals had a significantly greater prevalence of coronary heart disease compared to those who were physically active.

14. **Factors that may be involved in the increased incidence of hypertension in Blacks include the following except**
    a) High dietary salt intake.
    b) Genetic factors.
    c) Psycho-social stress.
    d) Obesity
    e) Elevated saturated fat intake.

15. **The following are true concerning the epidemiology of hypertension except**
    a) Blood pressure increases with age in all population groups.
    b) Hypertension is not always a risk factor of coronary heart disease.
    c) Weight reduction of obese hypertensives can decrease blood pressure significantly.
    d) The major clinical manifestations of hypertension are strokes, cardiac and renal failure.
    e) The Japanese, Caribbean and American Blacks exhibit the highest worldwide prevalence of hypertension.

16. **The prevalence of adolescent obesity in the U.S. is**
    a) 20–25%
    b) 10–15%
    c) 5%
    d) 30–35%
    e) None of the above

17. **The metabolic and nutritional factors associated with obesity include the following except**
    a) Hyperinsulinism
    b) Hypertriglyceridemia
    c) Carbohydrate intolerance
    d) Hypoferremia
    e) Hyperadrenalism

18. **Which of the following agencies are involved in the monitoring of nutritional products:**
    a) FTC and FDA
    b) FTC and EPA
    c) FDA and EPA
    d) HHS and NIH
    e) None of the above

19. **An average supermarket contains the following number of different food items from which the housewife must choose to build a nutritious diet for her family:**
    a) 1,000
    b) 500
    c) 5,000
    d) 15,000
    e) None of the above

20. **The use of wheat germ contributes the following to the daily meal pattern:**
    a) Substantial amounts of polyunsaturated fatty acids
    b) B vitamins, a small amount of polyunsaturated fatty acids and fiber
    c) Large amounts of trace minerals
    d) Large amounts of carbohydrates
    e) None of the above

21. **High intakes of the water-soluble vitamins (100 times RDA)**
    a) Are non-toxic at any level.
    b) Improve appetite and well-being in controlled studies.
    c) Only result in "expensive and colorful urine" (elevated levels of urinary riboflavin makes urine fluoresce).
    d) Have been known to cause death.
    e) Have been shown to improve schizophrenia in large controlled studies.

22. **Vitamin E**
    a) Has been proven to be non-toxic.
    b) May enhance blood coagulation.
    c) Improves virility.
    d) Can cure sterility.
    e) Is found in substantial amounts in lentils.

23. **Of the following current "folk-medicine" concepts, which has/have the most valid scientific bases?**
    a) Grapefruits catalyze the oxidation of other foods.
    b) Low carbohydrate diets are especially effective in weight loss.
    c) Garlic can decrease elevated blood pressure.
    d) (a) and (b)
    e) None of the above.

24. **Which of the following is true:**
    a) Freshly ground peanut butter has less saturated fat than commercially prepared peanut butter.
    b) There is a 70% loss of water-soluble vitamins in canned spinach and asparagus.
    c) Freezing fruits retains more of their Vitamin C content than canning them.
    d) Lentils have a very low protein content.
    e) None of the above.

25. **Regarding the treatment of obesity, which of the following is true:**
    a) Amphetamines have an important place in treatment.
    b) If the same number of calories (for example 1,200 per day) are derived from different sources of macronutrients (fats, proteins and carbohydrates) the weight loss after 3–4 weeks will be identical.
    c) There is about 50% recidivism of weight loss after one year when obesity is treated by internists.
    d) Behavior modification techniques usually involve in-depth probing of the psychogenic determinants of obesity.
    e) Group weight reduction provides no higher success rates than individual treatment regimens.

26. **Which is true regarding vegetarians:**
    a) Macrocytic anemias are rarely encountered.
    b) Use of vegetable sources of protein, excluding lentils and chickpeas, are adequate for the protein needs of children.
    c) Wheat as a source of protein can be adequate for adults.
    d) Vegetarianism is rarely linked to religious-philosophical beliefs.
    e) People who predominantly consume a high wheat diet develop more beri-beri than those consuming high intakes of rice.

27. **Which of the following additives is probably harmless:**
    a) Calcium proprionate
    b) Diethylstilbestrol
    c) Nitrates
    d) Cobalt
    e) Butylated hydroxy anisole

28. **Concerning cooking practices, the following are true except:**
    a) Cooking vegetables in a small amount of water conserves water-soluble vitamins.
    b) Parboiling rather than boiling rice conserves B vitamins.
    c) Frying pans with teflon surfaces reduce the need for oil in frying.
    c) Baking may severely oxidize water-soluble vitamins.
    e) Toasting bread decreases its caloric content by 10%.

29. **Good shopping practices include the following except:**
    a) Purchase of bread one-day old seriously impairs its nutritional value.
    b) It's wiser not to go shopping when you're hungry.
    c) Plan to shop on a weekly rather than a daily basis.
    d) Impulse buying usually increases the food bill.
    e) Using a shopping list is efficient and economical.

30. **Which of the following does not represent a "good buy" nutritionally for a low-income family?**
    a) Loaf of bread (whole wheat or white)
    b) Skim milk powder
    c) Protein-enriched spaghetti
    d) Peanut butter
    e) Lettuce

Prepared by the Ad Hoc Committee on Nutrition.

Appendix A
NUTRITION AND PHYSICAL FITNESS[1]

A Statement by The American Dietetic Association

With industrialization and mechanization, many individuals in the United States have become more sedentary. The decrease in physical activity and an abundant food supply have contributed to wider prevalence of obesity and reduced physical fitness. In turn, the risk of chronic disease, such as cardiovascular disease and diabetes mellitus, is increased. Members of The American Dietetic Association are obligated to influence a change in the fitness of the American public.

In our professional affiliations, it is our responsibility to promote programs that incorporate concepts of good nutrition and physical fitness. This statement by The American Dietetic Association is intended as a guideline to help dietitians and nutritionists achieve these goals. Recommendations are made for two levels of physical fitness: (a) For the general public and (b) for the more intense level of performing athletes.

Part I. Recommendations for the general public

The American Dietetic Association maintains that a nutritionally adequate diet and exercise are major contributing factors to physical fitness and health.

With a nutritionally adequate diet and an increase in the level of exercise, most persons will improve in their physical capacities until they

[1] Copyright 1980 by the American Dietetic Association. Reprinted by permission from the *Journal of the American Dietetic Association*, Vol. 76:437.

reach a genetically predetermined level. The nutritionally adequate diet is one that provides sufficient nutrients and energy to meet the metabolic needs for optimal functioning of the body. In addition, substantial evidence indicates that individuals who avoid excessive intakes of carbohydrates, fat, cholesterol, sugar, salt, and highly refined foods lacking in fiber can maintain better health and may reduce their risk of developing chronic diseases.

The many benefits of physical conditioning include: development of muscular strength, muscular endurance, and cardiovascular endurance; improved work capacity; increased muscle efficiency in handling oxygen; better muscle tone; greater flexibility and agility; and an improved sense of well-being. Also, blood pressure, pulse rate, and percentage of body fat may be modified. Aerobic exercise is one of many factors that may alter the lipid profile of the blood[1,2] and reduce the risk of coronary artery disease.

In addition to appropriate diet and exercise, physical fitness and health are influenced by other interdependent factors: genetic variables; endocrine balances; psychologic and emotional status; sleep; and the use of alcohol, drugs, and tobacco.

The American Dietetic Association recommends that weight maintenance and weight loss be achieved by a combination of dietary modification, change in eating behavior, and regular aerobic exercise.

The key to weight control is a balance of energy intake and energy output. Individuals must learn to adjust their energy intakes throughout life to correspond to their changing metabolic needs. Customarily, some reduction in caloric intake is recommended during the middle and later years of adult life to correspond to the generally reduced energy requirements for the maintenance of desirable body weight and body fatness. For the obese, a low-calorie diet will bring about weight loss. However, with dietary adjustments alone, the recidivism rate has been high.

Behavioral modification of food habits is based on the premise that food intake is a learned response that can be changed. The individual learns to focus attention on the environmental factors that influence his/her food intake and to modify them gradually so that desirable changes in eating behavior occur.

An increase in physical activity can be as important as a decrease in the caloric intake to enable an individual to maintain desirable weight with the advancing years or to reduce weight if obese. Energy expenditure varies from one individual to another, depending on body weight, efficiency of movement, and training. The energy equivalents of many kinds of exercise have been determined, and convenient guidelines are available[1,3,4]. With exercise, there is a slight increase in lean body mass which may result initially in a small increase in body weight since muscle tissue is heavier than fat tissue. Exercise will gradually reduce the percentage of body fat, even with weight maintenance, and to a greater extent with weight loss. When exercise is interrupted for an extended period, the percentage of body fat again increases[5].

Individuals are likely to achieve a higher success rate for long-term weight maintenance or weight loss if they take a three-phase approach: (a) Adjustment of the caloric intake to lose or maintain weight, (b) modification of inappropriate eating behavior, and (c) an increase in energy expenditure through regular aerobic exercise.

The American Dietetic Association recommends that skinfold measurements be used to determine the level of body fatness.

Traditionally, standard height-weight tables have been used to determine desirable body weight. However, individuals who conform to these standards actually vary widely in the proportions of lean and fatty tissue; that is, some persons who fall within the defined height-weight standards may have excessive deposits of fatty tissue.

Body composition is a better indicator of leanness than is body weight. A number of techniques have been used by investigators to determine body composition, including underwater weighing (body density), considered the most accurate technique; multiple isotope dilution (total and extracellular body water); total body potassium, using a whole body scintillation counter (lean body mass); and soft tissue roentgenography (width and thickness of adipose pads)[6,7].

Acceptable levels of body fat range from 7 to 15 per cent for men and from 12 to 25 per cent for women[8]. A fat content in excess of 20 per cent for men and 30 per cent for women is regarded as obesity[9]. With aging, total body fat for both sexes gradually increases, with the greater increase occurring in women[10,11].

None of the techniques used in research laboratories lends itself to clinical practice. Skinfold measurements with calipers applied at constant pressure at selected body sites—triceps, subscapular, abdominal, suprailiac crest, pectoral, and thigh and calf areas—are practical, reliable predictors of body fatness[12-14]. Changes occur with aging in the subcutaneous tissues. Occasionally, large errors in estimation of body fat can occur, especially with a single measurement, because of unusual fat distribution. Such errors are reduced with multiple measurements[15]. Tables based on several measurements show the interpretation of skinfold measurements of men and women in terms of percentage of body fat[8,14].

The triceps skinfold is a single measurement readily used for the estimation of body fatness, but, as mentioned, it does have limitations. The individual does not need to undress, as is necessary when several sites are measured. A table is available showing minimum values for skinfold thickness for men and women of various ages; above these levels, obesity is present[13].

The American Dietetic Association maintains that the generally healthy individual who regularly consumes a diet that supplies the Recommended Dietary Allowances receives all necessary nutrients for a physical conditioning program.

The Recommended Dietary Allowances[16] for each age/sex category afford a margin of safety for most individuals and will furnish the needs of persons entering on a physical conditioning program. Adjustments for energy intake are made to effect weight maintenance, weight loss, or weight gain as individually determined. For pre-adolescent and adolescent youth, the energy intake must be sufficient to cover growth needs.

A slight increase in the body's muscle mass occurs during the training period. Consequently, there is a small addition to the body's content of protein and water. Once the muscle mass has been developed, little addition to body protein and no increased catabolism of body tissues with continuing exercise occur. The recommended allowances for protein fully cover the increment to body tissues during the training period. Moreover, most Americans consume protein in excess of the recommended allowances. This additional protein consumption is not harmful and may be desirable, because many of the protein-rich foods are also excellent sources of the B-complex vitamins, iron, and other trace minerals.

The percentage of calories from protein varies somewhat with the level of caloric intake. For low-calorie diets, the protein intake may account for 20 per cent, and occasionally more, of total caloric intake. On maintenance diets, a protein intake representing 10 to 15 per cent of calories is customary. Nutritionally adequate diets can be planned with widely varying proportions of carbohydrate and fat. Many nutritionists, physicians, and athletic coaches recommend that the fat intake be kept to from 30 to 35 per cent of calories, with a corresponding increase in carbohydrate intake. The use of complex-type carbohydrates should be emphasized.

The new "Dietary Guidelines for Americans,"* developed by the Departments of Agriculture and of Health, Education, and Welfare, together with the food groups published in 1979 by the Department of Agriculture in the booklet, *Food***, are useful for planning the diet. One of the food groups, namely "Fats, Sweets, and Alcohol," includes foods that are generally low in nutrient density. If these foods are used in moderation and within the nutrient and caloric requirements of the individual, they may enhance the palatability of the diet. If the fat intake is restricted to 35 per cent of calories or less, food choices from the milk and meat groups should be modified and those from fats sharply restricted. Persons who have increased caloric requirements should give preference to additional servings from the bread-cereal and vegetable-fruit groups.

Protein, mineral, and/or vitamin supplements do not enhance physical performance or well-being if the healthy individual consumes a diet that meets the Recommended Dietary Allowances. For some individuals with chronic conditions, the physician may prescribe supplements to meet specific deficiencies or increased metabolic needs.

The American Dietetic Association recommends that the intensity, duration, and frequency of exercise should be determined according to the age, physical condition, and health status of the individual.

Before starting any exercise program, the individual should be advised to consult a physician. This is especially important for individuals over thirty-five years of age and for all persons in whom risk factors for cardiovascular disease, such as hypertension, smoking, or elevated blood lipids, are present[1]. When an individual enters into an exercise program, his/her cardiovascular fitness can be assessed by an electrocardiogram and by oxygen uptake levels during maximal and submaximal stress tests administered and interpreted by a cardiologist or physiologist (with a physician present for persons over thirty-five years of age).

The capacity of a person's body to take in, deliver, and use oxygen is measured by *maximum aerobic power* (abbreviated vo_2-max.). It is expressed as milliliters of oxygen consumed per kilogram body weight per minute (ml. 0_2 kilogram per minute)[4]. The vo_2-max. for women is from 70 to 85 per cent of that for men.

On the basis of the individual's medical history, physical examination, and stress tests, a planned program should be worked out for each person. The duration and intensity of each exercise period are increased

*USDA and DHEW: Nutrition and Your Health. Dietary Guidelines for Americans. 1980. (Available from: Off. of Governmental and Public Affairs, USDA, Washington, D.C. 20250.)

**Food. USDA Home & Garden Bull. No. 228, 1979.

gradually until the prescribed goal is reached. The goal for intensity is from 60 to 80 per cent of the person's vo_2-max. Below 60 per cent, there is little cardiovascular benefit; above 80 per cent, there is little added benefit and possible excessive stress. The goal should be from 15 to 60 min. of continuous aerobic activity three to five days a week. Low- to moderate-intensity exercise of longer duration is recommended for the non-athletic adult[17].

Aerobic exercises promote the improved utilization and consumption of oxygen in the body. The exercise should be continuous and of sufficient duration and intensity to condition muscles and the cardiovascular system without being excessively strenuous. Jogging, brisk walking, swimming, skating, cross-country skiing, cycling, jumping rope, aerobic dancing, rowing, and jumping on a trampoline are examples of aerobic exercises. Walking can be recommended for persons of all ages. Jogging may increase the risk of foot, leg, and knee injury in some individuals[17]. Such exercises as handball, tennis, squash, and volleyball are not considered aerobic for most people and may promote overexertion[18]. Golf and bowling are not effective aerobic exercises.

The heart rate provides a guide to aerobic activity. Each individual entering on a physical conditioning program should be taught how to measure the pulse rate *immediately* on beginning exercise, at the peak period, and at the end of each exercise period. Since the maximum heart rate declines with age, an appropriate guide to the maximum heart rate is to substract the age in years from 220. Exercise that achieves 70 per cent of the maximum heart rate is likely to be accompanied by from 55 to 60 per cent oxygen utilization. An intensity of exercise that achieves 85 per cent of maximum heart rate results in an aerobic response of from 75 to 80 per cent[1]. Within this range of response, improvement in physical conditioning can be expected.

The American Dietetic Association recommends that habits for a nutritionally balanced diet and physical fitness be established during childhood and maintained throughout life.

Food habits and patterns of activity are set in childhood. The establishment of good food habits requires consideration of the physical needs of the individual and the socioeconomic environment that pertains. Food habits are also affected by psychologic, ethnic, cultural, and religious factors. Desirable patterns of food behavior are fostered by nutrition education in the school and by continuing nutrition education throughout adult life.

Physical education in the schools can introduce the child to activities that may be pursued on an individual as well as a group basis throughout a lifetime. If physical fitness is to become a lifetime goal, the activities to achieve it must be enjoyable and adaptable to a variety of environments. Activities appropriate for a lifetime should be promoted by the schools, at camps and playgrounds, and in the home.

An integrated nutrition/physical fitness approach can be achieved in the elementary and secondary schools through the cooperation of classroom teachers, health and physical education teachers, school physicians and nurses, school foodservice dietitians, and nutrition specialists.

Part II. Recommendations for athletes involved in training or competition

The American Dietetic Association recommends that the athlete meet increased caloric and nutrient needs by increasing the number of selections from the "calories-plus-nutrients" foods.*

Athletes usually expend from 3,000 to 6,000 kcal per day. With the increased energy requirement, there is a proportionate increase in the need for thiamin (0.5 mg. per 1,000 kcal). The recommended allowances for riboflavin and niacin intake are also based on caloric intake[16].

The athlete can best meet the higher caloric requirement by increasing the number of servings from the "calories-plus-nutrients" food groups. Liberal intake of carbohydrates from the bread-cereal and fruit-vegetable groups should be emphasized. Moderate amounts of fats and sugars may be used to furnish energy and to enhance the palatability of the diet. When caloric requirements are from 5,000 to 6,000 kcal per day, five or six meals may be preferred to three.

The protein needs of performing athletes include tissue maintenance requirements, allowances for growth by adolescent athletes, and small increments for the development of muscle mass during the conditioning period. No satisfactory evidence exists that additional protein improves work performance or that activity leads to increased cellular destruction of protein[19-21]. Although the recommended allowances for protein are appropriate for the athlete in training, they may not be sufficient to cover the significant losses of nitrogen that occur from the skin during vigorous activity accompanied by profuse sweating in a hot, humid environment. Balance studies have shown that 100 gm. protein per day is adequate to cover all needs of men performing heavy work and perspiring profusely[19]. If protein furnishes from 10 to 12 per cent of the total caloric intake, it will be more than sufficient to cover the losses through the skin.

*Food. USDA Home & Garden Bull. No. 228, 1979.

The American Dietetic Association recommends that athletes maintain a hydrated state by consuming fluid before, during, and after exercise.

Water is the substance of primary concern when profuse sweating accompanies prolonged strenuous exercise. Some individuals may lose as much as 2 to 4 liters of sweat (from 6 to 8 lb. body weight) per hour when competing in endurance events[22-25]. In addition, with heavy exercise, the respiratory loss of water may exceed 130 ml. per hour, compared with a normal loss of 15 ml. per hour[26].

The effects of dehydration are: Fatigue; deterioration in performance; an increase in body temperature; reduced volume of extracellular fluid; reduced urinary volume; and a decline in circulatory function, including lower blood volume, lower blood pressure, increased pulse rate, and if the dehydration is severe enough, circulatory collapse[27,28]. A 3 per cent weight loss leads to impaired performance; a 5 per cent loss can result in some signs of heat exhaustion; a 7 per cent loss may produce hallucinations and put the individual in the danger zone[28]. A 10 per cent weight loss can lead to heat stroke and circulatory collapse.

Dehydration to accomplish weight loss prior to an event, as for wrestlers and boxers, is never acceptable[28,29]. When such athletes must lose weight, the loss should result from a caloric deficit so that body fat, not body water, is lost.

Ordinarily, thirst is a reliable guide to the need for water. But, because of tension and anxiety and because of large sweat losses, thirst is an inaccurate indicator of water need during competition. Athletes should be encouraged to weigh themselves before and after an event to determine the amount of fluid that needs to be replaced. Some forced drinking of fluid is essential.

About 2 hr. before an event, the athlete in endurance competition should try to drink about 600 ml. (21 oz.) fluid. Then 10 to 15 min. before the event, he/she should drink about 400 to 500 ml. (14 to 17 oz.) water. Small amounts of water—100 to 200 ml. (3 to 7 oz.)—at 10- to 15-min. intervals are better than copious amounts of water every hour or so. The maximum fluid intake is about 1 liter per hour, because this is the limit of gastric emptying time[22,23]. Cold drinks (5°C. or 41°F.) leave the stomach more rapidly than warm drinks (35°C. or 94°F.)[30].

Fluid taken before and during the event will not fully replace fluid losses, but partial replacement reduces the risk of overheating. After the event, the athlete should continue to drink water at frequent intervals until the weight has been regained. If the weight loss is from 4 to 7.5 per cent, up to 24 to 36 hr. are required for complete rehydration[26].

The glycogen stores built up with carbohydrate loading prior to endurance competition are a potential source of water to the body. With the breakdown of 1 gm. glycogen, 2.7 gm. associated water are released. Also, each gram of glycogen aerobically metabolized forms 0.6 gm. water. Thus, for each gram of glycogen released, more than 3 gm. water are available that can partially compensate for evaporative water loss[22,27].

The American Dietetic Association recommends that athletes meet their needs for additional electrolytes from the foods they ordinarily consume.

Sodium and chloride are the principal electrolyte deficits that must be corrected following profuse sweating. On occasion, potassium may also require replacement.

The concentration of electrolytes in sweat and the total losses that occur during an event vary widely from one individual to another, according to the degree of acclimatization, adrenal cortical activity, environmental temperature, and humidity[31]. The range of electrolyte concentrations in sweat is great: sodium, from 12 to 120 mEq; potassium, from 5 to 30 mEq; and chloride, from 8 to 80 mEq[32]. Sodium losses of 350 mEq per day are not uncommon as a result of profuse sweating[33]. With acclimatization, the losses are lower.

The precise requirements for sodium and chloride are not known. A suggested "safe and adequate intake" of sodium by adults is from 1,100 to 3,300 mg. (48 to 144 mEq) and of chloride, from 1,700 to 5,100 mg. (48 to 144 mEq)[16]. Typical mixed diets furnish from 6 to 18 gm. salt (100 to 300 mEq sodium and chloride)[33]. The production of 5 to 8 liters of sweat may necessitate an intake of from 13 to 15 gm. salt daily[26]. Athletes do not need to replace salt losses hour by hour but can correct these losses in the foods they consume following the event[26,27,34,35]. They may use more salt at the table and eat foods that have been prepared with a high salt content. One-half tsp. salt contains approximately 1 gm. sodium. Liberal amounts of fluid should accompany sodium replacement. *Caution:* Excessive sodium intake leads to potassium depletion.

A "safe and adequate intake" of potassium for adults is from 1,875 to 5,625 mg. (48 to 144 mEq)[16]. Typical mixed American diets furnish from 1,950 to 5,850 mg. (50 to 150 mEq) per day[33]. Acclimated athletes who perspire profusely need more than 3,000 mg. potassium daily, while those who are not acclimated require up to 5,000 to 6,000 mg.[36]. If the athlete selects foods to meet his additional energy requirements from foods that are also rich sources of potassium, he/she should be able to replace all but the most exceptionally heavy losses. With the substantial metabolism of glycogen during endurance competition, considerable amounts of potassium are released to help meet body needs. Each gram of glycogen metabolized releases 16.6 mg. (0.45 mEq) potassium[22,23].

The American Dietetic Association recommends that electrolyte supplements should be used only on the advice of the team physician.

Generally, the losses of sodium chloride and potassium can be made up at meals following the competition. If sweat losses exceed 4 liters, some electrolyte replacement during the competition may be indicated[33]. The team physician is best qualified to evaluate the conditions of temperature, humidity, and activity that require such supplementation.

Gastric emptying is controlled by the volume and osmolarity of the fluid administered. Hypertonic solutions should be avoided because they exert an osmotic effect, forcing water into the stomach. They can thus accentuate dehydration and cause a feeling of gastric fullness and distress. Gastric emptying will not occur until the stomach contents are isotonic. Not more than 20 to 30 mEq sodium chloride per liter and 50 to 60 gm. glucose per hour are well tolerated[22]. A solution that contains less than 10 mEq sodium per liter, less than 5 mEq potassium per liter, and up to 2.5 per cent of glucose is recommended[23].

Salt tablets are not recommended because they frequently cause nausea, vomiting, and gastric distress[37]. Excessive salt intake increases the load on the kidney, and without adequate fluid intake, a state of dehydration can be further aggravated.

The American Dietetic Association recognizes that a high carbohydrate intake prior to competition can be beneficial to some athletes engaging in endurance events.

It is generally agreed that the availability of muscle glycogen is the limiting factor in endurance competition[20,38-40]. When the muscle glycogen is exhausted, the athlete can no longer perform. Carbohydrate loading or glycogen loading is a dietary procedure whereby high-carbohydrate diets are used to build up muscle glycogen stores. A store of liver glycogen is also necessary to reduce the likelihood of hypoglycemia[22].

When muscles are first depleted of glycogen and then replenished by consumption of a high-carbohydrate diet, the glycogen content of muscle is about twice that achieved with a normal mixed diet[39,41]. The endurance time correlates with the glycogen content of the muscle. Carbohydrate loading entails these steps: (a) Depleting the muscle glycogen one week before the event by exercising to exhaustion, using the same type of activity that will occur in the competition; (b) consuming a high-protein, high-fat, low-carbohydrate (100 gm.) diet for three days; (c) consuming a moderate-protein, low-fat, high-carbohydrate (250 to 525 gm.) diet for three days immediately preceding the event[38,40-43]. The small amount of carbohydrate recommended during the depletion phase is necessary to prevent the effects of ketosis. During the repleting phase, complex carbohydrates are preferred since they are also useful sources of minerals and vitamins and are more gradually absorbed. Excessive amounts of sugar, candy, soft drinks, and honey are not needed[43].

Carbohydrate loading must not be used indiscriminately[4]. It is of no advantage to the athlete in short-time, high-intensity competition[4,22]. Because water is held with the glycogen that is stored, the weight gain may be as much as 2.5 to 3.5 kg.[27]. This can lead to a feeling of stiffness and heaviness that is a distinct disadvantage to the athlete in competition.

Carbohydrate loading should be used very selectively for high school and college athletes, and rarely, if ever, for early adolescent or preadolescent athletes[42]. Some athletes do not tolerate carbohydrate loading very well and should not attempt it for the first time prior to a competition. Probably the full loading sequence should be used no more than two or three times a year[43].

An athlete with diabetes or hypertriglyceridemia should consult his physician before adopting a carbohydrate loading program[43]. Occasional health impairments have been observed, including chest pains, changes in the electrocardiogram[44], and myoglobinuria, following persistent glycogen loading[45]. Although these changes are uncommon, athletes should seek medical advice if they encounter symptoms.

The American Dietetic Association does not recognize any unique ergogenic values of products such as wheat germ, wheat germ oil, vitamin E, ascorbic acid, lecithin, honey, gelatin, phosphates, sunflower seeds, bee pollen, kelp, or brewer's yeast.

An ergogenic aid is any substance that can increase the ability to work. Many athletes claim that one reason for a successful performance was the inclusion of a particular food or food supplement. This type of testimonial is purely anecdotal and is not supported by scientific studies[4,34,40]. Investigations with vitamin E supplementation[46,47] and ascorbic acid supplementation[48] showed that performance was no better with the supplement than with the placebo.

For those engaging in athletic events, The American Dietetic Association does not advocate the use of beer, wine, or distilled alcoholic beverages as a source of calories, as a muscle relaxant, or as an ergogenic aid.

Although alcohol is a ready source of energy for muscular work, its use by athletes is not recommended. Alcohol is a depressant of the central nervous system. It accentuates fatigue by increasing the production of lactate[49]. It interferes with the nervous system by slowing the reaction time; interfering with voluntary and involuntary reflexes; and reducing the responsiveness, reaction time, and coordination[49,50]. Alcohol has a diuretic effect that increases the loss of body water, thus contributing to dehydration.

The American Dietetic Association maintains that future research is needed on the usefulness of caffeine as a stimulus to fatty acid mobilization.

Initially, in endurance competition, carbohydrate furnishes about 90 per cent of the energy, and fat about 10 per cent. As the competition continues, less energy is derived from carbohydrate and more from free fatty acids. By the end of the competition, most of the energy is derived from free fatty acids[24].

With improved fat utilization, the depletion of glycogen is retarded, and endurance is enhanced[20]. Some claims have been made that caffeine ingested 1 hr. prior to exercise stimulates the release of free fatty acids[8,51], thus sparing glycogen; others do not support the use of caffeine[4].

The suggested intake is from 4 to 5 mg. per kilogram body weight. For a 70-kg. person, this is equivalent to about two cups of coffee (approximately 150 mg. caffeine per cup). For most persons, such moderate consumption probably has no harmful effect[4].

Some persons are more sensitive than others to the effects of caffeine. When a person ingests 1 gm. caffeine (six to seven cups coffee) or more, effects on the central nervous system and circulatory system include insomnia, excitement, restlessness, ringing of the ears, tachycardia, extrasystoles, and quickened respiration. Gastric irritation often occurs, and muscles become tense. Diuresis can accentuate losses of body fluids[49].

The American Dietetic Association recommends that a light pre-game meal be eaten 3 to 4 hr. prior to the competition.

The stomach should be empty at the time of competition. If an athlete begins to exercise immediately after ingesting food, he/she may experience gastrointestinal distress, including nausea, vomiting, stomach fullness, or cramping. The digestion of food and absorption of nutrients competes with muscle metabolism for the blood supply. The result may be a diminished blood supply to the working muscle. A 3- to 4-hr. interval between meal time and training or competition will minimize any gastrointestinal discomfort.

Athletes vary in their assimilation and tolerance of foods. These differences are accentuated during physical and mental stress. Thus, the best pre-game meal is one with familiar foods that the athlete tolerates well and is convinced will help him/her to win[4,8]. Some athletes experience discomfort when they eat foods that are gas-producing or that are highly spiced.

The pre-game meal should include some protein, a minimal amount of fat, and a liberal level of complex carbohydrates. It might include moderate amounts of lean meat, poultry, or fish, vegetables, fruits, and bread. Milk—long tabooed in the past—may be drunk[4]. There is no evidence that liquid meals are tolerated better than solid meals.

Small amounts of carbohydrate taken up to an hour before competition are not harmful but probably do no good. Large amounts of simple sugars are not recommended, for they may cause a surge in the release of insulin and subsequent hypoglycemia.

The American Dietetic Association recommends that athletes not currently involved in training or competition should reduce their caloric intake to balance their energy expenditure.

Caloric expenditure is substantially reduced when the athlete is not involved in training or competition. To maintain desirable body weight and levels of body fatness, the caloric intake must be substantially reduced. The recommendations made for diet and for exercise for the general public are appropriate during the interim or off-season period.

REFERENCES

1. FOX, S.M., NAUGHTON, J.P., and HASKELL, W.L.: Physical activity and the prevention of coronary heart disease. Ann. Clin. Res. 3:404, 1971.
2. GYNTELBERG, F., BRENNAN, R., HOLLOSZY, J.O., SCHONFELD, G., RENNIE, M.J., and WEIDMAN, S.W.: Plasma triglyceride lowering by exercise despite increased food intake in patients with type IV hyperlipoproteinemia. Am. J. Clin. Nutr. 35:716, 1977.
3. PASSMORE, R., and DURNIN, J.V.G.A.: Human energy expenditures. Physiol. Rev. 35: 801, 1955.
4. JENSEN, C.R., and FISHER, A.G.: Scientific Basis of Athletic Conditioning. 2nd ed. Philadelphia: Lea & Febiger, 1979.
5. PÂŘÍZKOVÁ, J.: Impact of age, diet and exercise on man's body composition. Ann. N.Y. Acad. Sci. 110:661, 1963.
6. KEYS, A., and GRANDE, F.: Body weight, body composition and calorie status. *In* Goodhart, R.S., and Shils, M.E., eds: Modern Nutrition in Health and Disease. 5th ed. Philadelphia: Lea & Febiger, 1973, pp. 1–27.
7. PIKE, R.L., and BROWN, M.L.: Nutrition: An Integrated Approach, 2nd ed. N.Y.: John Wiley & Sons, Inc., 1975, pp. 757–813.
8. FOX, E.L.: Sports Physiology. Philadelphia: W.B. Saunders Co., 1979.
9. DAVIDSON, S., PASSMORE, R., BROCK, J.F., and TRUSWELL, A.S.: Human Nutrition and Dietetics. 6th ed. London: Churchill Livingstone, 1975, p. 289.

10. YOUNG, C.M., BLONDIN, J., TENSUAN, R., and FRYER, J.H.: Body composition of "older" women. J. Am. Dietet. A. 43:344, 1963.
11. KEYS, A., and BROZEK, J.: Body fat in adult men. Physiol. Rev. 33:245, 1953.
12. EDWARDS, D.A.W., HAMMOND, W.H., HEALY, M.J.R., TANNER, J.M., and WHITEHOUSE, R.H.: Design and accuracy of calipers for measuring subcutaneous tissue thickness. Br. J. Nutr. 9:133, 1955.
13. SELTZER, C.C., and MAYER, J.A.: A simple criterion of obesity. Postgrad. Med. 38: A101 (Aug.). 1965.
14. DURNIN, J.V.G.A., and WOMERSLEY, J.: Body fat assessed from total body density and its estimation from skinfold thickness: Measurements on 481 men and women aged from 16 to 72 years. Br. J. Nutr. 32:77, 1974.
15. YUHASZ, M.S.: Assessment of Percentage Body Fat from Skinfold. Physical Fitness and Sports Appraisal. A Laboratory Manual. London, Ont., Canada: Univ. of Western Ontario.
16. FOOD & NUTR. BD.: Recommended Dietary Allowances. 9th rev. ed. Washington, D.C.: Natl. Acad. Sci., 1980.
17. AM. COLL. SPORTS MED.: Position paper: The recommended quantity and quality of exercise for developing and maintaining fitness in healthy adults. Med. Sci. Sports, 10: vii (3), 1978.
18. VAN HUSS, W.D.: Physical activity and aging. *In* Strauss, R.H., ed: Sports Medicine and Physiology. Philadelphia: W.B. Saunders Co., 1979.
19. CONSOLAZIO, C.F.: Protein metabolism during intensive physical training in the young adult. Am. J. Clin. Nutr. 28:29, 1975.
20. LEWIS, S., and GUTIN, B.: Nutrition and endurance. Am. J. Clin. Nutr. 26:1011, 1973.
21. IRWIN, M.I., and HEGSTED, D.M.: A conspectus of research on protein requirements of man. J. Nutr. 101:385, 1971.
22. BERGSTROM, J., and HULTMAN, E.: Nutrition for maximal sports performance. J.A.M.A. 221:999, 1972.
23. AM. COLL. SPORTS MED.: Position statement: Prevention of heat injuries during distance running. Med. Sci. Sports 7:vii(1), 1975.
24. COSTILL, D.L.: Physiology of marathon running. J.A.M.A. 221:1024, 1972.
25. WILLIAMS, M.H.: Nutritional Aspects of Human Physical and Athletic Performance. Springfield, Ill.: Charles C. Thomas, 1976.
26. COSTILL, D.L.: Water and electrolytes. *In* Morgan, W., ed.: Ergogenic Aids and Muscular Performance. N.Y.: Academic Press, 1972, pp. 293–320.
27. OLLSON, K., and SALTIN, B.: Diet and fluids in training and competition. Scand. J. Rehab. Med. 3:31, 1971.
28. COMM. ON NUTRITIONAL MISINFORMATION, FOOD & NUTR. BD.: Water deprivation and performance of athletes. Nutr. Rev. 32:314, 1974.
29. SMITH, N.J.: Gaining and losing weight in athletics. J.A.M.A. 236:149, 1976.

30. COSTILL, D.L., and SALTIN, B.: Factors limiting gastric emptying during rest and exercise. J. Appl. Physiol. 37:679, 1974.
31. CONSOLAZIO, C.F., MATOUSH, L.O., NELSON, R.A., HARDING, R.S., and CANHAM, J.E.: Excretion of sodium, potassium, magnesium and iron in human sweat and the relation of each to balance and requirements. J. Nutr. 79:407, 1963.
32. WEST, E.S., TODD, W.R., MASON, H.S., and VAN BRUGGEN, J.T.: Textbook of Biochemistry. 4th ed. N.Y.: Macmillan Publishing Co., 1966, p. 686.
33. FOOD & NUTR. BD.: Recommended Dietary Allowances. 8th rev. ed. Washington, D.C.: Natl. Acad. Sci., 1974, pp. 88–91.
34. MAYER, J., and BULLEN, B.: Nutrition and athletic performance. Physiol. Rev. 40:369, 1960.
35. MURPHY, R.J.: Heat illness and athletics. *In* Strauss, R.H., ed.: Sports Medicine and Physiology. Philadelphia: W.B. Saunders Co., 1979, pp. 320–26.
36. LANE, H.W., and CERDA, J.J.: Potassium requirements and exercise. J. Am. Dietet. A. 73:64, 1978.
37. SHILS, M.E.: Food and nutrition relating to work and environmental stress. *In* Goodhart, R.S., and Shils, M.E., eds.: Modern Nutrition in Health and Disease. 5th ed. Philadelphia Lea & Febiger, 1973, pp. 722–24.
38. BERGSTROM, J., HERMANSEN, L., HULTMAN, E., and SALTIN, B.: Diet, muscle glycogen and physical performance. Acta Physiol. Scand. 71:140, 1967.
39. CONSOLAZIO, C.F., and JOHNSTON, H.L.: Dietary carbohydrate and work capacity. Am. J. Clin. Nutr. 25:85, 1972.
40. HORSTMAN, D.H.: Nutrition. *In* Morgan, W., ed.: Ergogenic Aids and Muscular Performance. N.Y.: Academic Press, 1972, pp. 343–397.
41. KARLSSON, J., and SALTIN, B.: Diet, muscle glycogen and endurance performance. J. Appl. Physiol. 31:203, 1971.
42. SMITH, N.J.: Nutrition and the athlete. *In* Strauss, R.H., ed.: Sports Medicine and Physiology. Philadelphia: W.B. Saunders Co., 1979, pp. 271–81.
43. FORGAC, N.T.: Carbohydrate loading. A review. J. Am. Dietet. A. 75:42, 1979.
44. MIRKIN, G.: Carbohydrate loading. A dangerous practice (letter). J.A.M.A. 223:1511, 1973.
45. BANK, W.J.: Myoglobinuria in marathon runners. Possible relationship to carbohydrate and lipid metabolism. Ann. N.Y. Acad. Sci. 301:942, 1977.
46. LAWRENCE, J.D., BOWER, R.C., RIEHL, W.P., and SMITH, J.L.: Effect of α-tocopherol acetate on the swimming endurance of trained swimmers. Am. J. Clin. Nutr. 28:205, 1975.
47. SHARMAN, I.M., DOWN, M.G., and SEN, R.N.: The effects of vitamin E and training on physiological function and athletic performance in adolescent swimmers. Br. J. Nutr. 26:265, 1971.

48. GEY, G.O., COOPER, K.H., and BOTTENBERG, R.A.: Effect of ascorbic acid on endurance performance and athletic injury. J.A.M.A. 211:105, 1970.
49. GOODMAN, L.S., and GILMAN, A., ed: The Pharmacological Basis of Therapeutics. 5th ed. N.Y.: Macmillan Publishing Co., 1975, pp. 137, 373.
50. HANLEY, D.F.: Drug use and abuse. *In* Strauss, R.H., ed.: Sports Medicine and Physiology. Philadelphia: W.B. Saunders Co., 1979, pp. 396–404.
51. COSTILL, D.L., DALSKY, G., and FINK, W.J.: Effects of caffeine ingestion on metabolism and exercise performance. Med. Sci. Sports 10:155, 1978.

Reading list

ASTRAND, P., and RODAHL, K.: Textbook of Work Physiology. N.Y.: McGraw-Hill Book Co., 1970.

DARDEN, E.: Nutrition and Athletic Performance. San Marino, Calif.: Athletic Press, 1976.

MATHEWS, D.K., and FOX, E.L.: The Physiological Basis of Physical Education and Athletics. Philadelphia: W.B. Saunders Co., 1976.

NUTRITION FOR ATHLETES. A Handbook for Coaches. Washington, D.C.: Am. Assoc. for Health, Physical Education & Recreation (with cooperation from The Am. Dietet. Assoc. and The Nutr. Foundation), 1971.

SMITH, N.F.: Food for Sport. Palo Alto, Calif.: Bull Publishing Co., 1976.

WILLIAMS, M.H.: Nutritional Aspects of Human Physical and Athletic Performance. Springfield, Ill.: Charles C. Thomas, 1976.

ZOHMAN, L.R.: Beyond Diet . . . Exercise Your Way to Fitness and Heart Health. Englewood Cliffs, N.J.: Best Foods, 1974.

Appendix B

APPENDIX B.1. NUTRITIVE VALUES OF THE EDIBLE PART OF FOODS *(Continued)*

(Dashes show that no basis could be found for computing a value although there was some reason to believe that a measurable amount of the constituent might be present.)

Food, approximate measure, and weight (in grams)	Approx. Measure	Grams	Water %	Calories	Protein gm.	Fat (Total lipid) gm.	Fatty Acids: Saturated gm.	Fatty Acids: Unsaturated Oleic gm.	Fatty Acids: Unsaturated Linoleic gm.	Carbohydrate gm	Calcium mg.	Iron mg.	Vitamin A I.U.	Thiamine mg.	Riboflavin mg.	Niacin mg.	Ascorbic Acid mg.
MILK, CREAM, CHEESE; RELATED PRODUCTS																	
Milk, cow's:																	
Fluid, whole (3.7% fat)	1 cup	244	87	161	9	9	5	2	Trace	12	285	Trace	366	.07	.41	.2	2
Fluid, nonfat (skim)	1 cup	246	90	88	9	Trace	—	—	—	12	295	Trace	Trace	.10	.44	.2	2
Cheese																	
Cheddar	1 oz. slice	28	37	113	7	9	5	3	Trace	1	213	.3	372	Trace	.13	Trace	0
Cottage creamed	1 cup	225	78	239	31	10	5	2	Trace	7	212	.7	383	.07	.56	.2	0
Ice cream, vanilla	1 scoop	71	62	147	3	9	5	3	Trace	15	87	.1	369	.03	.13	.1	1
EGGS																	
Raw, whole	1 med	50	74	78	6	6	2	3	Trace	Trace	26	1.1	562	.04	.12	Trace	0
MEAT, POULTRY, FISH, SHELLFISH; RELATED PRODUCTS																	
Beef, cooked:																	
Rump Roast: Choice grade																	
Lean and fat	4 oz.	113	48	268	18	21	10	10	1	0	8	2.4	39	.05	.14	3.3	0
Lean only (visible fat removed at table)	4 oz.	113	60	120	17	6	3	3	Trace	0	7	2.2	11	.04	.13	3.0	0
Loin chop	1 thin slice	68	55	113	13	6	2	3	1	0	6	1.7	0	.48	.14	2.9	0
Lamb, cooked:																	
Roast leg, choice grade	4 oz.	113	54	206	19	14	8	5	Trace	0	8	1.2	0	.11	.20	4.0	0
Veal, cooked:																	
Cutlet, medium fat	3 oz.	85	60	235	28	13	6	5	Trace	0	9	3.6	0	.10	.27	5.4	0
Chicken, cooked:																	
Fryer, ¼ whole, med.		85	54	255	38	10	3	5	1	0	15	2.3	215	.08	.45	12	0
Fish, cooked:																	
Swordfish, broiled	3½ oz.	100	65	174	28	6	—	—	—	0	27	1.3	2,050	.04	.05	10.9	0
Tuna, packed in oil	½ cup	115	61	223	33	9	3	2	2	0	9	2.1	91	.05	.13	13	—
Shrimp	4 oz.	113	70	132	28	1	—	—	—	Trace	130	3.5	68	.01	.03	2.0	—
Bacon, broiled or fried	2 slices	14	8	96	4	7	2	4	1	Trace	2	.4	0	.08	.04	.8	0
Frankfurter, cooked	1 med	51	58	152	6	14	—	—	—	1	3	.8	—	.08	.10	1.3	—
Liver, calf, broiled	4 oz.	113	51	221	33	7	—	—	—	4	15	16.1	37,114	.27	4.73	19	42

APPENDIX B.1. NUTRITIVE VALUES OF THE EDIBLE PART OF FOODS *(Continued)*

(Dashes show that no basis could be found for computing a value although there was some reason to believe that a measurable amount of the constituent might be present.)

Food, approximate measure, and weight (in grams)	Approx. Measure	Grams	Water %	Calories	Protein gm.	Fat (Total lipid) gm.	Fatty Acids: Saturated gm.	Fatty Acids: Unsaturated Oleic gm.	Fatty Acids: Unsaturated Linoleic gm.	Carbohydrate gm	Calcium mg.	Iron mg.	Vitamin A I.U.	Thiamine mg.	Riboflavin mg.	Niacin mg.	Ascorbic Acid mg.
VEGETABLES AND VEGETABLE PRODUCTS																	
Asparagus, cooked	1 cup	181	94	36	4	Trace	—	—	—	7	38	1.1	1,629	.29	.33	2.5	47
Beans:																	
Lima, cooked	1 cup	166	71	164	10	Trace	—	—	—	32	33	2.8	382	.12	.08	1.7	28
Snap, green, cooked	1 cup	125	92	31	2	Trace	—	—	—	7	63	.8	675	.09	.11	.6	15
Baked, with tomato, molasses	1 cup	187	76	309	14	8	2	2	Trace	45	134	4.8	148	.16	.09	1.4	2
Beets, cooked	1 cup	167	91	52	2	Trace	—	—	—	12	23	.8	33	.05	.07	.5	10
Broccoli, cooked	1 cup	164	91	43	5	1	—	—	—	7	144	1.3	4,100	.15	.33	1.3	148
Cabbage:																	
Coleslaw, raw	1 cup	120	83	119	1	9	1	2	5	10	52	.5	180	.06	.06	.4	35
Cooked	1 cup	146	94	29	2	Trace	—	—	—	6	64	.4	190	.06	.06	.4	48
Carrots, cooked, diced	1 cup	160	91	50	1	Trace	—	—	—	11	53	1.0	16,800	.08	.08	.8	10
Cauliflower, cooked	1 cup	125	93	28	3	Trace	—	—	—	5	26	.9	75	.11	.10	.8	69
Celery, raw	1 stalk	40	94	5	Trace	Trace	—	—	—	1	12	.1	72	.01	.01	.1	3
Corn, sweet																	
Cooked	1 ear	100	73	91	3	1	—	—	—	21	3	.6	400	.12	.10	1.4	9
Canned	1 cup	169	81	140	5	2	—	—	—	32	5	1.0	676	.19	.17	2.2	12
Cucumbers, raw, whole	1 small	100	96	15	1	Trace	—	—	—	3	25	1.1	250	.03	.04	.2	11
Lettuce, leaf	1 med	10	94	2	Trace	Trace	—	—	—	1	4	.1	59	.01	.01	.1	1
Mushrooms, canned	1 cup	161	93	31	2	Trace	—	—	—	6	13	1.3	Trace	.03	.39	3.2	—
Onions, cooked	1 cup	197	92	57	2	Trace	—	—	—	13	47	.8	79	.06	.06	.4	14
Parsnips, cooked	1 cup	211	82	139	3	1	—	—	—	31	95	1.3	63	.15	.17	.2	21
Peas, cooked	1 cup	160	82	114	9	1	—	—	—	20	32	3.2	1,002	.45	.15	2.8	22
Peppers, sweet, green	1 shell	62	93	13	1	Trace	—	—	—	3	5	.4	239	.05	.05	.3	73
Potatoes, medium:																	
Baked, peeled	1 potato	99	75	93	3	Trace	—	—	—	21	9	.7	Trace	.10	.04	1.7	20
Peeled, boiled	1 potato	122	83	79	2	Trace	—	—	—	18	7	.6	Trace	.11	.04	1.5	20
French-fried	10 pieces	57	45	156	2	8	2	2	4	21	9	.7	Trace	.07	.05	1.8	12
Mashed with milk and margarine	1 cup	195	80	183	4	8	4	3	Trace	24	47	.8	332	.16	.10	2.0	18
Potato chips	10 med	20	2	114	1	8	2	2	4	10	8	.4	Trace	.04	.01	1.0	3

APPENDIX B.1. NUTRITIVE VALUES OF THE EDIBLE PART OF FOODS *(Continued)*

(Dashes show that no basis could be found for computing a value although there was some reason to believe that a measurable amount of the constituent might be present.)

Food, approximate measure, and weight (in grams)	Approx. Measure	Grams	Water %	Calories	Protein gm.	Fat (Total lipid) gm.	Fatty Acids: Saturated gm.	Fatty Acids: Unsaturated Oleic gm.	Fatty Acids: Unsaturated Linoleic gm.	Carbohydrate gm	Calcium mg.	Iron mg.	Vitamin A I.U.	Thiamine mg.	Riboflavin mg.	Niacin mg.	Ascorbic Acid mg.
Vegetables, cont.																	
Pumpkin, canned	1 cup	228	90	75	2	1	—	—	—	18	57	.9	14,590	.07	.11	1.4	11
Radishes	4 small	40	94	7	Trace	Trace	—	—	—	1	12	.4	4	.01	.01	.1	10
Sauerkraut, canned	1 cup	188	93	34	2	Trace	—	—	—	8	68	.9	94	.06	.08	.4	26
Spinach, cooked	1 cup	180	92	46	6	1	—	—	—	7	186	4.4	16,200	.14	.28	1.0	56
Squash, summer, cooked, diced	1 cup	136	96	19	1	Trace	—	—	—	4	34	.5	530	.07	.11	1.1	14
Sweet potatoes, baked	1 potato	110	64	169	3	1	—	—	—	39	48	1.1	9,720	.11	.08	.8	26
Tomatoes, raw	1 med	120	94	25	1	Trace	—	—	—	5	15	.6	1,021	.07	.05	.8	26
Tomato juice, canned	1 cup	242	94	47	2	Trace	—	—	—	11	17	2.2	1,976	.12	.07	2.0	40
FRUITS AND FRUIT PRODUCTS																	
Apples, raw	1 med	150	85	64	Trace	1	—	—	—	16	8	.3	99	.03	.02	.1	4
Apple juice	1 cup	249	88	116	Trace	Trace	—	—	—	29	15	1.5	—	.02	.05	.2	2
Apricots																	
Raw	1 med	40	85	21	Trace	Trace	—	—	—	5	7	.2	1,134	.01	.02	.3	4
Canned	4 halves; 2 tbsp. syrup	122	77	103	1	Trace	—	—	—	26	17	.5	2,777	.03	.03	.6	6
Avocados, raw, cubed	¼ cup	36	74	59	1	6	1	3	1	4	13	.2	103	.04	.07	.6	5
Bananas, raw	1med	150	76	88	1	Trace	—	—	—	23	8	.7	196	.05	.06	.7	10
Blackberries, raw	1 cup	144	84	84	2	1	—	—	—	19	46	1.3	288	.04	.06	.6	30
Cantaloupe	½ med	385	91	56	1	Trace	—	—	—	14	26	.8	6,290	.08	.06	1.1	61
Cherries, raw, sweet	1 cup	130	80	108	2	1	—	—	—	27	34	.6	169	.08	.09	.6	15
Cranberry juice	1 cup	250	83	161	Trace	Trace	—	—	—	41	12	.7	Trace	.02	.02	Trace	99
Fruit cocktail, canned	1 cup	229	80	137	1	Trace	—	—	—	36	21	.9	321	.05	.02	1.1	5
GRAIN PRODUCTS																	
Bread, rolls, etc.:																	
Biscuit, baking powder	1 (2½″ diam)	38	27	129	3	6	2	3	1	16	42	.6	Trace	.07	.07	.6	Trace
Corn muffin	1 muffin	48	33	141	3	5	2	2	Trace	21	47	.8	135	.09	.10	.7	Trace
White bread, enr.	1 slice	23	36	62	2	1	—	—	—	12	19	.6	Trace	.06	.05	.6	Trace
Whole wheat bread	1 slice	23	45	56	2	1	—	—	—	11	23	.5	0	.06	.03	.6	0

APPENDIX B.1. NUTRITIVE VALUES OF THE EDIBLE PART OF FOODS *(Continued)*

(Dashes show that no basis could be found for computing a value although there was some reason to believe that a measurable amount of the constituent might be present.)

Food, approximate measure, and weight (in grams)	Approx. Measure	Grams	Water %	Calories	Protein gm.	Fat (Total lipid) gm.	Fatty Acids: Saturated gm.	Fatty Acids: Unsaturated Oleic gm.	Fatty Acids: Unsaturated Linoleic gm.	Carbohydrate gm	Calcium mg.	Iron mg.	Vitamin A I.U.	Thiamine mg.	Riboflavin mg.	Niacin mg.	Ascorbic Acid mg.
Grain products, cont.																	
Rye bread, light	1 slice	23	36	56	2	Trace	—	—	—	12	17	.4	0	.04	.02	.3	0
Plain enriched roll	1 med	38	31	113	3	2	Trace	1	Trace	20	28	.7	Trace	.11	.07	.8	Trace
Hard roll	1 med	52	25	162	5	2	Trace	1	Trace	31	24	1.2	Trace	.14	.12	1.4	Trace
Sweet roll	1 med	55	32	174	5	5	1	2	Trace	27	47	.4	39	.04	.08	.4	Trace
Cakes:																	
Angel food	1 (2″ sector)	40	32	104	2	Trace	—	—	—	24	38	.1	0	Trace	.04	Trace	0
Chocolate, (chocolate frosting)	1 (2″ sector)	120	22	407	5	15	6	7	1	70	71	1.0	180	.04	.10	.4	Trace
Fruitcake, dark	2″ sq.	30	18	114	1	5	—	—	—	18	22	.8	36	.04	.04	.2	Trace
Cupcake, plain	1 med	60	24	204	2	7	1	3	Trace	34	32	.2	74	.01	.04	.1	Trace
Pound cake	1 slice	30	17	123	2	6	2	3	Trace	16	12	.2	87	.01	.03	.1	Trace
Doughnuts (cake type)	1 med	32	24	125	2	6	1	4	Trace	16	13	.4	26	.05	.05	.4	Trace
Cookies:																	
Plain and assorted	1 cookie	25	3	82	1	3	—	—	—	12	6	.1	14	.01	.01	.1	Trace
Bar cookie	1 bar	16	14	60	1	2	—	—	—	10	11	.2	19	.01	.01	.1	Trace
Crackers:																	
Graham, plain	1 sq.	7	6	27	1	1	—	—	—	5	3	.1	0	Trace	.01	.1	0
Saltine, 2″ sq.	2	8	4	28	1	Trace	—	—	—	5	2	Trace	0	Trace	Trace	Trace	0
Cereals (prepared):																	
Bran flakes (40%)	1 cup	38	3	115	4	1	—	—	—	31	27	1.7	0	.15	.06	2.4	0
Corn flakes	1 cup	28	4	108	2	Trace	—	—	—	24	5	.4	0	.12	.02	.6	0
Corn, wheat, rice flakes	1 cup	22	3	88	1	Trace	—	—	—	20	7	.4	0	.08	.01	1.2	0
Puffed wheat	1 cup	14	3	51	2	Trace	—	—	—	11	4	.6	0	.08	.03	1.1	0
Rice krispies	1 cup	28	4	109	1	Trace	—	—	—	25	13	.3	0	.09	—	1.3	0
Shredded wheat	1 biscuit	28	7	99	3	1	—	—	—	22	12	1.0	0	.06	.03	1.2	0
Wheat flakes	1 cup	28	4	99	3	Trace	—	—	—	23	11	1.2	0	.18	.04	1.4	0
Cereals (cooked):																	
Cream of wheat	1 cup	215	90	103	3	Trace	—	—	—	21	144	.6	0	.12	.07	1.0	0
Oatmeal	1 cup	236	87	132	5	2	—	—	—	23	22	1.4	0	.19	.05	.2	0

APPENDIX B.1. NUTRITIVE VALUES OF THE EDIBLE PART OF FOODS *(Continued)*

(Dashes show that no basis could be found for computing a value although there was some reason to believe that a measurable amount of the constituent might be present.)

Food, approximate measure, and weight (in grams)	Approx. Measure	Grams	Water %	Calories	Protein gm.	Fat (Total lipid) gm.	Fatty Acids: Saturated gm.	Fatty Acids: Unsaturated Oleic gm.	Fatty Acids: Unsaturated Linoleic gm.	Carbohydrate gm	Calcium mg.	Iron mg.	Vitamin A I.U.	Thiamine mg.	Riboflavin mg.	Niacin mg.	Ascorbic Acid mg.
Grain products, cont.																	
Cereal Products:																	
Macaroni, enr. cooked	1 cup	140	64	155	5	1	—	—	—	32	11	1.3	0	.20	.11	1.5	0
Noodles, egg, cooked	1 cup	160	70	200	7	2	—	—	—	37	16	1.4	112	.22	.13	1.9	0
Rice, white, enriched, cooked	1 cup	193	73	210	4	Trace	—	—	—	47	19	1.7	0	.21	.06	1.9	0
Spaghetti, enr., cooked	1 cup	160	72	178	5	1	—	—	—	37	13	1.4	0	.22	.13	1.8	0
PIES																	
Fruit	1/7 cut	135	48	343	3	15	4	9	1	51	15	1.1	416	.11	.09	1.4	3
Custard	1/7 cut	130	58	283	8	14	5	8	1	30	125	1.2	299	.10	.25	.8	0
Lemon Meringue	1/7 cut	120	47	306	4	12	4	7	1	45	17	1.0	204	.07	.13	.6	4
Mince	1/7 cut	135	43	366	3	16	4	10	1	56	38	1.9	Trace	.18	.11	1.2	1
Pumpkin	1/7 cut	130	59	274	5	15	5	7	1	32	66	1.2	3,211	.12	.18	1.3	Trace
FATS AND OILS																	
Butter	1 pat	7	16	50	Trace	6	3	2	Trace	Trace	1	0	230	—	—	—	0
Margarine	1 pat	7	16	50	Trace	6	1	3	1	Trace	1	0	230	—	—	—	0
Cooking Fats:																	
Lard	1 Tbsp	14	0	126	0	14	5	6	1	0	0	0	0	0	0	0	0
Vegetable fats	1 Tbsp	13	0	106	0	12	3	8	1	0	0	0	—	0	0	0	0
Salad Dressing:																	
Commercial, mayonnaise type	1 Tbsp	15	41	65	Trace	6	1	1	3	2	2	Trace	33	Trace	Trace	Trace	—
French	1 Tbsp	15	39	72	Trace	7	1	1	3	2	2	Trace	—	—	—	—	—
Mayonnaise	1 Tbsp	15	15	93	Trace	11	2	3	6	Trace	2	.1	36	Trace	.01	Trace	—
Salad or Cooking Oils:																	
Corn	1 Tbsp	14	0	125	0	14	1	4	7	0	0	0	—	0	0	0	0
Cottonseed	1 Tbsp	14	0	125	0	14	4	3	7	0	0	0	—	0	0	0	0
Olive	1 Tbsp	14	0	125	0	14	2	11	1	0	0	0	—	0	0	0	0
Safflower	1 Tbsp	14	0	125	0	14	1	2	10	0	0	0	—	0	0	0	0
Soybean	1 Tbsp	14	0	125	0	14	2	3	7	0	0	0	—	0	0	0	0

APPENDIX B.1. NUTRITIVE VALUES OF THE EDIBLE PART OF FOODS *(Continued)*

(Dashes show that no basis could be found for computing a value although there was some reason to believe that a measurable amount of the constituent might be present.)

Food, approximate measure, and weight (in grams)	Approx. Measure	Grams	Water %	Calories	Protein gm.	Fat (Total lipid) gm.	Fatty Acids: Saturated gm.	Fatty Acids: Unsaturated Oleic gm.	Fatty Acids: Unsaturated Linoleic gm.	Carbohydrate gm	Calcium mg.	Iron mg.	Vitamin A I.U.	Thiamine mg.	Riboflavin mg.	Niacin mg.	Ascorbic Acid mg.
SUGARS AND SWEETS																	
Chocolate, plain	1 oz.	28	1	147	2	9	5	4	Trace	16	65	.3	77	.02	.10	.1	Trace
Honey	1 Tbsp	21	17	64	Trace	0	0	0	0	17	1	.1	0	Trace	.01	.1	Trace
Jams, jellies, preserves	1 Tbsp	20	29	55	Trace	Trace	—	—	—	14	4	.3	Trace	Trace	.01	Trace	1
Syrup	1 Tbsp	20	24	58	0	0	0	0	0	15	9	.8	0	0	0	0	0
Sugar	1 Tbsp	12	Trace	46	0	0	0	0	0	12	0	Trace	0	0	0	0	0
MISCELLANEOUS ITEMS																	
Beer (3.6% alcohol)	1 bottle	340	92	171	2	0	0	0	0	16	15	0	0	Trace	11	.8	0
Carbonated beverage	8 oz.	240	90	90	0	0	0	0	0	23	—	—	0	0	0	0	0
Nuts:																	
Peanuts, roasted	1 oz.	28	2	160	8	13	3	6	4	5	10	.9	—	.07	.04	5.4	0
Peanut butter	1 Tbsp	16	2	87	4	7	1	4	2	3	9	.3	—	.02	.02	2.4	0
Pizza (cheese)	1 (5½″ pc)	75	45	184	7	5	2	3	Trace	27	117	.7	303	.05	.13	.8	5
Popcorn with margarine	1 cup	28	3	155	2	12	3	7	2	11	5	.4	462	—	.02	.3	0
Soups, canned:																	
Noodle type	1 cup	250	93	68	4	2	Trace	1	1	8	10	.8	113	.03	.05	1.0	Trace
Tomato	1 cup	245	90	88	2	3	—	—	—	16	15	.7	1,005	.05	.05	1.2	12

APPENDIX B.2. ANTHROPOMETRIC CHARTS FOR INFANT BOYS, INFANT GIRLS, BOYS AND GIRLS[1]

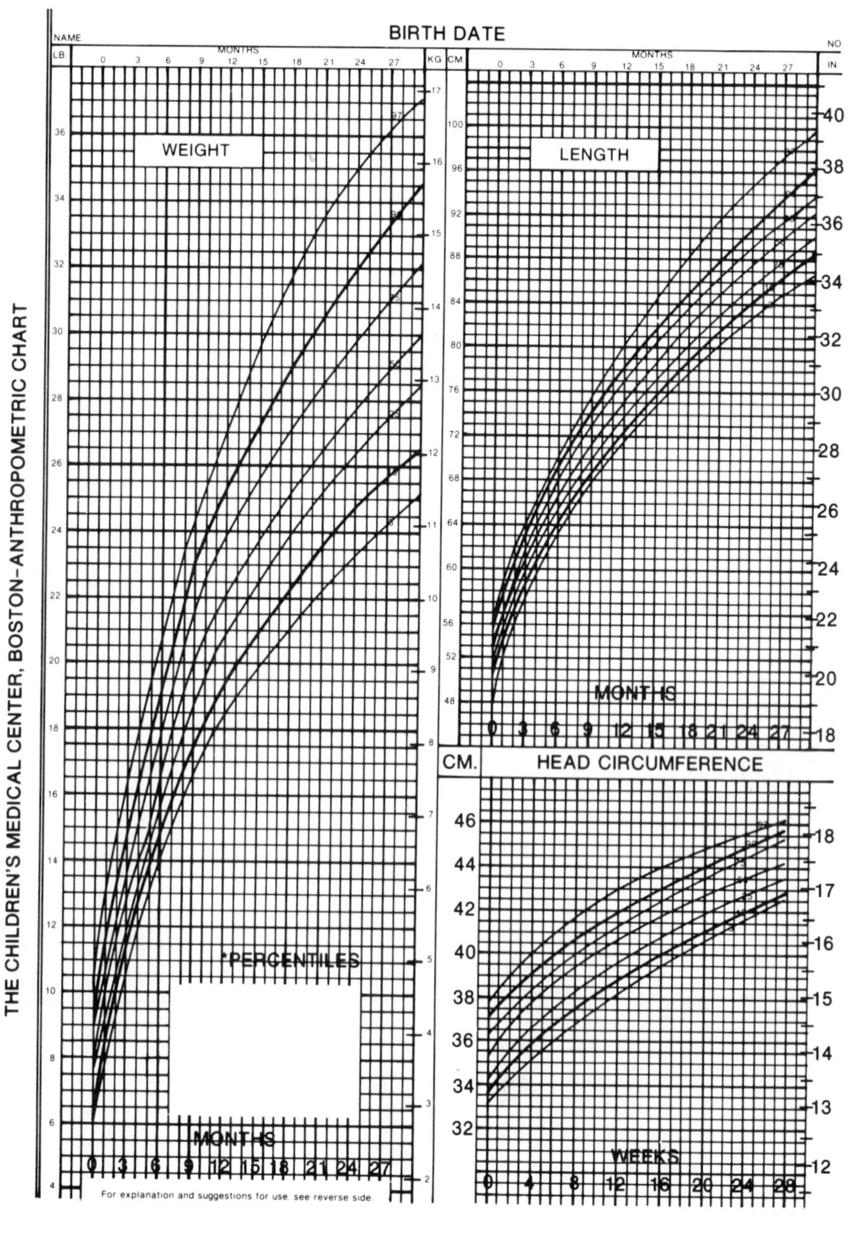

[1] From the Children's Medical Center, Boston, Massachusetts.

APPENDIX B.2. *(Cont'd.)*

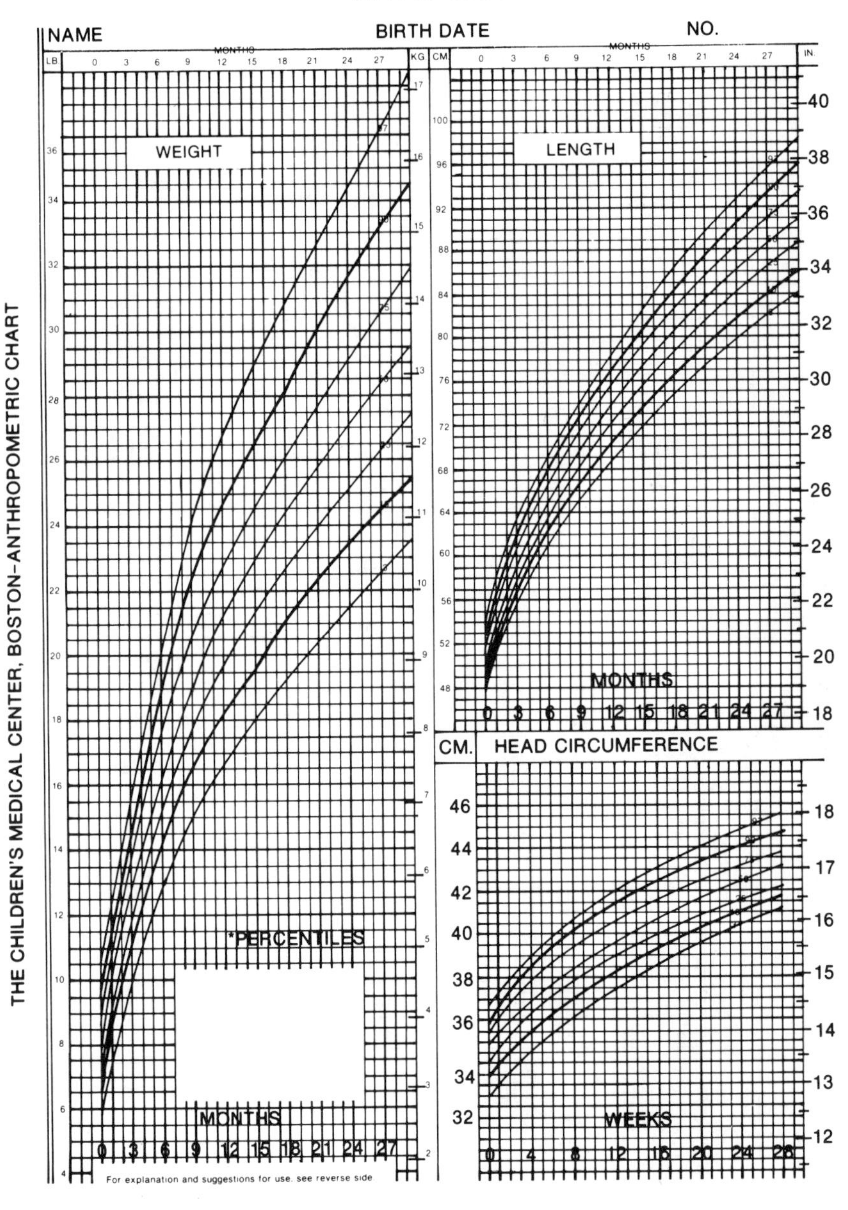

APPENDIX B.2. *(Cont'd.)*

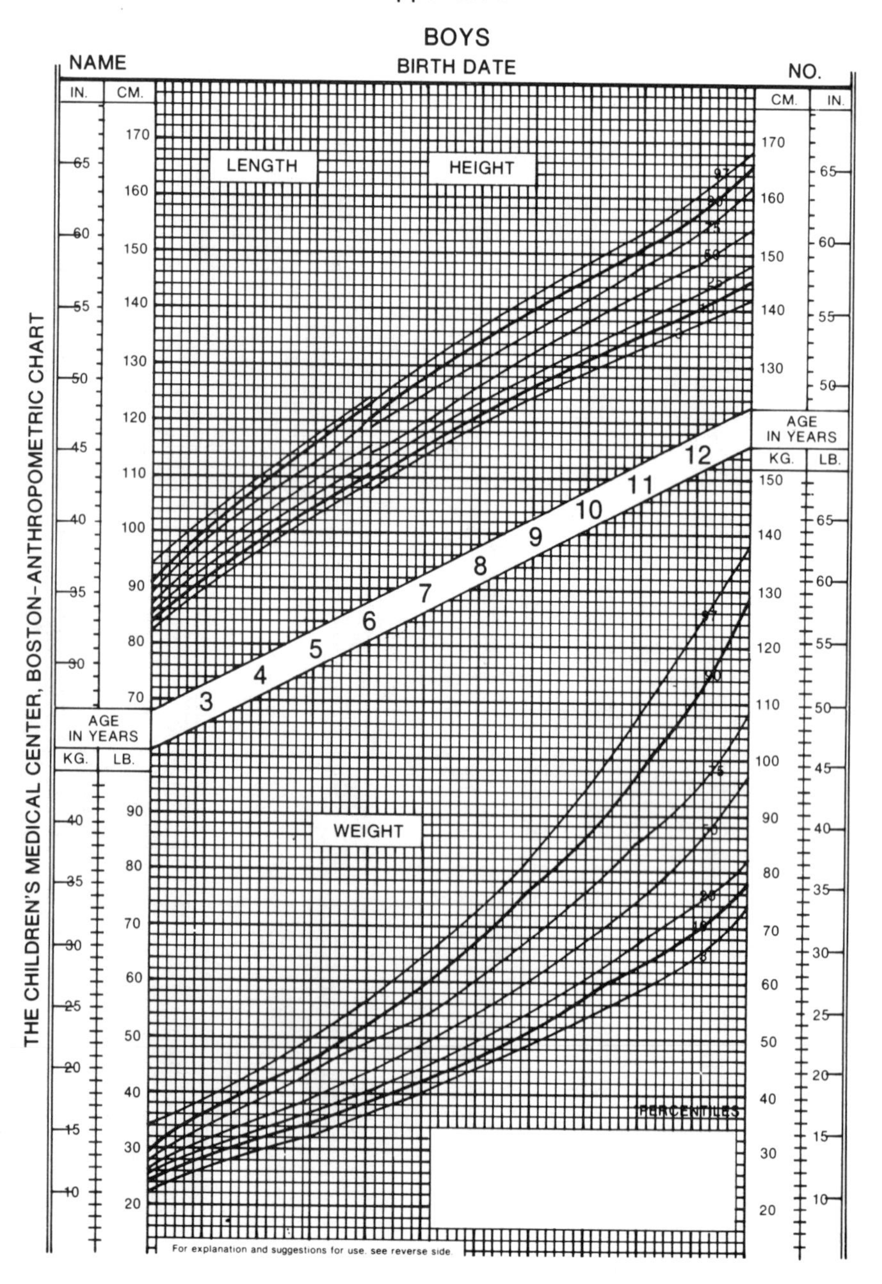

APPENDIX B.2. *(Cont'd.)*

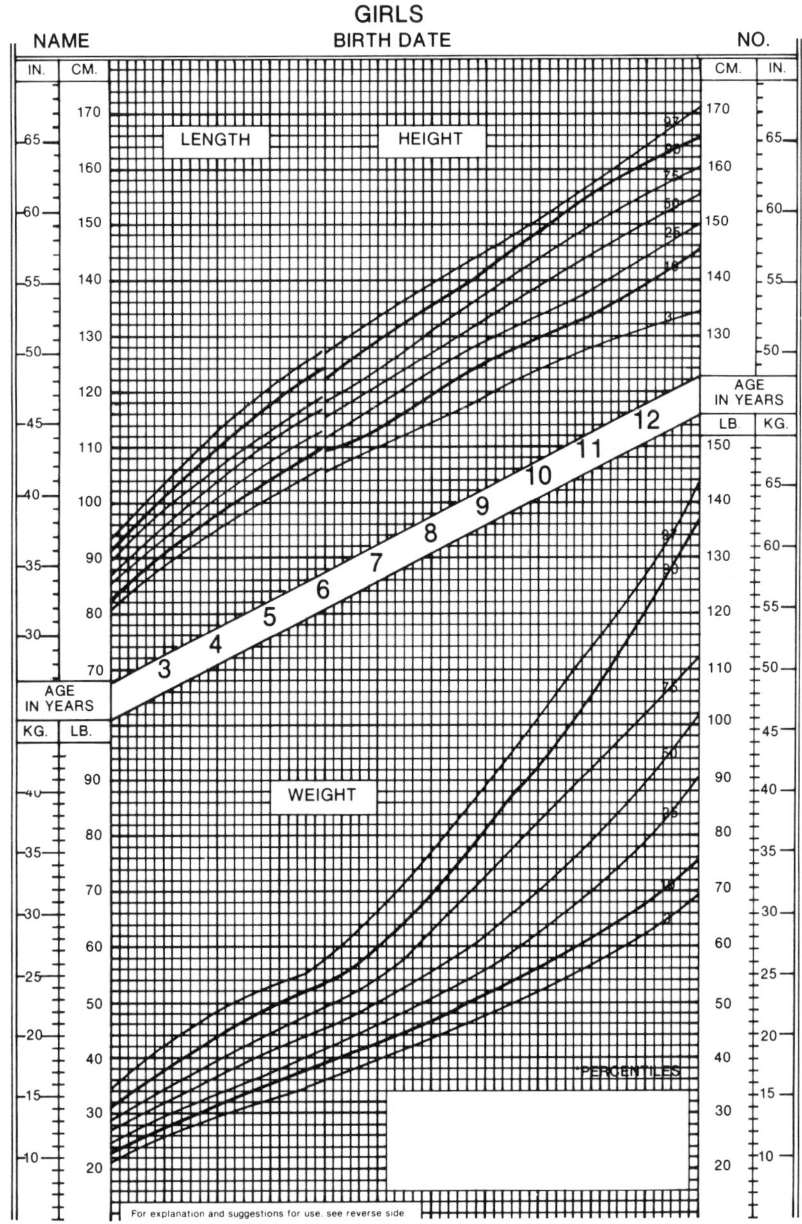

APPENDIX B.3. HEAD CIRCUMFERENCE GRAPHS FOR MALES AND FEMALES FROM BIRTH THROUGH 18 YEARS

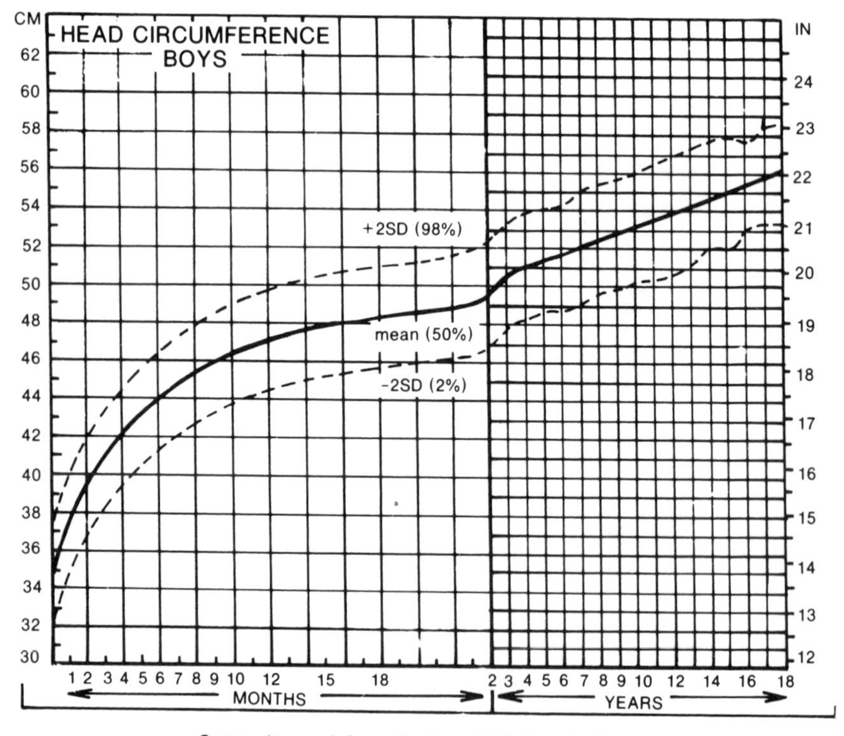

Composite graph for males from birth through 18 years

APPENDIX B.3. *(Cont'd.)*

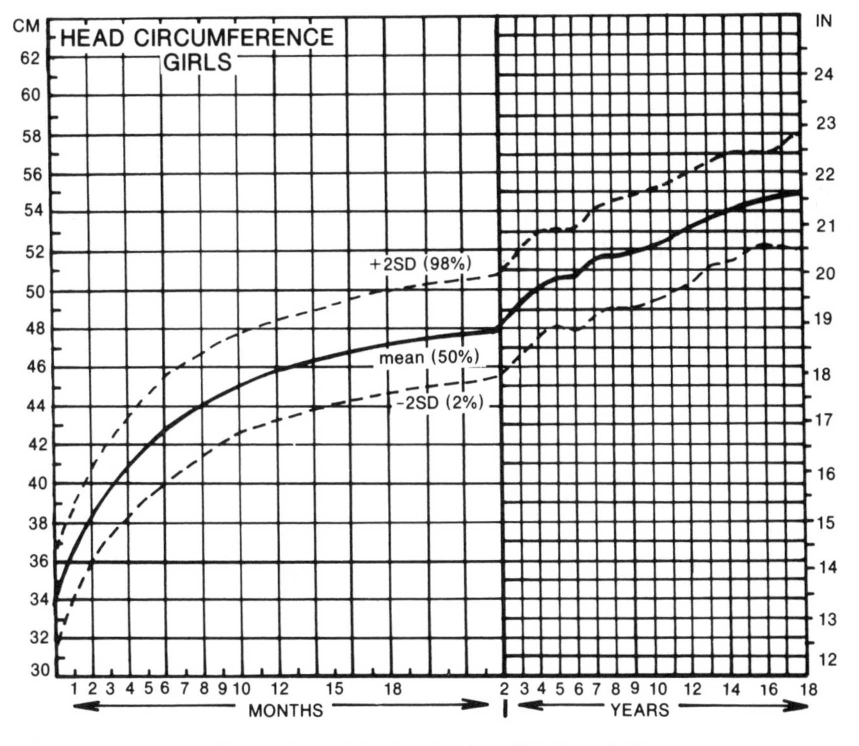

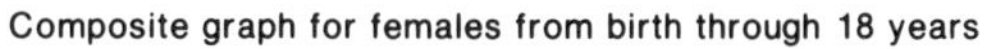

Composite graph for females from birth through 18 years

APPENDIX B.4. PERCENTILE DISTRIBUTION OF BIRTHWEIGHT FOR GESTATIONAL AGE

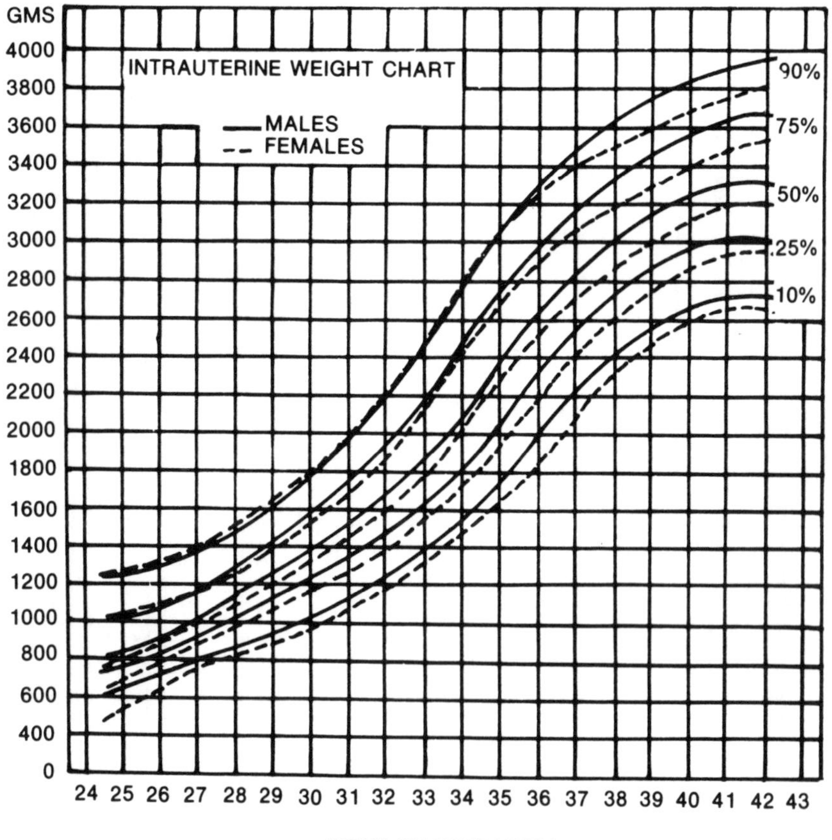

APPENDIX B.5. NATIONAL ACADEMY OF SCIENCE/NATIONAL RESEARCH COUNCIL TABLES OF IDEAL BODY WEIGHT FOR HEIGHT (1980)

TABLE 1. PERCENTILES FOR WEIGHT AND HEIGHT OF MALES AND FEMALES, 0-18 YEARS[a]

	Males						Females					
	Weight (kg)			Height (cm)			Weight (kg)			Height (cm)		
Age	5	50	95	5	50	95	5	50	95	5	50	95
(Months)												
1	3.16	4.29	5.38	50.4	54.6	58.6	2.97	3.98	4.92	49.2	53.5	56.9
3	4.43	5.98	7.37	56.7	61.1	65.4	4.18	5.40	6.74	55.4	59.5	63.4
6	6.20	7.85	9.46	63.4	67.8	72.3	5.79	7.21	8.73	61.8	65.9	70.2
9	7.52	9.18	10.93	68.0	72.3	77.1	7.00	8.56	10.17	66.1	70.4	75.0
12	8.43	10.15	11.99	71.7	76.1	81.2	7.84	9.53	11.24	69.8	74.3	79.1
18	9.59	11.47	13.44	77.5	82.4	88.1	8.92	10.82	12.76	76.0	80.9	86.1
(Years)												
2	10.49	12.34	15.50	82.5	86.8	94.4	9.95	11.80	14.15	81.6	86.8	93.6
3	12.05	14.62	17.77	89.0	94.9	102.0	11.61	14.10	17.22	88.3	94.1	100.6
4	13.64	16.69	20.27	95.8	102.9	109.9	13.11	15.96	19.91	95.0	101.6	108.3
5	15.27	18.67	23.09	102.0	109.9	117.0	14.55	17.66	22.62	101.1	108.4	115.6
6	16.93	20.69	26.34	107.7	116.1	123.5	16.05	19.52	25.75	106.6	114.6	122.7
7	18.64	22.85	30.12	113.0	121.7	129.7	17.71	21.84	29.68	111.8	120.6	129.5
8	20.40	25.30	34.51	118.1	127.0	135.7	19.62	24.84	34.71	116.9	126.4	136.2

Source: Hamill *et al.* 1979.

[a] Data in this table have been used to derive weight and height reference points in the present report. It is not intended that they necessarily be considered standards of normal growth and development. Data pertaining to infants 2–18 months of age are taken from longitudinal growth studies at Fels Research Institute. Ages are exact, and infants were measured in the recumbent position. The measurements were based on some 867 children followed longitudinally at the institute between 1929 and 1975. Data pertaining to children between 2 and 18 years of age were collected between 1962 and 1974 by the National Center for Health Statistics and involve some 20,000 individuals comprising nationally representative samples in three studies conducted between 1960 and 1974. In these studies, children were measured in the standing position with no upward pressure exerted on the mastoid processes. In the previous edition of this report, data for children up to six years of age were taken from longitudinal growth studies in Iowa and Boston, where children were measured in the recumbent position. This explains the systematically small heights for 2–5-year-old children in this current table compared with those represented in previous editions. In this table, actual age is represented.

APPENDIX B.5. *(Cont'd.)*

TABLE 1. PERCENTILES FOR WEIGHT AND HEIGHT OF MALES AND FEMALES, 0–18 YEARS[a]

Age	Males						Females					
	Weight (kg)			Height (cm)			Weight (kg)			Height (cm)		
	5	50	95	5	50	95	5	50	95	5	50	95
(Years)												
9	22.25	28.13	39.58	122.9	132.2	141.8	21.82	28.46	40.64	122.1	132.2	142.9
10	24.33	31.44	45.27	127.7	137.5	148.1	24.36	32.55	47.17	127.5	138.3	149.5
11	26.80	35.30	51.47	132.6	143.3	154.9	27.24	36.95	54.00	133.5	144.8	156.2
12	29.85	39.78	58.09	137.6	149.7	162.3	30.52	41.53	60.81	139.8	151.5	162.7
13	33.64	44.95	65.02	142.9	156.5	169.8	34.14	46.10	67.30	145.2	157.1	168.1
14	38.22	50.77	72.13	148.8	163.1	176.7	37.76	50.28	73.08	148.7	160.4	171.3
15	43.11	56.71	79.12	155.2	169.0	181.9	40.99	53.68	77.78	150.5	161.8	172.8
16	47.74	62.10	85.62	161.1	173.5	185.4	43.41	55.89	80.99	151.6	162.4	173.3
17	51.50	66.31	91.31	164.9	176.2	187.3	44.74	56.69	82.46	152.7	163.1	173.5
18	53.97	68.88	95.76	165.7	176.8	187.6	45.26	56.62	82.47	153.6	163.7	173.6

Source: Hamill *et al.*, 1979.

[a] Data in this table have been used to derive weight and height reference points in the present report. It is not intended that they necessarily be considered standards of normal growth and development. Data pertaining to infants 2–18 months of age are taken from longitudinal growth studies at Fels Research Institute. Ages are exact, and infants were measured in the recumbent position. The measurements were based on some 867 children followed longitudinally at the institute between 1929 and 1975. Data pertaining to children between 2 and 18 years of age were collected between 1962 and 1974 by the National Center for Health Statistics and involve some 20,000 individuals comprising nationally representative samples in three studies conducted between 1960 and 1974. In these studies, children were measured in the standing position with no upward pressure exerted on the mastoid processes. In the previous edition of this report, data for children up to six years of age were taken from longitudinal growth studies in Iowa and Boston, where children were measured in the recumbent position. This explains the systematically small heights for 2–5-year-old children in this current table compared with those represented in previous editions. In this table, actual age is represented.

TABLE 2. SUGGESTED DESIRABLE WEIGHTS FOR HEIGHTS AND RANGES FOR ADULT MALES AND FEMALES

Height[a]		Weight[b]							
		Men				Women			
in.	cm	lb		kg		lb		kg	
58	147	—		—		102	(92–119)	46	(42–54)
60	152	—		—		107	(96–125)	49	(44–57)
62	158	123	(112–141)	56	(51–64)	113	(102–131)	51	(46–59)
64	163	130	(118–148)	9	(54–67)	120	(108–138)	55	(49–63)
66	168	136	(124–156)	62	(56–71)	128	(114–146)	58	(52–66)
68	173	145	(132–166)	66	(60–75)	136	(122–154)	62	(55–70)
70	178	154	(140–174)	70	(64–79)	144	(130–163)	65	(59–74)
72	183	162	(148–184)	74	(67–84)	152	(138–173)	69	(63–79)
74	188	171	(156–194)	78	(71–88)		—		—
76	193	181	(164–204)	82	(74–93)		—		—

Source: Bray, 1975.
[a]Without shoes.
[b]Without clothes. Average weight ranges in parentheses.

TABLE 3. MEAN HEIGHTS AND WEIGHTS AND RECOMMENDED ENERGY INTAKE[a]

Category	Age (years)	Weight (kg)	Weight (lb)	Height (cm)	Height (in.)	Energy Needs (with range) (kcal)		(MJ)
Infants	0.0–0.5	6	13	60	24	kg × 115	(95–145)	kg × 0.48
	0.5–1.0	9	20	71	28	kg × 105	(80–135)	kg × 0.44
Children	1–3	13	29	90	35	1300	(900–1800)	5.5
	4–6	20	44	112	44	1700	(1300–2300)	7.1
	7–10	28	62	132	52	2400	(1650–3300)	10.1
Males	11–14	45	99	157	62	2700	(2000–3700)	11.3
	15–18	66	145	176	69	2800	(2100–3900)	11.8
	19–22	70	154	177	70	2900	(2500–3300)	12.2
	23–50	70	154	178	70	2700	(2300–3100)	11.3
	51–75	70	154	178	70	2400	(2000–2800)	10.1
	76+	70	154	178	70	2050	(1650–2450)	8.6
Females	11–14	46	101	157	62	2200	(1500–3000)	9.2
	15–18	55	120	163	64	2100	(1200–3000)	8.8
	19–22	55	120	163	64	2100	(1600–2400)	8.8
	23–50	55	120	163	64	2000	(1400–2200)	8.4
	51–75	55	120	163	64	1800	(1200–2000)	7.6
	76+	55	120	163	64	1600	(1200–2000)	6.7
Pregnancy						+300		
Lactation						+500		

[a] The data in this table have been assembled from the observed median heights and weights of children shown in Table 1, together with desirable weights for adults given in Table 2 for the mean heights of men (70 in.) and women (64 in.) between the ages of 18 and 34 years as surveyed in the U.S. population (HEW/NCHS data).

The energy allowances for the young adults are for men and women doing light work. The allowances for the two older age groups represent mean energy needs over these age spans, allowing for a 2-percent decrease in basal (resting) metabolic rate per decade and a reduction in activity of 200 kcal/day for men and women between 51 and 75 years, 500 kcal for men over 75 years, and 400 kcal for women over 75 years. The customary range of daily energy output is shown in parentheses for adults and is based on a variation in energy needs of ±400 kcal at any one age, emphasizing the wide range of energy intakes appropriate for any group of people.

Energy allowances for children through age 18 are based on median energy intakes of children of these ages followed in longitudinal growth studies. The values in parentheses are 10th and 90th percentiles of energy intake, to indicate the range of energy consumption among children of these ages.

Index

Other AVI Books

ALCOHOL AND THE DIET
Roe
DIETARY NUTRIENT GUIDE
Pennington
DRUG-INDUCED NUTRITIONAL DEFICIENCIES
Roe
ENCYCLOPEDIA OF FOOD SCIENCE
Peterson and Johnson
FOOD AND ECONOMICS
Hungate and Sherman
FOOD AND THE CONSUMER
Kramer
FOOD FOR THOUGHT
2nd Edition *Labuza and Sloan*
FOOD SERVICE FACILITIES PLANNING
Kazarian
FOOD SERVICE SCIENCE
Smith and Minor
MENU PLANNING
2nd Edition *Eckstein*
NUTRITIONAL QUALITY INDEX OF FOODS
Hansen, Wyse and Sorenson

The AVI Functional Medical Laboratory Technology Series:
CLINICAL BACTERIOLOGY
Scimone
CLINICAL CHEMISTRY
Scimone and Rothstein
HEMATOLOGY AND URINALYSIS
Lamberg and Rothstein
HISTOLOGY AND CYTOLOGY
Lamberg and Rothstein
CLINICAL MICROBIOLOGY
Diliello
SEROLOGY, IMMUNOLOGY AND BLOOD BANKING
Williams
SOURCEBOOK FOR FOOD SCIENTISTS
Ockerman